# Forensic Emergency Medicine

# Forensic Emergency Medicine

## Editors

**Jonathan S. Olshaker**, M.D., F.A.C.E.P., F.A.A.E.M.
*Director, Emergency Care Services*
*Baltimore Veterans Affairs Medical Center*
*Professor, Division of Emergency Medicine*
*Department of Surgery*
*University of Maryland Medical Center*
*Baltimore, Maryland*

**M. Christine Jackson**, M.D.
*Assistant Professor*
*Division of Emergency Medicine*
*Department of Surgery*
*University of Maryland Medical Center*
*Baltimore, Maryland*

**William S. Smock**, M.D., M.S., F.A.C.E.P.
*Associate Professor of Emergency Medicine*
*Department of Emergency Medicine*
*University of Louisville Hospital*
*Louisville, Kentucky*

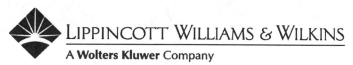

LIPPINCOTT WILLIAMS & WILKINS
**A Wolters Kluwer** Company
Phildelphia • Baltimore • New York • London
Buenos Aires • Hong Kong • Sydney • Tokyo

*Acquisitions Editor: Anne Sydor*
*Developmental Editor: Kerry B. Barrett*
*Production Editor: Emily Lerman*
*Manufacturing Manager: Colin J. Warnock*
*Cover Designer: Christine Jenny*
*Compositor: TechBooks*
*Printer: Edwards Brothers*

© 2001 by LIPPINCOTT WILLIAMS & WILKINS
530 Walnut Street
Philadelphia, PA 19106 USA
LWW.com

**Library of Congress Cataloging-in-Publication Data**
Forensic emergency medicine/ [edited by] Jonathan S. Olshaker, M. Christine Jackson, William S. Smock.
    p. ; cm.
Includes bibliographical references and index.
ISBN 0-7817-3144-5 (alk. paper)
    1. Assault and battery. 2. Emergency medicine. 3. Medical jurisprudence.
I. Olshaker, Jonathan S. II. Jackson, M. Christine. III. Smock, William S.
    [DNLM: 1. Emergency Medicine–methods. 2. Forensic Medicine–methods.
3. Expert Testimony. 4. Sex Offenses. 5. Violence. W 700 F7147 2001]
RA1122 .F67 2001
614'.1–dc21                                              00-067806

Care has been taken to confirm the accuracy of the information presented and to describe generally accepted practices. However, the authors, editors, and publisher are not responsible for errors or omissions or for any consequences from application of the information in this book and make no warranty, expressed or implied, with respect to the currency, completeness, or accuracy of the contents of the publication. Application of this information in a particular situation remains the professional responsibility of the practitioner.

The authors, editors, and publisher have exerted every effort to ensure that drug selection and dosage set forth in this text are in accordance with current recommendations and practice at the time of publication. However, in view of ongoing research, changes in government regulations, and the constant flow of information relating to drug therapy and drug reactions, the reader is urged to check the package insert for each drug for any change in indications and dosage and for added warnings and precautions. This is particularly important when the recommended agent is a new or infrequently employed drug.

Some drugs and medical devices presented in this publication have Food and Drug Administration (FDA) clearance for limited use in restricted research settings. It is the responsibility of the health care provider to ascertain the FDA status of each drug or device planned for use in their clinical practice.

10 9 8 7 6 5 4 3 2 1

*To my parents, Bennett and Thelma Olshaker, for their love, guidance, and goodness;
to my wife, Kelly, for her love and support and for being my partner and best friend;
and to my sons, Scott and Eric, for their spirit and their smiles
and for making my dreams come true.*

JSO

*I dedicate this book to the many survivors of sexual abuse and incest
and to the many people in the health profession,
law enforcement, and the judicial system who try to eradicate the problem of sexual violence.
And I thank all of the SAFE examiners at Mercy Medical Center
who are constantly teaching me about the sexual assault patients.
I also dedicate this book to my parents and to my extended family
whom I love dearly.*

MCJ

*To my loving wife, Cathy, and our children, Mariah, Skye and Forrest,
for their support, patience, encouragement, and understanding
in my academic pursuits.
To my grandfather, S. Spafford Ackerly, M.D.,
the kindest and wisest physician and teacher I have ever known.*

WSS

# Contents

# Contributing Authors

**Patrick E. Besant-Matthews, M.D.,**   *Self Employed, Dallas, Texas*

**John E. Douglas, Ed.D.,**   *FBI Unit Chief, National Center for the Analysis of Violent Crime, FBI Academy, Quantico, Virginia (Retired)*

**Carroll Ann Ellis, M.A.,**   *Director, Victim Services, Fairfax County Police Department, Fairfax, Virginia*

**Richard C. Fahlteich, Sr., B.S.,**   *Detective Lieutenant/Shift Commander, Criminal Investigation Division, Homicide Section, Baltimore Police Department; Adjunct Professor, Allied Human Services Department, Criminal Justice & Public Safety Programs, Baltimore City Community College, Baltimore, Maryland*

**Adam J. Geroff, M.D.,**   *Assistant Professor, Division of Emergency Medicine, University of Maryland School of Medicine; Attending Physician, Emergency Department, University of Maryland Medical Center; Attending Physician, Emergency Care Services, Baltimore Veterans Affairs Medical Center, Baltimore, Maryland*

**Georgina A. Groleau, M.D.,**   *Assistant Professor, Division of Emergency Medicine, Department of Surgery, University of Maryland Medical Center, Baltimore, Maryland*

**M. Christine Jackson, M.D.,**   *Assistant Professor, Division of Emergency Medicine, Department of Surgery, University of Maryland Medical Center, Baltimore, Maryland*

**V. Jill Kempthorne, M.D., M.S.,**   *Assistant Professor, Department of Pediatrics, University of Maryland at Baltimore; Staff Pediatrician, Department of Pediatrics, University of Maryland Health System, Baltimore, Maryland*

**Richard Lichenstein, M.D., F.A.A.P.,**   *Associate Professor, Department of Pediatrics, University of Maryland School of Medicine; Director, Pediatric Emergency Medicine, University of Maryland Medical Center, Baltimore, Maryland*

**Sharon May, J.D.,**   *Deputy State's Attorney, Baltimore, Maryland*

**Clare McCarthy, M.D.,**   *Clinical Instructor, Department of Emergency Medicine, University of Louisville School of Medicine; Attending Physician, Department of Emergency Medicine, Norton Hospital, Louisville, Kentucky*

**John S. O'Brien II, M.D., J.D.,**   *Clinical Assistant Professor of Psychiatry, University of Pennsylvania, Pennsylvania Hospital, Philadelphia, Pennsylvania*

**Jonathan S. Olshaker, M.D., F.A.C.E.P., F.A.A.E.M.,**   *Director, Emergency Care Services, Baltimore Veterans Affairs Medical Center; Professor, Division of Emergency Medicine, Department of Surgery, University of Maryland Medical Center, Baltimore, Maryland*

**Mark Olshaker,**   *Author, Novelist, Filmmaker, Washington, DC*

**Daniel J. Sheridan, R.N., Ph.D.,**   *State Abuse Investigator, Office of Investigations and Training, State of Oregon, MHDDSD, Salem, Oregon*

**William S. Smock, M.D., M.S., F.A.C.E.P.,**   *Associate Professor, Department of Emergency Medicine, University of Louisville School of Medicine and University of Louisville Hospital, Louisville, Kentucky*

**Adrienne Suggs, M.D.,**   *Assistant Professor, Department of Pediatrics, Division of Emergency Medicine, University of Maryland Medical Center; Attending Physician, Pediatric Emergency Department, University of Maryland Medical System, Baltimore, Maryland*

**DePriest W. Whye, Jr., M.D., J.D.,**   *Clinical Assistant Professor, Division of Emergency Medicine, Department of Surgery, University of Maryland; Chief Executive Officer, Maryland Medicine Comprehensive Insurance Program, University of Maryland, Baltimore, Maryland*

# Preface

Although total violent crime is currently on a decline in this country, acts of child and elder abuse and neglect, sexual assault, and domestic violence remain at epidemic levels. In 1998, three million referrals for child maltreatment were made. More than one-third of these cases were substantiated. At least four million women experience ongoing physical, psychological, sexual, or violent abuse from male intimate partners each year in the United States. The 1998 National Institute of Justice Center for Disease Control survey on violence against women documented that an estimated 302,100 women and 92,000 men are forcibly raped each year in the United States. The National Elder Abuse Incidence Study showed that at least 450,000 elders each year are victims of abuse or neglect.

Emergency physicians have frequent opportunities to play a major role in the identification, evaluation, and treatment of these patients whose care involves significant forensic issues. The emergency department is clearly the most likely place where the healthcare system will encounter the unfortunate victims just described. For many victims, this will be the only chance to identify a serious problem before more tragic results ensue.

In some cases of abuse or sexual assault, the diagnosis will be obvious. In addition to evaluation and treatment, our role includes insuring proper documentation and evidence chain of custody to maximize law enforcement's chances of successful prosecution. Most importantly, we must realize that we are among the victim's first encounters with "the system." Therefore, we must carry out our evaluation and treatment in a compassionate, supportive, nonthreatening manner that gives the victims the best chance of getting through their nightmarish experience as psychologically whole as possible.

Many cases of abuse and neglect, however, are subtle and go unrecognized. While healthcare professionals have become increasingly aware of the incidence of child abuse and its manifestations, until recently, domestic violence and elder abuse have been largely ignored. Physicians fail to make the diagnosis for a variety of reasons: for example, they may lack proper training as medical students or residents, or they may not consider the diagnosis in cases with nontrauma chief complaints. Hence, these serious issues go unnoticed because physicians have not been taught the significance of less obvious clues or do not think to ask some basic questions.

This book was developed with the goal of providing all emergency physicians with a reference that will give them the necessary information to perform the essential tasks of recognition, evaluation, treatment, documentation, and understanding of victims of acts of violence, abuse, or neglect.

Importantly, it is unnecessary for emergency physicians to become judge and jury or to spend inordinate amounts of time with individual patients in an already busy environment. First and foremost, we must simply recognize that a problem exists. This will lead to appropriate referrals and disposition. The various chapters in this text describe at length the myriad of victim services immediately available in most jurisdictions, including child and adult protective services, social workers, sexual assault nurse examiners, and police forensic technicians. In addition, we included chapters on the relevant aspects of the legal system and guidance to medical personnel on testifying in court. This discussion should prove beneficial not only to emergency care providers involved in criminal evidentiary matters, but also to anyone called upon to give expert witness testimony.

We are greatly indebted to the authors of *Forensic Emergency Medicine* for their informative and passionate contributions. We sincerely hope this text will significantly aid emergency physicians in providing compassionate treatment, thorough forensic support, and, most importantly, early recognition of victims of sexual assault and other acts of violence, abuse, and neglect.

*Jonathan S. Olshaker,* M.D.

# Acknowledgments

There are a number of people from Emergency Medical Services at the University of Maryland Medical Center whose efforts contributed significantly to *Forensic Emergency Medicine.* We first thank Brian Browne, M.D., Director of Emergency Medical Services. Brian's leadership and guidance played a major role in the initial plans for this book, as well as in the development of numerous forensic emergency medicine programs at the University of Maryland.

We also thank Sara Martin for the tremendous job she did as the administrative coordinator for this book. Her effort, skills, and sense of humor were crucial in successfully bringing together contributions from across the country. Linda Kesselring, our department's medical editor, provided significant help to many authors in the preparation and editing of their chapters.

We also are extremely thankful for the wonderful guidance we received from all the publishers and editors at Lippincott Williams & Wilkins, particularly Anne Sydor, Kerry B. Barrett, and Glenda Insua.

# Forensic Emergency Medicine

# 1

# Perpetrators

John E. Douglas and Mark Olshaker

## WHERE DO WE BEGIN?

Early in the 1980s, when one of the authors was conducting in-depth interviews with incarcerated serial offenders that would help form the basis for the FBI's behavioral profiling and criminal investigative analysis program (1), he interviewed an inmate of the Joliet Penitentiary in Illinois who had been convicted of murdering a woman by inflicting multiple stab wounds.

Throughout the extensive interview, the five-feet nine-inch white man in his mid-twenties maintained a soft, inappropriate affect, smiling frequently. He displayed what FBI special agents referred to as "the look"—darting eyes, nervous twitches, continual hand-rubbing. His primary concern was how he had looked in a CBS television interview the day before. When told he had come across well, he laughed, relaxed considerably, and was much more forthcoming.

After the interview, the special agent sought out the prison psychiatrist to find out how the inmate was doing. The psychiatrist gave a positive reaction, stating that the inmate was responding very well to medication and therapy, adding that he had joined a bible study group in prison and that if the progress continued he would be ready for parole.

The special agent asked the psychiatrist if he knew the specifics of the crime the inmate had committed. "No, I don't want to know," he replied. "I don't have the time, with all the inmates I have to deal with here." And, he added, he didn't want to unfairly influence his relationship with his patient.

But before the psychiatrist could protest, the agent related how this asocial person had joined a church group and how after a meeting, when everyone else had gone, he propositioned the young woman who hosted the meeting. She rejected his advances, at which point he knocked her to the floor, went to the kitchen and retrieved a knife, and stabbed her numerous times. Then, as she lay bleeding to death on the floor, he inserted his penis into an open wound in her abdomen and ejaculated.

"You're disgusting, Douglas!" the psychiatrist declared. "Get out of my office!"

"I'm disgusting?" the agent countered. "You're in a position to make a recommendation that this individual is responding to therapy and could be freed, and you don't know who in the hell you're talking to when you're dealing with these inmates. How are you supposed to understand them if you haven't taken the time to look at the crime scene photos or reports, to go over the autopsy protocols? Have you looked at the way the crime was committed? Do you know if it was planned? Do you understand the behavior leading up to it? Do you know how he left the crime scene? Do you know if he tried to get away with it? Did he try to establish an alibi? *How in the hell do you know if he's dangerous or not?*" (2).

At the heart of the dilemma is that much of psychiatric therapy is based on self-reporting, and while a patient coming to a therapist under normal circumstances has a vested interest in revealing his true thoughts and feelings, a jailed convict desirous of early release has a vested interest in telling the therapist what he wants to hear. To the extent that the therapist takes the report at face value without correlating it with other information about the subject, there is grave danger of a fundamental and perilous mis-evaluation. Edmund Kemper in California and Montie Rissell in Virginia, to name but two of the serial murderers the author has interviewed and studied, were in court-mandated therapy as a condition of parole while they continued committing new crimes. Both managed to remain undetected and both showed "progress" to their therapists. On at least one occasion, Kemper attended a meeting with state psychiatrists while the severed head of his most recent victim lay in the trunk of his car (3).

The point of this experience and research is clear. Neither the law enforcement nor the medical/health communities can effectively deal with violent, predatory, often repeat or serial criminals, or even evaluate the critical question of their current or future level of dangerousness, until the effort is made to *understand* the nature and type of each offender.

There can be many reasons why certain individuals—almost exclusively males—become violent sexually oriented predators, having do with both "nature" and "nurture," "hard wiring," and environment. But studies have shown common elements too prominent to ignore. Among these are family history of alcoholism and psychiatric disorders, instability of residence, mother as the dominant parent, and negative relationship with father or male caretaker. All of these factors came into play in significantly more than half of the instances in the author's study. In addition, such other important indicators as family members with criminal histories, father leaving before subject's twelfth birthday, negative relationship with mother, subject's ongoing perception of unfair treatment, and no older sibling role model all showed up in roughly 50% of the cases. About 40% of the subjects were physically abused as children or adolescents, and nearly 75% experienced some form of psychological abuse; various forms of sexual abuse were also common, but seen in lower percentages (4).

Not surprisingly, what this type of upbringing led to in the subjects studied was a tendency to failure in interpersonal relationships; aggres-siveness and other antisocial behavior patterns; inappropriate emotional responses, including absence of guilt or conscience, chronic lying, and rebelliousness; underperformance in school and underemployment; active fantasy life and preoccupation with fantasies of violence, domination, and control (5). It is therefore not difficult to see the type of background, combined with whatever is inherent in the child's physical/neurologic/emotional makeup, as part of a template for the adult violent offender.

Is early environment the only determining factor? Certainly not. Many have posed the question, in one form or another, of whether certain people are simply "evil." While each of us may have personal views on the subject, we are not qualified, nor is it relevant to this discussion, to pass judgment on that issue. The one thing we can state empirically is that there are many complexities to individual personality that we do not understand or know how to evaluate, some of which do seem to be "born in" and, together with other influences, unquestionably play a significant role in the formation of the adult criminal. Combining the environmental template with these inherent traits and characteristics, what we often see emerge is an individual whose personality incorporates deep-seated feelings of inadequacy with equally deep-seated feelings of grandiosity and entitlement—that he is better than anyone else and being held back by society and the people around him.

Once the antisocial behavior begins (often as fire-starting and/or cruelty to animals and other children), a series of "feedback filters" come into play: The subject justifies the act in his own mind; he sorts out errors in his performance of the act so that he can do it "better" and more efficiently next time; he finds that in performing the act he experiences an increased state of arousal; he discovers increased areas of dominance, power, and control in his life; he learns how to continue these acts without detection or punishment; he escalates to a larger, more elaborate and harmful acting out of his fantasies (6).

But let us add a word of caution here, because it would be easy to misinterpret the data. As with other aspects of medicine, it is critical to keep in mind that while nearly all of the affected subjects conform in greater or lesser degree to these and many other related traits, the *vast majority* of individuals who have suffered similar backgrounds and upbringings are in no way criminally motivated and, in fact, grow up to lead "normal," productive lives. This is true not only for this population at large but more specifically for the siblings of criminal offenders, many of whom experienced the same negative influences.

Stated simply, the various studies and our own experience have led us to conclude: While the background described above could certainly result in an adult with serious psychological problems and emotional unhappiness, it does not follow that this adult would then be compelled to perpetrate violent, predatory acts on others. Why, then, do serial predatory offenders do what they do? It is because this act of manipulation, domination, and control—be it rape, murder, arson, or any other criminal enterprise—gives them a feeling of power, satisfaction, and fulfillment that they achieve nowhere else in life. For this one moment, a "loser" or "nobody" who feels that he has no power or influence in normal life can exert the ultimate power over another human being, can make that other human being suffer and bend to his will, can decide whether that other human being will live or die. For this type of individual, there is no greater sense of empowerment.

Let us also remind our readers that this discussion applies primarily—almost exclusively—to male individuals. While a girl may appear to have an identical background to a boy who goes on to a troubled life of crime, she will almost never develop into the same type of sexual predator. Even the types of violent crimes committed by women are different in character, as are preference of weapons and means of murder. For reasons often speculated on but not yet clearly understood, girls and women from dysfunctional and abusive backgrounds tend to direct their rage, anger, and despair inward. Rather than being outwardly aggressive toward others, they often engage in self-destructive or self-punishing behaviors, such as alcohol or drug abuse, suicide attempts, prostitution, and attraction to abusive men (7).

What this means, of course, is that the violent predatory crimes with which we deal are almost always committed by men, and therefore men should be the focus of our examination.

Are individuals who derive satisfaction from forcibly controlling, assaulting, and killing *sick*? Depending on one's definition of the term, that can be a pretty safe bet. Are such individuals mentally ill? We would be more than willing to concede that anyone who derives his life's satisfaction from inflicting pain and suffering does have some pretty severe mental problems. But is this individual *insane*? In other words, is he incapable of understanding the wrongness of his actions and resisting the impulse to follow through on his fantasies? In almost all cases, we believe the answer to that question is no. To our knowledge, there are no recorded cases of the hypothetical "policeman at the elbow," for example, in which an individual is so compelled to perform a predatory criminal act that he does so knowing that a uniformed police officer is watching him.

Although this may be a rather glib restatement of an important and admittedly controversial issue, our conclusion is that the critical operative word is *choice*. Regardless of family background and all other formative influences, regardless of intelligence or level of emotional stability, the overwhelming number of predatory criminals *choose* to do what they do because of the way it makes them feel. They are fully aware of what they are doing, often plan it, and understand that it is wrong and contrary to society's rules. They simply don't care. Or if they do care, that care is outweighed by the desire to do it anyway.

It is important to keep in mind also that by definition a serial criminal is a successful criminal. The more times he is able to get away with a particular offense, the better able he will be to refine his *modus operandi* to continue getting away with the same crime. In any given case, this may be because the offender is above average in intelligence, despite his record of underachievement. Many serial offenders, particularly of the organized variety (a distinction explained later in this chapter), are reasonably bright. But success at avoiding detection and capture can also be due to the obsessive amount of time and energy the offender puts into fantasizing, planning, and evaluating the crime. When one of the authors was a teenaged agricultural intern, he noted with amazement the uncanny ability of cows to wander out of seemingly secure enclosures. He finally concluded that if the cow had nothing else on its mind, it could devote all of its mental resources to the task of finding a way out, however long it took. The situation of the sexual predator who spends an inordinate amount of his time, intellect, and emotional resources on his crimes turns out to be a somewhat analogous situation.

Thus armed with an understanding of the commonalities among criminal sexual predators, it is equally important to understand the differences. Because only then may we be equipped to evaluate the offender as an individual, to lend aid and support to his victims, to assist in his prosecution, and to make an attempt to predict his likelihood of future violence. The method and manner in which a crime is committed relates directly to the personality type of the criminal.

## SEXUAL VIOLENCE

One of the most common predatory crimes with which emergency medical personnel have to deal is rape, and so it is perhaps more important that they have a full understanding of the rapist than of any other type of perpetrator. We will therefore devote the largest share of our discussion to this subject.

There is an ongoing debate within and between the law enforcement community, the health care community, and the women's movement about whether rape should be classified as a crime of sex or violence, and this will not abate any time in the foreseeable future. From our own experience and knowledge of the subject, we can say that whatever the definition, anger is almost always a key component.

We have heard no better explanation than the one provided by the distinguished prosecutor Linda Fairstein, Esq., head of the New York County District Attorney's Office Sex Crimes Unit (8): rape is a crime of violence in which sex is the weapon. In an interview, Fairstein explained, "There is a sexual element to this that

isn't part of any other crime, and that can't be denied. It's very much the piece of the crime that the victim doesn't want to happen or is afraid of. And so to me, it was about the one weapon that this type of offender had that other offenders don't use and victims don't want used against them" (9).

Rape of any kind is a horrible event and any sexual assault leaves its victim, her partner, friends, and loved ones devastated. But we do a grave disservice to all victims and potential victims if we do not invest the time and effort to distinguish between types of rape and rapists. It may seem more sympathetic and caring to proclaim, for instance, that date rape is the same as stranger rape, but it is not true. So much depends on the circumstances of the assault. To assert that a date rape that does not involve a weapon and does not cause the victim to fear for her life is the same as a stranger abduction-rape at knife- or gunpoint in which the victim is brutally beaten dangerously oversimplifies the situation and hinders our ability to defend against both crimes and their different types of perpetrators. There are certain elements that all sexual assaults share. But what they do not share is, in some ways, even more important if we are to learn prevention strategies from them and help victims recover from their individual traumas. Many things are required of the diligent, sensitive emergency medicine practitioner when dealing with a victim of sexual assault (10). After excellent medical care, by far the most important of these are caring and empathy.

In 1992, after more than 10 years of investigation and study by the Behavioral Science and Investigative Support Units of the FBI Academy in Quantico, Virginia, together with the pioneering research of Dr. Ann Burgess, Professor of Psychiatric Nursing at the University of Pennsylvania, categories of sexual assault, with similar breakdowns of homicide and arson, were organized into the *Crime Classification Manual* (11). Critical research was also conducted by Special Agents Roy Hazelwood and Ken Lanning of the Behavioral Science Unit.

Research involved the review of numerous case files, victim statements, police reports, court testimony, school reports and psychiatric evaluations, parole and probation records, and records of family and developmental history. Following the analysis, rapists were broken down into four basic types, with the crime of rape further broken down into more than 50 subgroups. Over the years, different researchers have assigned their own labels to the typologies, but the behavior is so consistent within each that the types should be recognizable regardless of how they are named (12).

*The power-reassurance rapist* feels himself to be inadequate, not the type with whom women would voluntarily become involved. He compensates for these feelings of male inadequacy by forcing women to have sex with him. All the while, as the designation suggests, he is looking for reassurance of his own power and potency. This type has sometimes been referred to as the "gentleman rapist," or even classified as an "unselfish" rapist, in large part because his offenses, while traumatic, are usually less physically damaging to his victim than those of other types of sex offenders. Such a rapist may even apologize during the assault or ask the victim if he is hurting her—a question that serves his own need for reassurance more than it expresses a genuine concern for the victim. Therefore, the terms "gentleman" and "unselfish" are only applicable within the context of the full spectrum of rapist types (13).

This type tends to be a loner who fantasizes that his victim actually enjoys the experience and might even fall in love with him. He may go so far as to contact the victim after the assault and ask her to go out with him. Of course, the reality of rape cannot live up to his fantasies: instead of winning over a reluctant lover, he has terrorized, hurt, and angered an innocent person. Most rapists of the power-reassurance variety will admit later that they did not enjoy the sex with their victims. The experience did not satisfy the underlying obsession and, therefore, he will have to try again with another woman.

Victims of choice are generally about the same age as or younger than the perpetrator, and usually of the same race. If he dates at all, the women he dates will be younger and less sophisticated than he; this is the only way he can feel equal. Because of his feelings of inade-

quacy, he gains control by surprise; he doesn't have the self-confidence or skills to con his way into a victim's apartment smoothly and is more likely to break in the middle of the night, for example. When we delve into this type of perpetrator's past, we generally see a history of unusual or bizarre masturbatory fantasies, often voyeurism, exhibitionism, cross-dressing, and/or obscene phone calls. He frequents adult bookstores or movies and collects pornography. If he has a specific sexual dysfunction, it is likely to involve premature ejaculation, which would be exhibited in consensual relationships he may have and which he would report as a problem (from his point of view only) in his rapes.

He will tend to prefer the night and operate in his own residential or work area—in other words, within a very prescribed comfort zone—and will usually travel to the crime scene on foot. If he is a serial offender, this is particularly true of his first offenses. He uses a weapon of opportunity, often something he found at the crime scene. His patterns of crime are generally consistent, and the entire act, from the time he overpowers his victim until the time he leaves, is relatively brief, sometimes as little as 5 or 10 minutes. He will not use profanity or try to demean or humiliate his victim to the extent that the other rapist types will, but may require her to recite a "script" in which she praises his lovemaking or expresses desire for him. He might cover the victim's eyes or mask his own features, both for the self-preservation motive of preventing identification and the possibility that he knows he should be ashamed of his actions. He is timid and will do whatever the victim allows him to. Rather than tear off her clothes or force her to strip, he may only expose the parts of the victim's body he intends to assault.

He is apt to keep a journal, news clippings, or some other record of his assaults to reassure himself of his potency. For the same reason, he may take souvenirs, such as pieces of the victim's underwear. Afterward, he may feel guilty or remorseful. But unless he is a first-timer who tries it, doesn't like it, and decides never to do it again, he *will* do it again. He will keep raping until he is caught or stopped in some other way, such as being arrested and incarcerated, or killed or seriously injured in another crime or other un-related incident. He lives alone or with parents or in some other type of dependent relationship. His mother probably was—or is—very domi-neering. He is employed below his ability level in a job that does not require a lot of contact with the public. While this is the least physically dangerous type of rapist, if he is successful over a series of attacks, his confidence can be boosted and he may become more physically aggressive.

Numerically, this is the most common type of rapist.

*The exploitative rapist* is a more impulsive predator. His crimes result from seizing an op-portunity that presents itself rather than by fan-tasizing about the act ahead of time. He might approach a potential victim with a ruse or con, or it could be a direct, overpowering, blitz-style attack. Unlike the power-reassurance rapist, this type will not appear in any way concerned with the victim's welfare. He is selfish—verbally, physically, and sexually. He may suffer from some form of sexual dysfunction, and if he does, it will be just as apparent with his wife, girl-friend, or any other consenting partner as it will be with a victim of force. Such sexual dysfunc-tion often has to do with retarded ejaculation or difficulty in reaching climax.

Victims of preference will tend to be around his age. He is on the prowl for a victim of op-portunity, and this activity could take place in a bar or neighborhood he has targeted. Once he has a woman under his control, his only concern is getting her to submit sexually to him. That is the real thrill for him—the sex act is satisfying as an act of domination and control rather than for providing what we think of as sexual grati-fication. Once he has forced submission, as far as he is concerned, the experience is over. But during that encounter, he can be expected to in-flict multiple assaults on the victim. Anal assaults are common. Masks or attempts at disguise or hiding his face are uncommon. With this type of offender, there will often be an interval between rapes—a day, a month, 6 months—until he once again goes on the hunt; however, unlike the power-reassurance rapist, he will not try to maintain any contact with or come back to a victim once he has left her, although he often

threatens to return if she reports the assault to police.

This type will be very body-conscious. He will want a macho reputation, to be known as a man's man, and therefore is likely to have some physically oriented employment. He is inter-ested in sports. His vehicle will reflect that im-age, too. In some regions of the country, it would be a Corvette or other muscle car; in others, it might be a pickup truck, well-equipped for hunt-ing. He does not take well to criticism or au-thority. He probably did not do well in high school or go to college. If married, he will have a history of cheating on his wife and paying scant attention to his children. When we look into the background of offenders like this, we very often find that his father treated his mother in the same way the offender treats women.

Next to the power-reassurance rapist, this is the most common type of rapist.

*The anger rapist* is just what the name im-plies. Also referred to as the anger-retaliatory rapist, his sexual assault is a displaced expres-sion of rage and anger within him. For this type of rapist, the victim represents a person—or group of people—the offender hates. This could be a mother, wife, or girlfriend, even women in general. But his anger and resentment need not be rooted in an actual or legitimate wrong ever perpetrated against him.

It would not be unusual for this type to be in-volved in an ongoing relationship with a woman. Because he is driven by rage, the consequences of the anger rapist's attack can be anything from verbal abuse, to severe beating, to murder, though the fact that his conscious or subcon-scious intention is to get the anger out of his sys-tem means that this type usually will not kill. His attacks will be episodic, not at predictable intervals, triggered by precipitating stressors in-volving the woman or women to whom his rage is actually directed. In almost all cases, the dis-placement means that he will not attack that per-son. He may attack someone else he knows, us-ing weapons of opportunity such as kitchen knives or even his own fists if he is strong enough. Because he wants not just to overpower but to humiliate his target, there could be anal sex followed by oral sex and a great deal of profanity, and the context of his behavior will be an intention to degrade, such as by ejaculating on the victim's face or clothing.

Therefore, it is important for the examiner to realize that crucial DNA and other evidence can be found on many parts of the patient's body and her clothes. Whenever this is a possibility, a delicate but thorough line of questioning on this topic is indicated, with the twin goals of preserving the chain of evidence while ensuring the victim's emotional well-being.

This type is far less common than either of the previous two, possibly as little as 5% of rapists.

*The sadistic rapist* is in many ways the most dangerous sexual predator of all. The purpose of his attack is to live out his sadistic sexual fantasies on the unwilling victim. With this type, sexual fantasy and aggression merge, which is why he is also referred to as an anger-excitation rapist. Aggression and sadistic fantasy feed on each other, so as the level of aggression rises, his level of arousal rises accordingly. His aggression is not anger-based, as it is with the previous category. In fact, he can be quite charming and seductive as he lures intended prey into his web. He is completely self-centered. The only thing he cares about is his own pleasure and satisfaction. And he derives satisfaction from hurting people, of having them in his power (14). Therefore, with this type, we expect to see various forms of mental and physical torture, and the physical torture may be directed particularly at sexually significant parts of the body such as mouth, breasts, genitals, buttocks, and rectum. His weapon of choice is frequently a knife, because it is so intimidating and causes mental anguish on the part of the victim. He often cuts or tears off his victim's clothing because he figures she will not need it after he has finished with her. Depending on his preferences, there may be much sexual activity, probably highly perverse in nature, or even none. He could, for example, prefer to penetrate with a sharp object rather than with his penis. His language will be commanding and degrading, but impersonal. The victim is merely there as an actress in his self-scripted drama, and her role is to show fear and respond to pain. Thus, there is

often a victim of preference, symbolic to him in some way, be she old or young, white, black, or Asian, slim or full-figured, black-haired or blonde, redhead or brunette.

The sadistic rapist anticipates his crime and has perfected his *modus operandi* over the course of his criminal career. As his fantasy evolves and he gains more experience with different victims, he will take more time planning ahead for successive crimes. He brings his weapon(s) with him and may have a torture kit made up in advance, including pliers or other sharp instruments, whips, manacles, needles, or whatever he needs to fulfill his fantasy. Since his assault unfolds over a long period of time, he will have a place to which he can take his victim where he knows they will not be disturbed. This might be an obscure cabin in the woods, or a specially outfitted and soundproofed van. He may tell the victim that if she does what he tells her he will not hurt her further or will let her go, but this is only a ruse to control her and get her to cooperate. Because his satisfaction lies in the act of tormenting and dominating his victim, he may take photographs or record the scene as it unfolds on either audio- or videotape. For the same reason, he may also take souvenirs to help him relive the experience and demonstrate to himself that he "owns" the victim. These souvenirs might include jewelry, items of clothing or underwear, or even body parts.

The attack itself will tend to be highly symbolic. There will be no remorse because the rapist has totally depersonalized his victim; he does not even think of her as a human being. This is the type of rape that most often ends in murder. In fact, killing the victim may be an integral part of the sadistic fantasy scenario. He may even continue to engage in activity with the body after death. It is generally impossible for the victim to play on his sympathy, because he has none. He wants her to suffer. The only instance in which he might relent is if the victim can somehow break through the depersonalization and get him to regard her as an individual. This occurred, for example, in one instance in which a victim stated that her husband had cancer. It happened that the rapist's brother was battling cancer, and he let her go. Another time, a sadistic rapist revealed in a prison interview that one of his victims reminded him of his mother so he released her. Unfortunately, this is a very uncommon scenario with the sexual sadist.

The sadistic type is usually white, with above-normal intelligence, and may be college-educated with a good middle-class job. He has a dominant personality and likes to collect bondage and sado-masochistic pornography. He may also collect related items, such as knives, guns, or Nazi memorabilia, and read military, law enforcement, or survivalist literature. He may have a large attack-type dog, such as a German shepherd, Doberman, or Rottweiler. Because of his intelligence and planning, he will be difficult to apprehend.

This is the least common type of rapist.

As we all know, human nature is not exact, and not every rapist fits neatly into one of these four categories. There is often a mixed presentation, with elements of one classification grafting onto the general description of another, which is why it is so difficult to give specific advice to potential victims as to how to react to a sexual criminal, particularly under the acute stress of the attack itself. But in the great majority of cases, one category will dominate, and our reaction should be molded around the understanding of what motivates that specific type of rapist and what he is after (15).

In any discussion of criminal personality, the cautions and cautionary tales hold equal importance with the conclusions. This only serves to underscore why we say it is so difficult to give ironclad advice. Montie Rissell, mentioned earlier, was in some ways an unusual rapist. He attacked and murdered five women near his home in Alexandria, Virginia, while still in his teens, later blaming his criminal behavior on having to live with his mother rather than his father after his parents' troubled marriage broke up when he was age 7. By the time he was in high school, he had a rap sheet detailing driving without a license, burglary, car theft, and rape.

Rissell's first killing was savagely instructive of the dangers of misinterpreting offender behavior. Still in high school, on probation and receiving psychiatric counseling as a provision of that probation, he heard from his girlfriend—a year ahead of him and then away at college—that their relationship was over. A trigger emotional event of this nature is generally the precursor to a serial sex crime. Rissell promptly drove to the college, where he spotted the young woman with her new boyfriend. Rather than express his rage on the person he felt hurt by, he drove back home, fortified himself with beer and marijuana, and spent hours sitting in his car in the parking lot of his apartment complex. Several hours later, another vehicle appeared, driven by a single woman. On the spur of the moment, Rissell decided to get back what he had just lost. He approached the other car, pulled a handgun on the woman, and forced her to go with him to a secluded area nearby.

As it happened, Rissell's victim was a prostitute, which is significant for two reasons: She would not have the same fear having sex with a stranger that someone outside the profession would; and, though frightened, she would probably draw on a strong and well-developed survival instinct. Her behavior, according to the prison interview with Rissell, reflected this. When she was alone and defenseless and it was clear that her attacker intended to rape her at gunpoint, she attempted to diffuse the situation by hiking up her skirt, asking him how he liked it and in what position he wanted her.

Rather than making him gentler or more sensitive to her, this behavior enraged him. As an anger (or anger-retaliatory) rapist, Rissell was set off by what he perceived as his victim's attempt to *control* the situation. In fact, when she subsequently feigned orgasm in an attempt to gratify him, he became greatly upset that she was "enjoying" the experience. This reinforced in him the notion that all women are whores. He was able to depersonalize her and it was easy for him to think about killing her, an idea that was solidified in his mind when she attempted to run away, thereby further "controlling" the situation (16).

Had the attacker been a power-reassurance rapist, resistance or struggle might have prevented the attack, and acquiescence might have mitigated its severity. However, in the case of this anger-retaliatory rapist, the opposite was true. And once this type has killed, found the act satisfying, and realized he can get away with it, his escalation to serial rapist-murderer takes place. He will not stop until something stops him.

In light of these and other considerations, the only nearly absolute advice we feel comfortable imparting to victims relates to a few key behavioral indicators on the part of the rapist or potential rapist. If an offender wears a mask or otherwise attempts to disguise his identity, that is a "good" sign. In most cases, it signifies that he intends to get away with the crime, leaving his victim alive but unable to identify him. If he does not attempt to prevent identification, this could signify at least two scenarios, neither of them good. The first is that he is disorganized, "making it up as he goes along," which means that his actions may be unpredictable even to himself. The second, even more dire, is that while he plans to get away with his crime, to ensure this outcome he does not intend to leave a victim alive to identify him. That being the case, resistance of whatever kind the victim can muster would be indicated. Unfortunately, this does not mean she might not be hurt, just that the consequences of not resisting are even riskier. Likewise, another indication to resist by any means possible would be if an offender orders his victim into a car, intending to take her away from the abduction point, because once in the vehicle she loses all control, all possibility of alerting others, and therefore all possibility of intervention (17).

In terms of evaluating a perpetrator of sexual assault for amenability to "rehabilitation" or future dangerousness, it is critical to look at the behavior exhibited during the crime and whether that behavior is representative of a pattern.

Rehabilitation and dangerousness are inextricably intertwined. On the general subject, we can do no better than to quote the distinguished clinical psychologist Dr. Stanton E. Samenow. With the late psychiatrist Samuel Yochelson, Samenow undertook a pioneering study of violent criminals at St. Elizabeth's Hospital in Washington, D.C., and published the landmark *The Criminal Personality* (18). In his own penetrating book, *Inside the Criminal Mind,* Samenow writes, "Rehabilitation as it has been practiced cannot possibly be effective because it is based on a total misconception. To rehabilitate is to restore to a former constructive capacity or condition. *There is nothing to which to rehabilitate a criminal.* There is no earlier condition of being responsible to which to restore him" (19).

In an interview, Samenow further stated, "If you've worked with sex offenders—people who have committed these offenses again and again and again—you know that we do not in psychiatry and psychology have a way to change sexual orientation. People who molest kids, for example, they've done it and they've done it and they've done it, and they haven't been caught for a fraction of what they've done. To turn these people back in to the community knowing that we have nothing to offer them that is going to ensure the safety of kids is unconscionable" (20).

Are there, then, any good candidates for *rehabilitation*? As a matter of fact, there are—a notion with which Samenow agrees (21). In terms of rapists, these would fall overwhelmingly into the power-reassurance category. An exploitative rapist also might possibly see the error of his ways and atone if he has committed only one offense that was highly opportunistic in nature. In his case, such factors as age and the sophistication of the crime would enter into the evaluation.

The far better candidate is the power-reassurance rapist, but again, we look closely at the individual indicators: Is this a first offense or has he already raped several times? With each crime, the likelihood of turning him around decreases substantially. Were there extraordinary stressors in his life at the time? Was his behavior overtly violent? What was his post-offense behavior? Did he readily admit his crime or did he immediately establish an elaborate alibi? Did he show remorse? All of these considerations are critical in determining whether rehabilitation is even possible, or if the possibility of future dangerousness is simply too great (22).

## VICTIMIZERS OF CHILDREN

If there is any crime more odious than sexual violence against women, it would be sexual violence against children. Children are "ideal victims":

curious by nature, trusting and easy for adults to manipulate and influence, hungry for affection and attention, anxious to assert independence from parents, and taught to obey adults (23). Again, offenders display varying personality types and a continuum of behaviors, all of which go into the evaluation of the individual case.

As with other such criminals, predators against children often represent a cycle of abuse. They themselves may have been victims of abuse as children, and their young victims may, in turn, become either future victimizers or chronically victimized by others (24).

Some pedophiles, like other sexual predators, spend enormous amounts of time and energy planning and executing an abduction. Others might be relatively harmless until placed in a situation of opportunity. For example, a shy, timid individual without social skills or deep, peer-oriented interpersonal relationships may seem "creepy" if we notice him gazing at young children on the pony ride at the local fair, possibly even photographing them. But he would not steal a child from such a public environment and attempt to take him or her away with him. Let's change the scenario. Now let us say that a young girl of his interest rings his doorbell selling Girl Scout cookies. If, upon answering the door, the man sees that a parent or some other competent adult is right there or watching from a car, nothing will happen. If, on the other hand, the child appears to be by herself, it is quite possible that on the spur of the moment, on impulse, the man might pull her inside, close the door, and commit a horrible crime. Prior to that moment, it might not have occurred to him that he might someday act on his fantasies. But when the situation presents itself, he does so. The added risk is that, as in the feedback loop of the rapist, if the subject gets away with the crime, he may be encouraged to continue and escalate his behavior.

Predators of children possess and use their advantages (25). They are bigger and stronger than their victims. They may impersonate police officers, teachers, or priests to legitimatize themselves. They may manipulate a child's emotions by showering him or her with attention and then threaten to isolate the child from parents and others. Like the hunting lion surveying an entire herd of antelope at a watering hole, the sophisticated, experienced predator will identify and target the one vulnerable potential victim, the emotionally needy child. Therefore, we cannot stress strongly enough that the best single defensive strategy is for parents to instill a sense of self-esteem and confidence in their children. These are not the ones the predator will choose to victimize if he can help it.

Along with this, it is critical to teach children age-appropriate safety skills, and for parents to take careful note of any changes in their child's attitudes, behavior, or self-confidence. These could include withdrawal or fearfulness; sleep disturbances, such as nightmares or bed-wetting; sexual "acting out" or unusual interest in sex; aggressiveness or rebelliousness; regression or infantile behavior; fear of specific people, places, or activities; and/or pain or injury in private regions (26).

Basic survival and safety skills involve teaching the child how to be something of a profiler. By that we mean if a child becomes lost or separated from parents or other guardian, she must know how to profile the types of adults most likely to be safe and to give aid. These would include an adult wearing a uniform or name tag, someone working behind a store counter, a bus driver, a pregnant woman or mother with her own children, or an elderly woman. Certainly, each of these has been used as a disguise by a child molester in an attempt to fool a potential victim. But here, the odds have shifted considerably in the distressed child's favor since she is the one doing the selecting; she is choosing the authority figure to go to, rather than the other way around. And as we have cautioned rape victims, children should be taught never to get into anyone's car unless a parent or guardian has specifically approved.

Children should be taught to be instantly wary if an adult stranger asks them for help or offers to take them somewhere or show them something (like a puppy). They should know it is good, not disobedient, to run away from anyone who tries to take them somewhere, and they should scream for attention (27).

As with predators of adults, child molesters fall into several categories and subcategories, and it is important to understand the distinctions. It is also important to note that not all pedophiles molest children; we suspect that the majority of them manage to keep their feelings in check. Pedophiles may have sexual relationships with adults and satisfy their urges in other ways, such as through fantasy, masturbation with dolls, or choosing lovers who are in some way childlike, such as a small and/or flat-chested woman, or one who engages in baby talk or other similar behavior (28). But like other fetishes, pedophilia has the potential for danger if and when the fantasy element is no longer enough.

First, we must distinguish between the true pedophile—someone who prefers sex with children and has them as the subjects of his fantasies—and the situational pedophile, whose primary sexual drives and fantasies are directed at adults, but who will have sex with a child to fulfill some other need (29). For example, this second type may feel too inadequate to approach the true object of his desires and uses a child as a substitute.

We believe there to be a considerably greater number of situational than preferential child molesters, although a pedophile who molests will likely molest far more children over the course of his life because that is where his primary sexual urges lie. This is what he thinks about all the time. It is possible for a situational offender to molest only one child, one time, or it may become a long-term behavior for him.

In *Child Molesters: A Behavioral Analysis for Law Enforcement Officers Investigating Cases of Child Sexual Exploitation,* published by the National Center for Missing and Exploited Children in Arlington, Virginia, Special Agent Kenneth Lanning of the FBI's Behavioral Science Unit outlines four types of situational child molesters: repressed; morally indiscriminate; sexually indiscriminate; and inadequate (30).

The *repressed molester* may be found abusing his own children because they are most readily available. Not surprisingly, he tends to have low self-esteem and has sex with children as substitutes for adults he does not feel he can approach. This subject is likely to use a lure or con rather than force to get a child to go with him, and the incidents are usually linked to some precipitating stressor in his life.

The *morally indiscriminate molester* would also molest his own children, although he will manipulate, lure, or even use force to obtain other victims. This subject tends to be abusive in virtually all areas of his life: he abuses his wife and friends, is a liar and a cheat at home and at work, and has no qualms about stealing something he wants. Because this type has no conscience, it is not difficult for him to act on impulse. If asked why he molested a child, he might think, "Why not?"

The *sexually indiscriminate molester* would answer the question in the same manner but takes the thought a step further. He abuses children because he is bored and the experience seems new, exciting, and different to him. Lanning has described this type as a "try-sexual," meaning he will try anything (31). These offenders might pursue group sex with adults, spouse swapping, bondage—acts that are not criminal among consenting adults—but then may involve a child (even his own) in that sexual experimentation. Compared with the other types of situational child molesters, these subjects generally come from a higher socioeconomic level and are more prone to molest multiple victims. Whereas the other types indulge in child pornography, this type might have a much more diverse collection of "erotica."

The *inadequate molester* is much like other inadequate subjects. He is a social outsider, has few friends his own age as a teenager, and may continue to live with his parents or an older relative as he grows older. For this subject, children are nonthreatening, like his other potential targets—the elderly and prostitutes. His victim could be a child he knows well or a stranger whom he can use as a substitute for an unapproachable peer. The subject is not so much naturally sexually attracted to children as he is sexually curious but insecure around adults. If he collects pornography, it likely involves adults, not children. Because he is so withdrawn from society, the danger is that hostility and anger could build up until he finds an outlet for them. This subject can be very dangerous, then, if his rage explodes, often leading him to torture and kill his victim.

Lanning classifies preferential molesters into three categories: seduction, introverted, and sadistic (32).

The *seduction molester* courts his victim with attention and gifts, attempting to slowly win trust and lower inhibitions. He is adept at communicating with children and at choosing the most vulnerable targets. This type is insidious, and may be involved with children as a popular teacher, coach, or scout or youth group leader. Alert parents may be able to spot the potential for trouble.

The *introverted molester,* the closest to the stereotype of the creepy stranger in a raincoat, does not possess the interpersonal or social skills to lure or con potential victims. His sexual activity is limited to brief encounters, and he usually targets strangers or much younger children.

The *sadistic molester* is the most physically dangerous type because, like a sadistic rapist of adults, his satisfaction derives from having total control and seeing the victim's response to inflicted suffering. He must cause physical and/or psychological pain to become sexually aroused. This molester uses trickery or force to obtain victims, and then tortures them when they are under his control. He is the type of molester most likely to abduct and murder his victims.

Like other sexual predators, child molesters are often difficult to recognize. In most cases, they look like the rest of us. However, there are a number of indicators that could arouse suspicion—particularly if, taken together, they form a long-term pattern of behavior. A teenager with unusual interest in children and little social contact with his peers would be a prime example. An adult who tends to move frequently and unexpectedly, or has a less than honorable military discharge with no reason given, would be another. Additional pedophile behavioral traits might include extreme relationships with women—either domineering or weak, dependent, and childlike; sexual problems with any women in his life; collecting child pornography; hanging out in malls, playgrounds, and other places frequented by

children; and idealization and objectification of children (33).

Child abductors tend to be social misfits who showed signs of trouble as children themselves. Usually unmarried—too incompetent socially to maintain a relationship with a woman even as a cover—they have no regular contact with children. Their poor social skills would make it difficult for them to manipulate, lure, or seduce a child, so they might carry weapons to intimidate or control a victim. They are also likely to harm the victim.

Let us note here that while we do see female child abductors, their motivations and behaviors are distinct from those of their male counterparts. A woman who abducts a child on her own—as opposed to being the compliant victim of a male offender—almost always does so not as a result of sexual urges but because of her emotional need to have a child. Therefore, the remainder of our discussion of molesters and abductors applies to men.

Lanning describes four phases of child abduction: buildup; abduction; post-abduction; and recovery/release (34).

In the buildup and abduction phases, the fantasy creates the need, and the precipitating stressor or stressors fuel the action. The level of planning and chance for success will depend on the type of abductor. The *thought-driven* abductor plans ahead, weighs risks, and exercises discipline in victim selection, whereas the *fantasy-driven* abductor answers his specific emotional needs and follows his own ritual, even though this might increase his risk of being caught.

In the post-abduction and recovery/release phases, the treatment of the child depends on motivation for abduction and competence of the offender, because as pressure grows the abductor must somehow rid himself of the victim. The longer a child is missing, the smaller the chances of a positive outcome.

As with other types of violent criminals, we categorize abductors as organized, disorganized, and "mixed." Behavior and physical evidence help us to make these determinations. A fuller discussion appears later in this chapter, but it is important here to understand these distinctions:

The *organized* abductor likely possesses average or above-average intelligence and social skills, targets strangers as victims, and plans ahead. He may transport his victim—alive or dead—over a significant distance. Body dump-sites are difficult to find, and evidence may be destroyed. He may try to make a statement, go-ing for shock value in disposing of the body. He is likely to be aggressive in sexual activity and may kill either for thrill or to avoid detection.

The *disorganized* offender is of lower intelli-gence, chooses victims he knows personally or has observed closely, and does not plan well. He may kill inadvertently or if he loses control of the situation. Sexual assault may occur after the child is unconscious or dead. Bodies are not moved far from the crime scene—the subject may not have the means to transport a body—and are not well covered or hidden, and so tend to be found quickly (35).

Incestuous molesters can cross the spectrum of types. An introverted pedophile may marry with the intent of producing children whom he can molest. A seduction molester may marry a woman with children so as to become a "father figure" and have access to them (36). One tip-off would be that he would engage in sex with his spouse only as often as necessary to preserve the illusion. Incestuous molesters, of course, are not limited to fathers. They may be grandfathers, uncles, or any other relative.

This can be a particularly difficult problem for health care and social workers and law en-forcement alike, as children are often hesitant or reluctant to report incest and molestation. The sad fact is that society can inadvertently punish the victim. Consider the best case: when a child reports the abuse and corrective action is taken. In addition to shame and embarrassment—including taunts from some people and disbelief from others—there is the potential for separa-tion from everything important and familiar to the victim. As Peter Banks, Director of Outreach at the National Center for Missing and Exploited Children, observes: "Think of what happens when you report that you've been abused by a family member. Your whole entire life is dis-rupted . . . You're taken out of your home. You lose your friends, your school, your dog, every-thing." Banks notes, too, that sometimes in the face of all this disruption and pressure, victims

even recant. Then, on top of the problems in the current situation, the child essentially becomes a victim for the rest of his life, suffering long-term damage from the trauma of the abuse, as well as from the stigma of being branded a liar (37). And if a child reports abuse to someone who cannot or will not help, the abuser's threats are reinforced. There is also the issue of emo-tional blackmail: the child's original feeling of being flattered by attention turns to fear, confu-sion, and humiliation.

Children need to be reminded that their feel-ings are important—that they have the right to say "no" to things that feel bad or wrong to them. They must know that if someone touches them in a way they don't like—or makes them touch someone else in a way they don't like—it is not their fault; and if they tell an adult who does not help them, they should tell another adult.

If a molester is accused, particularly for the first time, there are certain behaviors that we see frequently. He will deny, acting shocked, sur-prised, and indignant. He may blame the accu-sation on the child's misunderstanding, saying something like, "Is it a crime to hug a child?" Depending on his social support structure, he may bring in character witnesses to back him up. He will try to minimize events, and may ac-tually be aided inadvertently in this by the victim's reluctance to admit the extent of the molestation due to his or her own embarrassment or discom-fort. The molester often attempts to justify or rein-terpret what happened, or patently falsify the truth. He may pursue a strategy to lessen the impact or punishment, such as agreeing to plead to a lesser crime, or claim temporary insanity. It should also be noted that accused molesters in this phase tend to be high suicide risks (38).

Unfortunately, it is far from unknown in our society for parents to kill children. Though cer-tainly not an ironclad rule, investigators find that the younger a child victim, if forensic evidence does not indicate otherwise, the more likely a relative rather than a stranger was involved. Re-gardless of cause, the behavioral indicators for parental involvement with a homicide are often clear to a trained investigator. Parents are not usu-ally as detached about body disposal as strangers are, taking care with the body, wrapping it up, and showing it tenderness. Parents are also far more likely than strangers to feel remorse, leading investigators to recovery of the body for proper burial (39).

More common than murder by parents, of course, is the less extreme but more chronic type of harmful behavior. The nature of the offense tells us much about the perpetrator and probability of future violence.

In the case of certain types of situational abusers of children, we believe that rehabilitation through education and coping strategies is possible. This is almost strictly limited to abuse by parents, guardians, or other regular caretakers and would apply more to physical and psychological than to sexual abuse. Sometimes, mistreatment is caused by an overload of stress and responsibility on the part of the adult. For example, a single working mother who beats her misbehaving child out of frustration and physical and mental exhaustion may be very amenable to intervention that might alleviate some of her burden without removing the child. In such instances, the chances for cessation of the cycle are more positive.

This may also be true for those who mistreat the elderly—our next topic of focus.

## VICTIMIZERS OF THE ELDERLY

People are often surprised when we group children, prostitutes, and the elderly together as victims. But it is a fact that these three groups are uniquely linked because of their vulnerability. A given predator may view children (boys, girls, or either), or prostitutes, or elderly women as his preferential victim. But he may also use any of these three groups as a "warm-up," a practice before moving on to more challenging victims. A young (probably teenaged) beginning rapist, for example, may target an elderly woman because, at this point, such a victim is all he can handle. Once he learns what to do, he will then go after his true victim of preference.

An elderly woman is particularly vulnerable, not only because of physical weakness or infirmities, but also because of her dependence on others for maintenance and repairs around the house, running errands and doing chores, providing transportation, and the like. Often, the individual providing such service is not well known to her. A stranger let into the house or apartment to deliver something or make a repair can gather valuable intelligence information for a future assault, burglary, or scam. Since it is often difficult for senior citizens to get to a bank regularly, they may keep relatively large amounts of cash at home—an attractive target to a young, unsophisticated offender.

An early case in which the author was called to consult involved the 1977 murder of an elderly woman, Anna Berliner, in her home in Oregon. Local police had also sought help from a clinical psychologist about the type of offender they were dealing with in this crime. Among the victim's injuries were four deep pencil wounds in the chest. The psychologist had conducted interviews with approximately 50 men charged with or convicted of homicide. Most of these examinations had been done in prison. Based on his experience, he predicted that the offender would be someone who had spent a fair amount of time in prison, probably a drug dealer, because only in prison is a sharpened pencil widely considered a deadly weapon.

The author disagreed, believing that the age and vulnerability of the victim, the overkill, and the facts that it was a daytime crime and nothing of great value was missing suggested an inexperienced juvenile offender. The pencil was there—a weapon of opportunity requiring no great analysis or skills to employ.

The killer turned out to be an inexperienced 16-year-old who had gone to the victim's house scheming to get a contribution to a walk-a-thon in which he was not actually participating.

The key feature of this crime scene was that all behavioral evidence suggested an offender who was unsure of himself. An experienced felon attacking an elderly woman in her home would be very sure of himself. Merely picking up on a single piece of evidence does not give the entire picture. This is something we must keep in mind throughout our evaluations of offenders in crimes against the elderly (40).

## DOMESTIC VIOLENCE

Domestic violence cuts across all socioeconomic, cultural, and racial groupings and the rates of recidivism are sickeningly high.

A more detailed discussion of the entire problem takes place later in this volume. Therefore, for the present discussion, we will limit ourselves to an examination of the most critical aspect from the perspective of the perpetrator—that is, his emotional need to have total control over another human being. In this regard, it is informative to look closely at stalking behavior, a particular type of domestic violence that has far-reaching implications (41).

Simple obsession stalking is so intimately related to domestic violence that the two are virtually inseparable—different extensions of the same controlling, dominating behavior. Like love obsession stalkers who begin by obsessing from a distance and often focus on celebrities, the time during which the offender's emotional dependence blossoms into a full-blown obsession can range from years down to weeks—or even just a few dates. And dangerousness can escalate remarkably quickly.

In cases where there has been a long-term relationship between victim and stalker, the history of the offender's abusive behavior makes him all the more menacing. He knows his victim as celebrity or love obsession stalkers cannot; he knows which emotional buttons to push. He knows his victim's vulnerabilities. Even more frightening and dangerous, his past relationship with his victim has given him the intelligence data he needs. He already knows her patterns, her schedule, where she keeps her money, who her doctor is and whom she would count on and where she would go in an emergency.

There are warning signs but, unfortunately, they are often not revealed until the victim is already somewhat involved with the potential offender, which is why intelligent, otherwise self-protective women can find themselves in this type of situation. These offenders can be quite charming at first, creating a favorable initial impression. However, as time goes by, they reveal their true nature. They do not believe that ordi-

nary social rules apply to them and therefore have no problem lying, cheating, or breaking the law to get what they want.

It is a common misperception that stalkers, indeed domestic violence abusers in general, are typically undereducated, unemployed or holding menial jobs, and living close to the poverty level. In fact, this is yet another crime where anybody can be an offender or a victim, including people of all races, socioeconomic backgrounds, and even genders. According to one assessment, approximately one-third of men undergoing counseling for physically abusing a wife or girlfriend held respectable, professional occupations and often enjoyed high status in their community as executives, doctors, even ministers (42).

Whether the case of a successful businessman who stalks his estranged wife, or a high-school teen who cannot let go of his first serious girlfriend, the offender's criminal behavior grows out of a need to control and dominate his victim to boost his own self-esteem. This offender suffers from extreme insecurity and often is unable to develop and maintain personal and love relationships as others do. Some may have psychological problems but, for the majority, the problem is a personality disorder that manifests itself in inappropriate behavior and impaired social skills. Such persons often feel powerless in everyday situations and this, coupled with their inadequacies, makes them invest their emotions and sense of self-worth in the relationship with the other person.

In a sense, these offenders operate in the world of a fantasy relationship. Although they actually had a relationship with their victim, what they are really obsessed with is the feeling of power they got from the relationship, not the victim herself.

Before any physical and/or emotional abuse begins, the offender may appear very attentive, which is soon revealed to be possessiveness and jealousy rather than caring. He tries to control aspects of his mate's or girlfriend's life—from picking out her clothing, to trying to limit the time she spends away from him. An abusive husband or boyfriend may humiliate his victim, criticizing her appearance, downplaying her skills as a homemaker, mother, student, successful professional—whatever roles she holds within and outside their relationship that give her a sense of self-worth. He has more strength if he can keep her off balance.

His most successful gambit involves switching moods: loving and tender one moment, angry and violent the next. His partner never knows with whom she is dealing, and though she fears and loathes the one side of his behavior, she cares for the other and thrives under his attention.

To increase his control, the abuser tries to put his victim in a situation in which she is economically dependent on him. If there is a child involved, this makes it even easier for him to keep her under control because she may not feel capable of supporting herself and her child on her own. She may also be afraid that if she leaves he will get custody of—or outright kidnap—her children, and she will never see them or be able to protect them from him again. There have even been cases in which terrified mothers have escaped to a community "safe house," only to have the court force them to reveal their location when the abuser sued for visitation rights. Thus, the same system to which a victim of domestic violence may turn for protection can also be used by her abuser/stalker to exercise further control over her and maintain his presence in her life even after she has physically fled their home. Sadly, it is easy to see why some victims, lacking the financial resources to fight what seems to them an endless legal war, either give up and return to face more abuse or disappear underground in desperation, giving up jobs, family, and friends.

As an abusive relationship continues, the offender grows increasingly critical of his victim's friends and family, and more and more jealous and controlling of the time she spends away from him. She may get to the point where she feels it is not worth the fight to see them and, if he has beaten her and the marks are visible, she may be too embarrassed to see them. There are cases where abusers force their victims to keep records of every minute of their day. Such abusers may check the mileage on the car, even count the change in the victim's purse, thus micromanaging every aspect of the victim's life and wearing her down completely. Abusers do not acknowledge the true reason for their dependence on this relationship—or that they are in a position of dependence at all—but will project any blame for their actions on the victim. They may see their need to control as either their duty as a "good" husband or their right. In the offender's mind, violence occurs not because he is unable to cope with his emotions and lacks self-control, but because the victim did something wrong that set him off.

When a woman escapes such a relationship, the abuser may rationalize subsequent stalking behavior as efforts to win her back—often trying first the charm, flowers, and candy routine he used to win her the first time—or as punishment she deserves for leaving and treating him so unfairly.

All of the abuser's personality defects and pathologic rationalizations combine to make conditions extremely dangerous for a woman when she leaves a man like this. Overwhelmed with his own inadequacy and impotence, his emotions at that point also include rage over her rejecting him and trying to assert control, fear that he has been abandoned, and the drive for revenge. Threatened with losing the only aspect of his life that makes him feel powerful and in control, the abuser grows desperate. These are the cases in which we hear variations on the practically stock phrase, "If I can't have her, nobody will." As the stalker grows more frustrated by what he perceives as his victim's unwillingness to give him what he needs, he becomes increasingly harassing and threatening, in keeping with the abusive behavior he is accustomed to inflicting. If the victim tries to remove him permanently from her life at this stage, he may become violent in a last-ditch effort to reassert control over the relationship (43).

By the time a woman leaves an abuser, the two have often been through the cycle of courtship, intimidation, and violence more than once (44). It is almost as if they are programmed in their roles. This is partly why it is so threatening to the abuser when the victim breaks the pattern. He doesn't like her to call any play changes—

that's up to him—and he doesn't like the play she's called.

If, in fact, the offender's identity is so tied up with his victim that he has no other means to possess her than to kill her, once he has done that there is nowhere else for him to go emotionally, hence the frequency of murder-suicides.

Stalking is a terribly difficult crime for a victim to deal with because it can be both long term and unpredictable. Unlike any other domestic crime, this one can involve the perpetrator and victim for years rather than minutes, hours, or days. Imagine waking up every day for 20 years—or even 20 days—and having as your first thought, "Is this the day he gets me?" or "Is this the day he kills my kids?" Everywhere you go, you look around and expect to see him. Even if he isn't standing outside the window, watching you make the kids' lunch, you know he is always somewhere out there. Every time the phone rings, you know who it could be. The mail could bring just bills and advertisements, or a photo of you taken when you thought he wasn't around. Perhaps you secured a restraining order and police threatened to arrest him, so he has been quiet lately. That is no guarantee that he isn't still watching and waiting. Statistically, overwhelmingly, he will be back.

Victims suffer all sorts of problems as a result of their experiences, ranging from depression, anxiety attacks, and physical ailments brought on by prolonged feelings of anger, stress, fear, and helplessness, to recurring nightmares and even posttraumatic stress disorder (45). Just as some rape victims suffer from rape trauma syndrome, stalking survivors subjected to repeated and unpredictable acts of personal terrorism against them may go through life in a permanently stressed state, traumatized by their experiences.

The first step for any stalking victim should be getting in touch with someone local, because stalking laws vary from state to state and what constitutes grounds for an arrest in one jurisdiction may be outside the arm of the law in another. In some cases—especially if the stalking behaviors cross jurisdictions, or threatening phone calls are made from one state to another—federal charges may apply under stalking and/or antiterrorism laws. Working alone, victims may be unaware of the procedures involved in filing a stalking or related complaint (46).

In many cases, early intervention is key. David Beatty of the National Center for Victims of Crime notes: "The potential positive outcomes at the early stages of a stalking case are far better than at the last stages. If someone is overtly threatening you with violence, the options are pretty narrow." By then, Beatty adds, probably the best that can be done is to press charges and get the offender locked up. But the chances are great that he will be back out again and even angrier for having spent some time in prison or suffering some other punishment (47).

In any type of domestic violence situation, the potential for continued or renewed violence does not abate until a means is found to keep the abuser permanently away from his victim. Even then, it is likely that he will continue his abusive behavior in subsequent relationships with other victims.

## HOMICIDE

*Behavior reflects personality.*

This is one of the guiding principles of criminal investigative analysis. It is equally true that behavior often reveals the true nature of the crime. To illustrate this point, let us consider the case of Linda Haney Dover in Cartersville, Georgia, who was murdered the day after Christmas in 1980 (48).

The 27-year-old woman was separated from her husband Larry but remained on reasonably cordial terms with him. On the day of her murder, she was cleaning the house she used to share with her husband—a favor she did regularly—while Larry took their young son out for a day in the park. But when father and son returned from their outing, Linda was not there, and the bedroom appeared to have been ransacked. There were red stains on the carpet. When police arrived after Larry's frantic call, they found Linda's body wrapped in the comforter from the bedroom, with only her head exposed, in the crawl space under the house. As they unwrapped the body, they noted that her shirt and bra had been pushed up above her breasts, her jeans were around her knees, and her panties were pulled down to just below her pubic area. There was blunt-force trauma to the head and face and multiple stab wounds. The crime scene indicated that she had been assaulted initially in a bedroom; then her body had been moved outside. The presence of blood drops on her thighs indicated that the killer had handled and positioned her.

The author was called in on the case in his capacity as profiler for the FBI. Based on crime scene photos and information forwarded by the Cartersville Police Department, he stated that the unknown subject, or UNSUB in law enforcement parlance, would be one of two types. Possibly, he would be a young and inexperienced, inadequate loner who lived nearby and essentially stumbled into this crime of opportunity while attempting a burglary. Police then mentioned problems with a neighborhood thug, of whom many of the residents were afraid.

But the crime had too many "staging" elements, which more strongly indicated the second type: someone who knew the victim well and therefore wanted to divert attention from himself. The only reason a killer would have felt the need to hide the body was what we classify as a "personal cause homicide." The trauma to the face and neck also seemed highly personal.

The author told police he thought this UNSUB was intelligent, though only educated through high school, and had a job requiring physical strength. He would have a history of assaultive behavior and a low frustration level. He would be moody, unable to accept defeat, and was probably depressed at the time of the murder, most likely due to money problems.

The staging had its own internal logic and rationale. Whoever brutalized Ms. Dover did not want to leave her body in the open where another family member—particularly her son—might find it. That was why the UNSUB took the time to wrap her in a blanket and move her to the crawl space. He wanted to make it look like a sex crime—hence the raising of the bra and exposure of the genital area—though there was no forensic evidence of rape or sexual assault. He thought he had to do this but still felt uncomfortable with police seeing her bare genitals and breasts, so he covered them with the blanket. The behavior, therefore, suggested a domestic homicide disguised as a sex crime, pointing to the estranged husband, who fit the FBI profile in every significant aspect.

Unbeknown to the author, police had already arrested Dover for the murder and were using the profile to assure themselves that they were on the right track. In any event, justice was served. On September 3, 1981, Mr. Dover was convicted of the murder of Linda Haney Dover and sentenced to life imprisonment.

Let us contrast this with a different type of homicide. Beginning in the summer of 1979, a number of victims—mostly women—disappeared while hiking and were subsequently found murdered in the area of Mount Tamalpais Park, north of San Francisco. The UNSUB was dubbed the Trailside Killer by the local media (49).

In these cases, victims were stabbed and/or strangled and shot to death on remote park trails, which would, in the case of female victims, suggest an intention on the offender's part for sexual assault. There were conflicting witness sightings of possible suspects, which is not unusual. The fact that each murder site was remote and heavily wooded, accessible only on foot and involving a considerable hike, suggested that the killer was local and intimately familiar with the area.

To the author, the multiple stabbings and blitz-style attacks from the rear indicated an asocial type who was withdrawn, unsure of himself, and incapable of engaging his victims in conversation with the intent of seducing or conning them. The victims were physically fit hikers, and the blitz attack was an indication that the only way he could control an intended victim was to devastate her before she could respond. In contrast to the previous case discussed, these were not the crimes of someone who knew his victims. The sites were secluded and protected from view, which meant the killer essentially had as much time as he wanted to act out his fantasy with each victim. Yet he still felt the need for a blitz attack. There was handling of the bodies post mortem, and probably masturbation in addition to any sexual assault. The victims represented a range of ages and physical types, indicating a nonpreferential killer. The profile concluded with the prediction that the killer would have a speech impediment. This was met with considerable skepticism by the investigating task force.

Yet when the suspect, David Carpenter, was apprehended after a complex investigation that included the tracing of eyeglass frames the killer had inadvertently left at one of the murder scenes, the 50-year-old industrial arts teacher did indeed have a stutter, which became pronounced under stress. The reason for including such an odd trait in the profile was that this subject clearly did not feel comfortable taking his time or striking up a conversation with his intended victim. Despite the unlikelihood of interference in so secluded a setting, he did not have confidence in his ability to control the victim through words and manner. This suggested someone with a serious self-image/self-confidence problem. The most logical reason for this would be some sort of disfigurement or speech problem. Had there been disfigurement, it is likely that one or more witnesses would have made mention of a subject fitting this description. As none had, a speech impediment became the more likely factor.

Upon his arrest, Carpenter was found to be the product of a domineering and physically abusive mother and an at least emotionally abusive father. He was a child of well above average intelligence who was picked on because of his severe stuttering. His childhood was also marked by chronic bed-wetting and cruelty to animals. In adult life, his anger and frustration turned into fits of unpredictable, violent rage. He had been convicted of a previous attack on a woman using a knife and hammer, which occurred following the birth of his child into an already strained marriage. During the brutal assault itself, that victim reported, the terrible stutter disappeared.

What we hope to emphasize with these two cases is that while violent perpetrators can be classified according to type and manner of crime, as well as motive, it is critical to evaluate each incident and each offender on an individual basis, just as it is critical to so evaluate and support each victim.

The *Crime Classification Manual* organizes homicide into four main groupings based on motive (50):

*Criminal enterprise homicide* entails murder committed for material gain. This may include money, goods, territory, favors, or anything else perceived to have value to the individual. This category is further subdivided into contract (third-party) killing, gang-motivated murder, criminal competition homicide, kidnap murder, product tampering homicide, drug murder, insurance inheritance-related death (individual profit murder and commercial profit murder), and felony murder (indiscriminate felony murder and situational felony murder).

*Personal cause homicide* ensues from interpersonal aggression and results in death to a person or persons who may not be known to each other. This homicide is not motivated by material gain or sex and is not sanctioned by a group. It is the result of an underlying emotional conflict that propels the offender to kill. This category is divided into erotomania-motivated killing, domestic homicide (spontaneous domestic homicide and staged domestic homicide), argument/conflict murder, authority killing, revenge killing, nonspecific motive killing, extremist homicide (political extremist homicide, religious homicide, and socioeconomic extremist homicide), mercy/hero homicide, and hostage murder.

*Sexual homicide* involves a sexual element as the basis for the sequence of acts leading to murder. Performance and meaning of this sexual element vary with the offender. The act may range from rape (either before or after death) to a symbolic sexual assault. This category is divided into organized sexual homicide, disorganized sexual homicide, mixed sexual homicide, and sadistic murder.

*Group cause homicide* pertains to two or more people with a common ideology that sanctions an act, committed by one or more of its members, that results in death. This category is divided into cult murder, extremist murder (paramilitary extremist murder and hostage extremist murder), and group excitement homicide.

According to this classification, we can see clearly that the Dover murder would be considered a personal cause, staged domestic homicide (51).

The Trailside murders would be mixed sexual homicides because (a) the sexual element is the motivating factor and (b) while planning and stalking of the victim are traits of an organized offender, the style of attack was a blitz and no attempt was made to conceal the bodies—traits of a disorganized offender.

For the purposes of this chapter, it is not necessary to delve into each of the homicide classifications and subgroupings; most are self-explanatory, and the overview itself is sufficient to give understanding and insight to the emergency physician and health care worker. However, that understanding and insight can be enhanced through a brief look at the concept of organization versus disorganization of the perpetrator, which transcends individual crime classifications. This distinction was instituted as a result of research conducted under the auspices of the FBI in an attempt to get away from essentially psychiatrically based nomenclature and to come up with descriptive terminology that would be specifically helpful to law enforcement personnel directly involved in solving cases.

As the author and his collaborators pointed out in the *Crime Classification Manual,* profiling is a form of retroclassification (classification that works backward). Typically, we classify a *known* entity into a discrete category, based on presenting characteristics that translate into criteria for assignment to that category. In the case of homicide investigation, we have neither the entity (e.g., the offender) nor the victim. It is thus necessary to rely on the only source of information that typically is available: the crime scene. In essence, we are forced to "bootstrap," using crime scene-related data to make our classifications (52).

Developmentally speaking, the *organized type* externalizes hurt, anger, and fear through aggressive, often senseless acts. He has a superior attitude and may be described by others as a troublemaker. He generally will have had multiple sex partners; is angry with himself, his family, and society in general; and begins acting out that anger in a manifest way in his teens or early twenties, through such means as cruelty to animals and serious arson (e.g., to occupied buildings or causing large monetary damages).

He selects victims whom he can manipulate, dominate, and control.

This individual will be irresponsible and self-centered, methodical and cunning, indifferent to the welfare of society, with a chameleon-like personality; that is, he fits well into a given society. He is likely to be above average in intelligence, middle class, with a neat appearance and good communication skills but has a history of sporadic employment. He will possess criminal sophistication, and his criminal history may include financial or property crimes. When he escalates to murder, his choice of victims will be seemingly random; he will "cruise" for them, often many miles from where he lives or works.

The *disorganized type* internalizes hurt and anger and therefore becomes secluded, isolated, and withdrawn. He rejects society, which he feels has rejected him, and therefore feels lonely. He is frequently described as shy, quiet, and cooperative, and he finds interpersonal relationships difficult. He is an underachiever with a poor self-image, emotional inadequacies, and/or physical ailments and disabilities. His appearance may be disheveled. He is unemployed or involved in some menial type of job. As a surrogate for normal sex, he substitutes such activities as voyeurism, fantasy drawings and writings, pornography, and theft of fetish items, such as underwear. His behavior may be masochistic and his crimes tend to be committed against those weaker or more helpless than himself, such as the young, the elderly, and animals. He might also indulge in arson, but his crimes will be more of a nuisance variety than those with serious human or monetary consequences.

When he escalates to murder, he kills in close proximity to his home or some other zone of security. He lacks cunning and sophistication and is likely to kill in a frenzy. Unlike the organized type, who closely follows the media coverage of his crime and may actually change jobs or leave town, the disorganized type shows a minimal change in lifestyle after the crime (53).

The crime scene itself gives us many clues to the perpetrator's level of organization.

The organized offender may alter or stage the scene and will likely remove personal items belonging to the victim. He will use this souvenir to help him relive the crime in his own mind, or he may give it to a significant person in his life. This is common with jewelry. Because he has planned the crime, he will bring his weapon and other implements to the scene and not leave them. If it is an outdoor homicide, there will be a concerted effort to hide the corpse, or an equally concerted effort to display the body in some sort of symbolic manner, depending on his motive. If the murder is a first or second for this offender, the scene may be close to home. But as he refines his methods, he will move farther and farther from his zone of comfort so as to minimize the possibility of detection. By the same token, he might kill in one location, then methodically move the corpse to another. He may cut up the body, amputate limbs, or remove clothing in an attempt to delay identification of the victim.

The disorganized offender's crime is more spontaneous. There is likely to be a blitz style of attack and little or no communication with the victim, whom he may have difficulty controlling. The weapon is one of opportunity, and there is little attempt to destroy evidence or conceal the corpse, with which he may engage in post-mortem activity. Since he does not own a vehicle and relies on rides or public transportation, he will not move the body from the kill site to a dumpsite. If he takes a souvenir, it will be as a remembrance to help fuel a fantasy rather than to relive the crime, and he may later return it to the victim's grave or home.

The corpse may reflect a frenzy of uncontrolled stabbing or slashing, with post-mortem bite marks on breasts, buttocks, neck, thighs, or abdomen. The offender might attempt to dissect the body after death or even once the victim has been rendered unconscious, as a matter of curiosity and exploration, not to obliterate evidence. This curiosity can extend to cannibalism and vampirism, in which the perpetrator smears the victim's blood on himself or another surface, or insertion of foreign objects into the anal or vaginal cavity. This last activity takes the place of penile penetration. The body may be left in a ritualistic or symbolic way, but the meaning will probably be obscure to all but the killer.

Following the crime, an organized offender changes his clothing and cleans himself and his car. He immediately establishes an alibi. We should note a difference in his demeanor and behavior, including tension, insomnia, depression, episodes of explosive rage or anger, increased use of alcohol or drugs, renewed interest in religion, and a preoccupation with media. He may attend the funeral or burial of the victim and, if approached, will appear cooperative with investigators. Colleagues at work will notice a change in work habits, use of sick leave, irritability, perhaps quitting or being fired. He may return to the murder or disposal site and, if he feels police pressure, might seek a legitimate reason to leave the area.

The disorganized offender may also return to the scene or grave site, but it will be to engage in further mutilation or to "communicate" with the victim. He will become even more withdrawn, move or lose his job, and feel remorse over the victim being gone but not over his own act of killing. He may become fanatically religious and is far less likely to kill again than the organized offender.

We can see that there are some common elements between the two types of offenders, though often for different purposes. For example, both types may "experiment" with the victim, but the organized individual is more likely to do so ante-mortem while the disorganized will do so post-mortem. Both may show rage in the evidence of overkill, but the organized killer's rage will be controlled, whereas the disorganized offender will be uncontrolled, random, and sloppy. Both may display a victim's body for symbolic purposes, but the organized offender may do so to degrade his victim whereas the disorganized person is going for some arcane symbolism discernible only to himself.

Having said this, it is possible for an organized killer to become disorganized at the scene. Factors for this transformation might include the youthfulness and inexperience of the offender, use of alcohol or drugs, presence of more than one offender, an unexpected turn of events (such as another person showing up at the scene), or mental decompensation. However, it is extremely rare for the reverse transformation to occur and the scene to go from disorganized to organized.

As indicated with respect to the Trailside murders, human beings seldom fit neatly into rigid, predetermined niches. Therefore, we use the term "mixed" to describe a scene that has elements of both the organized and disorganized perpetrator (54). By weighing and evaluating the relative percentage of each type of behavior, we can go a long way to describing the likely profile and behavior of the UNSUB.

## SUMMARY

The forensic considerations of emergency physicians and practitioners dealing with the effects of violent crime will necessarily cut across a broad horizon of issues and procedures—from the physical and emotional treatment of victims, to gathering and handling evidence, to interaction with law enforcement authorities during the investigative process, to testifying in court. Although each of these activities requires its own special knowledge, talents, skills, and approach, the foundation and root cause of everything in forensic science is the perpetrator of the crime, because without his transgression there would be no need for the rest. For this reason, a basic understanding of the types and motivations of perpetrators is at the heart of all that we must do.

## ACKNOWLEDGMENT

The authors gratefully acknowledge the contribution of Ann E. Hennigan to the preparation of this work.

## REFERENCES

1. More information on offender study in Ressler RK, Burgess AW, Douglas JE. *Sexual homicide: patterns and motives.* New York: Lexington Books, 1988:ix–xiii, 15.
2. Douglas J, Olshaker M. *Mindhunter: inside the FBI's elite serial crime unit.* New York: Scribner, 1995: 335–337.
3. Newton M. *Hunting humans: an encyclopedia of modern serial killers.* Port Townsend, WA: Loompanics Unlimited, 1990:185.
4. Ressler RK, Burgess AW, Douglas JE. *Sexual homicide: patterns and motives.* New York: Lexington Books, 1988:17–26.
5. Ressler RK, Burgess AW, Douglas JE. *Sexual homicide: patterns and motives.* New York: Lexington Books, 1988: 28–43.
6. Ressler RK, Burgess AW, Douglas JE. *Sexual homicide: patterns and motives.* New York: Lexington Books, 1988:70.
7. Douglas J, Olshaker M. *The anatomy of motive.* New York: Scribner, 1999:34–35.
8. Bouton K. The prosecutor: Linda Fairstein vs. rape. *New York Times Magazine* 1990 Feb 25:21–23, 58–60.
9. Personal interview with Linda Fairstein, July 8, 1997. See also Fairstein L. *Sexual violence.* New York: William Morrow, 1993:13–18.
10. Zeccardi JA. Medical exam of the live sexual assault victim. In: Hazelwood R, Burgess A, eds. *Practical aspects of rape investigation: a multidisciplinary approach,* 2nd ed. Boca Raton: CRC Press, 1995: 253–262.
11. Douglas JE, Burgess AW, Burgess AG, Ressler RK. *Crime classification manual.* New York: Lexington Books, 1992. See also Burgess AG, Burgess AW, Hazelwood RR. Classifying rape and sexual assault. In: Hazelwood R, Burgess A, eds. *Practical aspects of rape investigation: a multidisciplinary approach,* 2nd ed. Boca Raton: CRC Press, 1995:193–203.
12. Information on the different rapist typologies described in the following section from Douglas J, Olshaker M. *Obsession.* New York: Scribner, 1998:93–99.
13. Hazelwood RR. Analyzing the rape and profiling the offender. In: Hazelwood R, Burgess A, eds. *Practical aspects of rape investigation: a multidisciplinary approach,* 2nd ed. Boca Raton: CRC Press, 1995:155–160.
14. Hazelwood RR, Dietz PE, Warren JI. The criminal sexual sadist. In: Hazelwood R, Burgess A, eds. *Practical aspects of rape investigation: a multidisciplinary approach,* 2nd ed. Boca Raton: CRC Press, 1995:361–371.
15. Additional information on prevention/protection strategies based on offender type can be found in Douglas J, Olshaker M. *Obsession.* New York: Scribner, 1998: 358–363.
16. Douglas J, Olshaker M. *Mindhunter: inside the FBI's elite serial crime unit.* New York: Scribner, 1995: 137–142. Also, Ressler RK, Burgess AW, Douglas JE. Rape and rape-murder: one offender and twelve victims. *Am J Psychiatry* 1983;140(1):36–40.
17. Douglas J, Olshaker M. *Obsession.* New York: Scribner, 1998:358–361.
18. Yochelson S, Samenow SE. *The criminal personality.* Vol. I and II. New York: Jason Aronson, 1979.
19. Samenow SE. *Inside the criminal mind.* New York: Times Books, 1984:203–204.
20. Personal interview with Dr. Stanton E. Samenow, July 11, 1997.
21. Samenow SE. *Straight talk about criminals.* Northvale, NJ: Jason Aronson, 1998:155–168.
22. Douglas J, Olshaker M. *Obsession.* New York: Scribner, 1998:114–115.
23. Lanning KV. *Child molesters: a behavioral analysis for law enforcement officers investigating cases of child sexual exploitation,* 3rd ed. National Center for Missing and Exploited Children, December 1992:41–44.
24. Lanning KV. Child molestation: a law enforcement typology. In: Hazelwood R, Burgess A, eds. *Practical aspects of rape investigation: a multidisciplinary approach,* 2nd ed. Boca Raton: CRC Press, 1995:330.

25. See also Finkelhor D, Dziuba-Leatherman J. Victimization of children. *Am Psychologist* 1994;49(3):173–183.
26. Meegan S. *Kids and company: together for safety, teacher's guide—a comprehensive manual for grades K–5/6,* 4th rev. ed. National Center for Missing and Exploited Children, 1988:18–19.
27. Douglas J, Olshaker M. *Journey into darkness.* New York: Scribner, 1997:178–186.
28. Lanning KV. *Child molesters: a behavioral analysis for law enforcement officers investigating cases of child sexual exploitation,* 3rd ed. National Center for Missing and Exploited Children, December 1992:3.
29. Lanning KV. Child molestation: a law enforcement typology. In: Hazelwood R, Burgess A, eds. *Practical aspects of rape investigation: a multidisciplinary approach,* 2nd ed. Boca Raton: CRC Press, 1995:324. Also Dietz PE. Sex offenses: behavioral aspects. In: Kadish SH, ed. *Encyclopedia of crime and justice.* New York: Free Press, 1983.
30. Descriptions of situational child molesters in this section from Lanning KV. *Child molesters: a behavioral analysis for law enforcement officers investigating cases of child sexual exploitation,* 3rd ed. National Center for Missing and Exploited Children, December 1992:6–7.
31. Lanning KV. *Child molesters: a behavioral analysis for law enforcement officers investigating cases of child sexual exploitation,* 3rd ed. National Center for Missing and Exploited Children, December 1992:7.
32. Descriptions of preferential molester types in this section from Lanning KV. *Child molesters: a behavioral analysis for law enforcement officers investigating cases of child sexual exploitation,* 3rd ed. National Center for Missing and Exploited Children, December 1992: 8–9.
33. Lanning KV. *Child molesters: a behavioral analysis for law enforcement officers investigating cases of child sexual exploitation,* 3rd ed. National Center for Missing and Exploited Children, December 1992:16–17.
34. Descriptions of four phases of abduction in Lanning KV. Investigative analysis and summary of teaching points. In: Lanning KV, Burgess AW, eds. *Child molesters who abduct: summary of the case in point series.* National Center for Missing and Exploited Children, March 1995:26–28.
35. Douglas J, Olshaker M. *Journey into darkness.* New York: Scribner, 1997:157–158. Also, Lanning KV. Investigative analysis and summary of teaching points. In: Lanning KV, Burgess AW, eds. *Child molesters who abduct: summary of the case in point series.* National Center for Missing and Exploited Children, March 1995:32.
36. Lanning KV. *Child molesters: a behavioral analysis for law enforcement officers investigating cases of child sexual exploitation,* 3rd ed. National Center for Missing and Exploited Children, December 1992:12.
37. Personal interview with Peter D. Banks, July 8, 1996.
38. Lanning KV. *Child molesters: a behavioral analysis for law enforcement officers investigating cases of child sexual exploitation,* 3rd ed. National Center for Missing and Exploited Children, December 1992:37–40.
39. Lanning KV. Investigative analysis and summary of teaching points. In: Lanning KV, Burgess AW, eds. *Child molesters who abduct: summary of the case in point series.* National Center for Missing and Exploited Children, March 1995:32.
40. Douglas J, Olshaker M. *Mindhunter: inside the FBI's elite serial crime unit.* New York: Scribner, 1995: 349–350.
41. Information in this section in Douglas J, Olshaker M. *Obsession.* New York: Scribner, 1998:265–289. Also Schaum M, Parrish K. *Stalked: breaking the silence on the crime of stalking in America.* New York: Pocket Books, 1995:53–77.
42. Douglas J, Olshaker M. *Obsession.* New York: Scribner, 1998:265–267.
43. *Stalking–questions and answers.* INFOLINK: A Program of the National Victim Center, No. 43, 1995:3–4.
44. Schaum M, Parrish K. *Stalked: breaking the silence on the crime of stalking in America.* New York: Pocket Books, 1995:63–65.
45. Schaum M, Parrish K. *Stalked: breaking the silence on the crime of stalking in America.* New York: Pocket Books, 1995:115–131.
46. See also *Helpful guide for stalking victims.* INFOLINK: A Program of the National Victim Center, No. 44, 1995, and *Stalking and the law.* INFOLINK: A Program of the National Victim Center, No. 67, 1995.
47. Personal interview with David Beatty, July 22, 1997.
48. Case details in Douglas J, Olshaker M. *Mindhunter: inside the FBI's elite serial crime unit.* New York: Scribner, 1995:284–287.
49. Case details in Douglas J, Olshaker M. *Mindhunter: inside the FBI's elite serial crime unit.* New York: Scribner, 1995:152–159. Also Graysmith R. *The sleeping lady—the Trailside murders above the Golden Gate.* New York: Penguin Books, 1991; and Newton M. *Hunting humans: an encyclopedia of modern serial killers.* Port Townsend, WA: Loompanics Unlimited, 1990:52–54.
50. Information on homicide in the following section from Douglas JE, Burgess AW, Burgess AG, Ressler RK. *Crime classification manual.* New York: Lexington Books, 1992:17–161.
51. See Douglas JE, Burgess AW, Burgess AG, Ressler RK. *Crime classification manual.* New York: Lexington Books, 1992:80–85.
52. Douglas JE, Burgess AW, Burgess AG, Ressler RK. *Crime classification manual.* New York: Lexington Books, 1992:21–22.
53. Organized/disorganized offender characteristics, etc., in this and next section, in Ressler RK, Burgess AW, Douglas JE. *Sexual homicide: patterns and motives.* New York: Lexington Books, 1988:121–133.
54. Douglas JE, Burgess AW, Burgess AG, Ressler RK. *Crime classification manual.* New York: Lexington Books, 1992:133–136.

# 2

# The Victims of Violence

## Carroll Ann Ellis

Violence is the creation of a medical/biological problem by the infliction of physical injury on a person by a person. This would include both lethal injuries and those injuries serious enough to be life threatening, mutilating, or disabling. From that standpoint, violence can be seen as a problem in public health and preventive medicine (1). In the aftermath of violence, medical professionals have the opportunity to invoke their power, strength, science, compassion, technology, and proximity to victims and thus enhance their role as key responders to the epidemic of violence in our nation.

Victims are those who experience the physical, mental, and emotional anguish of crime; those who witness the crime episode and are affected by it; and the community that is left reeling with fear and disgust in the wake of criminal behavior. Violent crime in our society must be considered in relationship to its subsequent impact not only on the tens of thousands of victims who suffer from the willful acts but also on the agents of the medical profession, criminal justice system, and all other responsible agents and systems, including the community at large.

This chapter discusses sexual assault, domestic violence (violence inflicted by one intimate partner on another, including adolescents), family violence (any violence within a family unit), elder abuse, and child victimization. Practical strategies for the care of victims will be offered as a general guideline to their rights, needs, and desires as human beings. Crime victims need to be informed about their rights as victims, as guaranteed by law, in terms and ways they understand. They also need to be informed about the services available to address their needs. They must be provided with access to those services as well. They need help in understanding the criminal justice system as well as the physical, emotional, and mental reactions they may experience as a consequence of victimization. And certainly, they have a need for safety, which can come only when they can seek protection through well-constructed processes. Their needs are fundamental: the ability to obtain services; some assurance of safety from the offender and from revictimization; and participation, when possible, in the justice process. Crime victims in every category need to know that the individual or individuals responsible for their victimization are being held accountable for their crimes by a competent criminal justice system. Medical examinations, when necessary, must be carried out in a nonthreatening manner by competent, compassionate, trained professionals. Finally, victims need to know that they and their experiences are valued in helping to ensure that others are not subjected to the same kind of criminal events or to failures of the systems intended to help and protect.

According to Judith Herman, M.D., the common denominator among trauma victims is a feeling of intense fear, helplessness, and loss of control and a threat of annihilation (2). Aphrodite Matsakis, Ph.D., says, "Just as the body can be traumatized, so can the psyche. On the psychological and mental levels, trauma refers to the wounding of your emotions, your spirit, your will to live, your beliefs about yourself and the world, your dignity, and your sense of security" (3). This chapter is about victims—individuals who become the targets of violent behavior—who experience trauma and what they encounter as a result of that experience. The chapter offers suggestions to health care providers who are the gateway to treatment, comfort, support, and relief for victims of crime.

## THE VICTIM'S EXPERIENCE

I provide supportive services to victims of crime, from the vantage of a Victim Services Division within the Criminal Investigations Bureau of a large police department. The painful, chilling, and humiliating abuse of the human body and spirit is a major element of my daily journey. I have witnessed firsthand the pollution that violent crime leaves in its wake. I often feel as though I am trapped in the belly of the whale—some large, powerful animal that thrashes about—while I try to help small fish wash out into safe waters. Through police-based victim service programs, human service professionals provide immediate and direct service and possible solution of a victim's conflict. Working from within the system, one sees what victims of crime—most of them solid citizens, ordinary people living each day, just like you and me—encounter when faced with traumatic situations. For unsuspecting victims, crime is an ugly reality of circumstance that landed them in their own personal chamber of horror.

Imagine what a rape victim experiences in being forced by a rapist to submit to a physical act so degrading and abusive that one frequently disconnects from all previous coping techniques for survival. The criminal act is animalistic, nauseating, frightening, controlling, injurious, and painful. Rape victims experience the criminal act on several levels: the rapist not only invades and destroys the victim's innermost privacy, body parts, and concept of self but also is a robber who damages and steals property. And the criminal act is only the beginning. Rape victims must submit to an investigation that is not always sensitive and often begins with being told not to wash, shower, rinse, urinate, or remove their clothing until their body (which is evidence) and their clothing (which is evidence) can be "processed." Injury, disease, and pregnancy are immediate concerns and all too often

become reality for victims. The rape victim, regardless of age or gender, is again forced to submit, this time to an examination, which generally includes consenting to the photographing of one's intimate body areas. The victim is made aware that the photographs may be used as evidence in a court of law. A rape victim must submit to being touched by a medical examiner in bodily places that the rapist defiled and degraded. This early medical procedure is the victim's introduction to the legalities of the criminal justice system. Victims become aware that they are "cases" who require study, examination, and analysis. All of this must occur before the victim can finally retreat to the privacy of a shower stall or bathtub to wash away the ravage of the event and the strain and stress of the examination. This process is stressful and dehumanizing, yet it is also a necessary component of the total response to rape victims, one that can be conducted with sensitivity and expertise. Still, there is no preparation, planning, or training for the rape victim, who is at the center of the process and of all subsequent system responses.

It is not enough to deal with the trauma of physical injury from violence. Victims must also cope with the aftermath of the experience, and effective systems must work together to intervene with support, solution, and justice. Victims of crime experience extended trauma, which must be recognized as an area for scientific study leading to a systematic approach that will enhance our current methods of addressing the needs of victims.

Victims of domestic violence withstand bodily injury in the form of bruises, lacerations, broken noses, loss of eyesight, burns, broken limbs, punctured eardrums, and other disfigurements. The victims of these crimes are seen most often in emergency departments, by family doctors, and in health clinics. Yet, too many physicians treat only the illnesses and injuries associated with the violence; in some cases, physicians never identify the violence. Even when violence has been recognized, too many physicians do not have adequate training or education that enables them to respond appropriately to the insidious problem of violent relationships. The victim sometimes is unable to share information with the physician because the batterer may be present. The victim may be unaware of the principle of patient confidentiality, and she is probably operating under the batterer's constant threat to her life. Domestic violence victims have generally been kept isolated from supportive information regarding the pervasive problem of abuse and access to help. These victims suffer from feelings of shame and humiliation; as a consequence, they are frequently reluctant to discuss the abuse in some instances, particularly with a physician who they believe is not knowledgeable or does not care about domestic violence.

One of the most tragic examples of system failure involved a woman who was systematically tortured by her husband. He inserted objects into her vagina and pulled large chunks of her hair from her head, leaving her with sparse patches of hair on parts of her scalp. He punched, kicked, and slapped her, particularly in the lower back area, where she was treated often for what they both described as her tendency to fall due to clumsiness. This victim was treated for kidney problems and other complaints over a 2-year period without any inquiry regarding the issue of domestic violence. The victim finally left her abuser, but he stalked her. As she entered the parking lot at her place of employment one morning, her husband inflicted a fatal stab wound to her abdomen. The victim had sought help from local authorities, used the system for protective orders, attempted to discuss her frequent fractures with her doctor, informed her place of employment, and developed safety plans. Her life could have been saved through a combined effort of professionals working together to help her through the early detection of danger, recognition of indicators, appropriate court intervention to address the abuser's behavior, and safety plans that included collaborative efforts by allied professionals. This case also represents an unresponsive system that failed to remove the abuser from the home, recognize his behavior as criminal, and support the victim's attempts to escape the situation. All too often, such abuse is undetected by the system until it reaches monumental proportions.

Victims of domestic violence seek medical help more often than any other type of support and care.

Health care professionals are in a prime position to identify those dynamics through careful examination of certain symptoms, reactions, and indications, which will alert them not only to the physical violence but also to emotional and sexual abuse. Recognizing that medical illness and physical injury can result from domestic violence and that proper medical intervention can prevent further violence and its consequences, the American College of Physicians has taken the position that (a) physicians should become more sensitive to the possibility of domestic violence as a cause of illness and injury, and (b) hospitals and organized medical staffs should develop protocols for the identification and treatment of domestic violence victims (4).

The health care approach of prevention, prevention/intervention during the early stages of a medical condition, followed by treatment/prevention is now being applied successfully to combat the global problem of domestic violence. To this extent, great strides have been made in educating the public regarding the gravity of this form of criminal behavior. Special programs have been developed to meet the needs of victims of domestic/family violence, yet more effort is needed to overcome centuries of the acceptance of violent behavior toward women. The goal is to permeate and saturate cultural thinking to a state of intolerance to violent behavior of any sort. The enormous problem of domestic/family violence still is fueled by its cultural entrenchment (attitudes that foster and perpetrate violence toward women) and the lack of consistent response to the violence. Consistent health care responses by professionals along with all other responding agents (including protocols, procedures, and policies for victim care) must be in place throughout the nation.

The elderly are victims of crime less often than other age groups. When they are abused, they are subjected to a dehumanizing denial of dignity as they strive to adjust to the aftermath of crime. They can suffer forms of exploitation coupled with physical and sexual abuse and neglect imposed by caregivers, who are frequently family members. Is there a greater insult than to live a long life with an expectation for peace, safety, contentment, and integrity in the final stages of life, only to have those life longings destroyed by callous, violent behavior? Erikson's identification of the core crisis of the elderly—integrity versus despair—takes on greater dimension in the face of crimes against the elderly. Those who feel few regrets achieve ego integrity; they have lived productive and worthwhile lives and have coped with their failures as well as their successes (5). The failure to achieve integrity leads to feelings of despair, hopelessness, guilt, resentment, and self-disgust. In the aftermath of violent crimes, elderly victims can experience intensified feelings of isolation, be hampered in their ability to care for their spouse, face reduced income, and feel increasingly dependent on others.

Recognition of elderly crime victims and interventions for their care have increased, and as a result the specific problems of this group of victims are now being addressed. Domestic violence, sexual assault, and even murder are still often overlooked because of factors commonly associated with age. The medical profession must lead in the effort to ensure that the elderly population is understood. Elderly victims may be forced to live with family members or in respite care following victimization. For the elderly, such major life changes can affect their independence and concept of self. Diminished physical abilities, frailty, decreased financial resources, and loss of mobility are all issues to be considered when treating elderly victims.

Children also are victims of physical assault and emotional trauma. They suffer neglect and abuse at the hands of parents (male and female), relatives, caregivers, and strangers. Witnessing violent episodes in the home also victimizes them. Without therapeutic intervention, many abused children will grow up to become abusers or candidates for serious revictimization (6). It is intolerable that so many children witness rape, assault, domestic violence, and even murder. Their lives are affected by what they see and, unless intervention occurs at an early stage, the effects can be long lasting. According to Deputy Attorney General Eric Holder, "Children who are victims of or witness crime are at an increased risk for delinquency, adult criminality, and violent behavior" (6). He indicates that national studies show that neglected, abused, and otherwise victimized children grow up with an increased risk of criminal behavior, substance abuse, mental illness, and suicide. No longer a secret, child sexual abuse is perpetrated by large numbers of individuals who themselves were sexually exploited.

## The Aftermath of Crime

For victims, crime is a process endured from its conception throughout its execution and eventual aftermath, which is often a continuum of reverberating pain and anguish. Individuals who endure criminal insult often develop certain health conditions, which can be directly linked to the stress associated with the crime event. The insult of crime extends to the financial inconvenience of replacing stolen and destroyed items, living with continuous pain and discomfort, and being forced to readjust one's life to accommodate the havoc and stigma caused by another.

At the moment of the crime event, a relationship erupts between the offender and the victim—the victim/offender dyad. Experiences, interactions, reactions, feelings, injuries, and events born of the dyad constitute the core of both the injury and insult to the human body and spirit. Those relationships form the experience and are in essence the victim episode. It is vital to the healing of crime victims to have their experience receive sensitivity, validation, and support from people charged with the responsibility for responding to their special needs. Responders must recognize the effects of crime on victims, be aware of the victim's tremendous needs in the aftermath of the crime, and take measures that will address those needs.

## Services for Victims

There are still pockets in this nation where victim services are unavailable. Even more amazing is that in areas where services to victims can be interlocked, customized, and guaranteed, the major components and agencies have failed to adopt a multidisciplinary, collaborative approach that would ensure the provision of vital services. Health care, mental health, religious, and social service agencies must work closely with police officers and detectives, prosecutors, judges, court personnel, correction professionals, and victim assistance providers to create a holistic approach to the many needs of victims. In the past, these professionals have not necessarily shared the same goals, nor were they necessarily amenable to working together. Turf issues, lack of knowledge and understanding of each other's roles and responsibilities, and limited knowledge regarding victims' issues and concerns were all responsible for inadequate systems. Law enforcement, criminal justice agencies, and allied professionals are beginning to recognize that they must cooperate and understand each other's functions when responding to criminal victimization (6).

The victim episode, in many instances translated and recounted by victims themselves, serves as a guide for developing specialized programs, fostering collaboration, and ensuring professional association in a system response to the victims of crime. As stated by Schornstein, "Doctors must treat the injuries and address the cause. Otherwise, the treatment is superficial and ineffective to prevent future injury" (4). Whether from medical expertise required in legal or criminal investigation, treatment, education, medical science, or research and technology, there is an overriding need for the health care community to provide front-line services for victims of crime. McAfee (7) emphasized the role of physicians in this effort:

> The AMA can bring its organizational resources to bear on a national agenda [of violence prevention through publications and advocacy] . . . . However, the true success of our commitment will come when we as physicians, treating patients one at time, make a difference by breaking the cycle of violence that engulfs people's lives.

There is increasing evidence that crime-related trauma takes a toll on the long-term physical health of victims. Doctor Dean Kilpatrick, a national expert on victimization and trauma, notes that crime victims have higher rates of health care utilization than people who have not been victimized (8). Compared with nonvictims, female victims have higher rates of

several behaviors and problems that jeopardize well-being: heavy alcohol and drug use, drunk driving, smoking, bulimia, and obesity.

## Victimology

The attention given to crime victims, their issues and concerns, and the responsibility of our institutions and agencies, including legislation that guarantees rights for victims, has given birth to *victimology,* the study of the victims of crime. Victimology examines the relationships experienced by victims as a result of encounters with systems and agencies during the aftermath of crime. Victimology is concerned with family; community; criminal justice; legal, mental, and health care systems; the media; and defender relationships, which are the core of the victim episode. It is now a recognized discipline, conducting exciting research and holding great promise for improved support of the victims of crime.

## THE VIOLENCE PARADOX

Violence "speaks" of an intolerable condition of human shame and rage, a blinding rage that speaks through the body.

*James Gilligan, M.D.* (9)

In their book *The Anatomy of Motive,* Douglas and Olshaker proclaim that every crime is a mystery story with a motive at the heart, which can often explain violent sociopathic behavior (10). They expose the devious nature of violence and its irreversible harm to its recipients. In their discussion of predatory behavior, they conclude that criminals, despite family background, intelligence, or emotional stability, choose to commit their acts of violence. Certainly, deviant behavior, as a choice that results in abuse and injury, is as old as recorded history. The magnitude of those choices continues to be grave, complicated, distressing, and of tremendous concern to society. Human violence remains the same: a manifestation of senseless, bizarre, incomprehensible acts inflicted on people who become victims of heinous crimes. From a historical perspective, most societies developed basic response systems for the management of violent behavior. However, early response systems were never adequate to address the length and breadth of violence in any society. Today, because of the combined efforts of criminal justice agencies, medical and mental health professionals, and members of the faith, business, educational, and legal communities, our response systems are making a difference in the lives of crime victims.

Violence, even as a means to achieve socially acceptable ends, is destructive, deprecating, dominating, painful, and, most importantly, unnecessary in any context. Criminologists, forensic psychiatrists, and correctional professionals can help us understand violence, but they often view the problem from their own field of concentration, which tends to preclude awareness of the lasting effect of violence on its victims. Doctor James Gilligan, former medical director of Bridgewater State Hospital for the Criminally Insane, believes that the different forms of violence are motivated by shame. The purpose of violence is to diminish the intensity of the perpetrator's shame and replace it with shame's opposite, pride (9). Conversely, victims of violence frequently experience feelings of shame, anger, rage, low self-esteem, helplessness, and defeat as result of perpetrators' efforts to eliminate their own uncomfortable feelings at the expense of the victim. For victims, the exposure creates a lasting relationship with perpetrators and their deeds. Such an injustice is not singular but is perpetrated on all of society and is, quite simply, an outrage. Further outrage is that for every reported case of violence there are countless numbers of cases and instances of violent crimes in these categories and others that are not reported through the established gates of entry for help. The medical profession should be the gatekeeper for those victims who of necessity seek medical help. Early detection of abuse, particularly of children, will diminish the numbers of children forced to live with the pathology of criminal behavior. The insult of victimization demands not only moral and legal consideration but also response to the causes of violence, treatment for those causes, and utilization of that knowledge to prevent further violence.

## SEXUAL ASSAULT

[Sexual assault] is a metamorphosis. Although the event is external, it is quickly incorporated into the mind, where it replicates itself, like a virus. There is no defense. And yet life goes on.

*Nancy Venable Raine* (11)

### Consider

By the age of 34, Karen had undergone a mastectomy and reconstruction breast surgery, earned a law degree, and was balancing a successful career. She was also raped in her home by a 19-year-old man. He entered her garden apartment through an open window around 2 o'clock in the morning and subjected her to 3 hours of physical, emotional, and psychological torture engineered through painful and humiliating acts. He raged and tormented her, calling her unspeakable names and demanding that she "shut up." He defiled and destroyed her apartment while demanding that she give him cash. He ripped the earrings from her ears and hurled items about the room in search of money. His sexual violence was engineered through vaginal penetration and forced anal and oral sodomy. She sustained vaginal tearing and anal injury. She had facial and neck bruises and swelling due to slaps, blows, and choking. Her back and buttocks were scratched, and she had multiple superficial stab wounds to her upper torso. A front tooth was chipped when her head was forced against the edge of the bathtub. Karen was kicked repeatedly in the lower back and side. She underwent extensive surgery to repair the internal damage to her spine and kidneys. In addition, her hands bore the cuts and slashes from the knife used to force her into submission. Karen still bears the scars of upper chest stab wounds. She was beaten and threatened with death if she reported the incident. Before fleeing Karen's apartment, the rapist promised to return. When Karen finally received help, the rapist made good his promise and returned to Karen's apartment, in the early hours of the next morning, expecting to continue his rampage of violence. When he returned, he was arrested and

Karen underwent nearly 2 years of court trials before the rapist was finally sentenced to a prison term of 65 years. Part of his conviction was based on the effective collection of evidence by SANE (Sexual Assault Nurse Examiner). After several surgeries and ongoing medical attention, Karen describes her life today as having been derailed from its former track; she has disconnected from previous relationships, and her activities have diminished in scope. No longer living alone, she describes her fear of being left alone in her parents' large house. "I cannot sleep until everyone is in the house. My windows must be closed at all times and I am afraid of the dark. I still wake up in the night terrified that I will be attacked again and no one will hear my cries for help. I avoid men, particularly young men." Karen is no longer with a law firm but is now working as a sales clerk in a bookstore. She is quick to offer that she considers herself lucky to be alive and is grateful for encounters with a criminal justice system and allied professionals who were knowledgeable about the "victim episode." The physical injuries sustained during Karen's fateful ordeal have long since healed. What remains is the insult of injury; it is an infestation of conflict. One of the major residuals of violence for victims is the stigma associated with the crime. Karen's residuals are manifested by her vow of celibacy, inability to resume her former career, medical expenses, financial needs, lingering legal matters, and safety issues. Karen's needs were addressed by a continuum of care and support, which began from the moment the call for help was received by police emergency services. The call set into motion a response system that included criminal justice agencies and trained allied professions working together to achieve common goals. After 5 years, Karen is just entering therapy.

The system of response worked for Karen. She was interviewed by knowledgeable detectives and treated at the hospital emergency department by sensitive medical professionals. A medical examination was conducted promptly, procedures were explained, and hospital protocol was followed. Karen received a nonjudgmental approach from examining practitioners, which helped to reduce her anxiety and support empowerment. She received individual care and treatment, which took into consideration her physical history with all of its complications. During this initial phase of Karen's aftercare, a victim service provider arrived at the hospital to ensure that Karen was receiving psychological support, to serve as a liaison with family and friends, and to provide information regarding victims' rights, the criminal justice system, and available services. Karen received a full explanation of all procedures, as well as reasons for and protocols associated with evidence collection. The examination was conducted, and Karen was referred for physician evaluation and treatment regarding her other injuries. However, this interaction with the health care system was only the beginning.

## Victims' Reactions to Rape

Professor Ann Burgess, a psychiatric nurse, along with Lynda Lytle Holmstrom, a sociologist, first described the reactions of rape victims as *rape trauma syndrome* (12). The short-term effects include denial, shock, disbelief, disruption, and feelings of guilt, shame, blame, and hostility. The long-term effects may be more deeply rooted, causing phobias and sexual problems and affecting the victim's ability to "function."

Rape victims have very specific concerns (13):

- Safety of self
- Safety of children
- Mistrust of men/husband/dating
- Frustration with impaired sexuality
- Frustration with impaired emotional intimacy
- Loss of self-esteem, self-respect, and level of functioning
- Perceptual distortion
- Marriage/dating problems
- Divorce
- Concern about the rapist being released and looking for them
- Fear of being revictimized

In addition, subsequent events occur in the lives of many rape victims, leading to additional emotional trauma and financial expense. These constitute secondary victimizations:

- Divorce
- Loss of sexual desire
- Cost of home safety equipment
- Cost of self-defense classes
- Cost of counseling (both victimization and marriage/family)
- Change of job
- Lack of information about legal procedures
- Fear of acquired immunodeficiency syndrome (AIDS)

## Definition of Sexual Assault

Each crime category has its distinct markings. Rape is a violent crime engineered through sexual acts that are forced and degrading. The idea is to control, humiliate, force, harm, and overpower the victim. We have long since moved beyond the old myths surrounding rape and sexual assault as being invited, confined only to women, stranger motivated, and uncommon. Sexual assault does not always transpire between a female victim and a stranger lurking in the dark. Rape occurs between acquaintances, which makes the act no less disgusting and degrading. Rape defies age and gender. Victims are children, elderly people, people with physical or mental disabilities, and anyone who falls prey to the predator. Women are the victims of rape and sexual assault most often, but men are also raped.

Current definitions of sexual assault and rape include male and female children and adolescents as well as men and women as victims. Rape by acquaintance and forced oral or anal sex are also considered to be rape and sexual assault. These more recent expansions have come about after years of definitions that have varied widely from state to state. The Illinois Criminal Sexual Assault Statute is now considered the national model for broadly defining rape. It has the following characteristics:

- Rape is defined as "gender neutral," which broadens the earlier definition of rape so that it now includes men as well as women.
- It includes acts of sexual penetration other than vaginal penetration by a penis.
- It distinguishes types of sexual abuse on the basis of the degree or threat of force, similar

to the "aggravated" versus "simple" distinction of physical assaults.
- Threat as well as overt force is recognized as a means of overpowering the victim.
- In addition, a new category of rape victim, "taking advantage of an incapacitated victim," is included. This category includes the mentally ill as well as victims under the influence of drugs or alcohol. (Some states require that the perpetrator had to give the victim the intoxicant in order to obtain sexual access.)

A 1986 federal statute defines two types of sexual assault:

- Sexual abuse: causing another person to engage in a sexual activity by threatening or placing that person in fear or engaging in a sexual act if that person is incapable of declining participation in or communicating unwillingness to engage in that sexual act.
- Aggravated sexual abuse: when a person "knowingly causes another person to engage in a sexual act . . . or attempts to do so by using force against that person, or by threatening or placing that person in fear that the person will be subjected to death, serious bodily injury, or kidnapping; when a person knowingly renders another person unconscious and thereby engages in a sexual act with that person, or administers to another person by force or threat of force, or without the knowledge or permission of that person, a drug, intoxicant, or other similar substance and thereby substantially impairs the ability of that person to appraise or control conduct and then engages in a sexual act with that person" (8).

### *Male Rape*

Sexual assault and abuse are not restricted to women and children; men are also sexually assaulted and therefore require services designed to meet their specific needs arising from sexual assault and domestic violence. Male victims also experience the debilitating aftermath with the added dimension of myths, gender stereotyping, and the stigma associated with male vulnerability to victimization. Men and boys are reluctant to report the crime of rape; as a consequence, male rape is grossly underreported and undertreated.

Most male rape victims are raped by other men, in the sense that they are forced to submit to anal intercourse, oral sex, mutual masturbation, masturbation of the offender, or other sex acts. Fear of bodily harm can cause a man to have an erection; therefore, a man can be raped by either a man or a woman. In addition, men can be raped by women in that they can be coerced or intimidated into sexual behavior they do not desire. Furthermore, a percentage of sexual abuse is perpetrated by adult females on young boys. It is a myth that only gay men are raped. Most male rape victims do not report their assaults, nor do they receive medical attention or counseling. Male victims suffer from feelings of shame and a sense of guilt, associated with the stigma of sexual contact with another male.

Data regarding the reactions to and specifics of male sexual assault are limited; however, it is believed that the shock of sexual assault is greater in male rape victims than women because of societal conditioning, which prepares a female for the possibility of rape. Male victims may be led to question their sexual orientation based on being subjected to what is considered a nonmasculine episode. Male victims may suffer sexual malfunctions due to sexual assault. They are often isolated and their needs for victim services go unmet because of lack of information regarding the problem, reluctance of providers to commit to services, lack of trained and skilled personnel to adequately address their needs, and system insensitivity to male victims of sexual assault. Medical sensitivity, public education, and training of professionals who deal with victims constitute a start toward greater initiatives in treatment, research, and program development.

### Stranger Rape

Stranger rape is among the most feared of all crimes. It is a rape executed by a person or persons who have had no previous contact with the victim. Gang rape usually falls into this category. Actually, fewer stranger rapes are committed than rapes by an offender known to the victim.

### Acquaintance Rape

Acquaintance rape transpires between individuals who know each other casually. Acquaintance rape occurs among college students more than any other age group. In a large survey, one in four college women reported being the victim of rape or attempted rape, and 84% of their assailants were dates or acquaintances. They may have a close relationship, may have dated steadily, may even have been sexual partners. Acquaintance rapes are most commonly not reported because of the difficulty in prosecuting, the stigma, and the lack of information regarding the right to receive victim services. Many victims of acquaintance rape do not label their experience of being forced to have sex as "sexual assault." However, the fact that a gun or knife was not used does not eliminate the trauma that acquaintance rape victims experience. The shame of rape in any context is so overwhelming that victims may not report it, particularly acquaintance rape. Victims wonder who will believe them. In giving voice to their experience, victims are sometimes met with telling reactions from the listener, which mirror shame to victims. Victims of acquaintance rape are often blamed for the incident, resulting in placement of responsibility for the rape on the victim. Acquaintance rape may account for the majority of rapes committed each year, but its incidence cannot be measured because of the failure of victims to report it.

### Date Rape

Date rape is rape in which a more defined relationship exists between the individuals at the time of the event. This type of rape contains all of the elements of acquaintance rape: it is underreported, difficult to prosecute, and extremely prevalent. Date rape is made more comple by dating norms and the extent of the relationship between the people involved. Victims may take responsibility for the event because they chose to date the offending individual. They experience the additional burdens of betrayal, self-accusation, and personal failure regarding their ability to select dating partners. Like acquaintance rape, date rape is common and difficult to prosecute. Dating behavior is defined by dating expectations. Men may expect that sex will be part of the dating experience; women may want a sense of commitment before they become intimate in a relationship.

### Marital Rape

Recognition of a woman's right to say no to sex within the state of marriage is responsible for the term *marital rape.* Many states have adopted a proactive stance regarding this underreported type of sexual assault. The Virginia Department of Criminal Justice Services provided the following definitions: Marital rape occurs when the victim is living separate and apart from her husband or if she has suffered serious physical injury, and if her husband is guilty of acts committed by force, threat, or intimidation of sexual intercourse against her will; forcible sodomy against her will; and object sexual penetration of vagina or anus against her will. Even if the victim is still residing with her husband and has not suffered serious physical injury, the husband is still guilty of marital sexual assault if he forces his wife to have sexual intercourse, oral sex, or anal sex; forcibly penetrates his wife's vagina or anus with an object; or forces his wife to penetrate herself with an object. Approximately 40% to 45% of physically abused women are also forced into sex (14,15).

### Reporting of Sexual Assault

The effects of rape are far-ranging, far-reaching, long-lasting, and late-arising.

*Cynthia Carosella* (16)

Most sexual assaults are never reported to law enforcement; consequently, there is no apprehension of many perpetrators for prosecution and incarceration. The rapist remains at large, free to assault again. In many instances, victims of rape are young, unsuspecting, frightened girls. They become prey to dates, employers, customers, relatives, and strangers. In surveys that asked victims why they did not report the rape, they gave the following reasons: shame; embarrassment; fear of rejection, exposure, or ridicule; fear of the rapist; distrust of the system; and lack of information regarding victims' rights.

Very often, when cases are reported to law enforcement, the report comes from some source other than the victim. A victim who arrives at an emergency department for help following a sexual assault is asked if she wants to report the crime to law enforcement. In most states the victim is allowed to make that decision but is encouraged to cooperate with the police investigation. It is generally believed that the best interest of the victim is served through her ability to make decisions. Victims who at least reach an emergency department have a chance of receiving an examination by a medical professional, information about pregnancy and disease prevention, and treatment for injury. Sexual assault victims who require medical attention and fail to receive it are left with unattended issues of great magnitude.

We will never know how many of those who have been raped lost their jobs, ended relationships, or experienced sexual dysfunction or addictions or eating disorders or procrastination or loss of hope, etc., all as effects of being raped. The effects of rape range from subtle to extreme and can be both physical and emotional. They are seen in the male victim who cannot bear to be spoken to in a certain way by his boss because it reminds him of his rapist's demanding voice, and in the woman who cannot bear to lose the protective covering of weight she gained after she was raped (16).

### A Measure of the Problem

Obtaining accurate measurements of the incidence of rape and other types of sexual assault poses many challenges. The number of reported rapes and other types of sexual assault reflects how these crimes are defined and how they are measured. The following statistics are derived from different sources, which often measure different factors using different methodologies.

- In 1996, the National Crime Victimization Survey found that more than two thirds of rapes/sexual assaults committed in the nation remained unreported (17).
- Using a definition of rape that includes forced vaginal, oral, and anal sex, the *National Violence Against Women Survey* found that 1 of 6 U.S. women and 1 of 33 U.S. men experienced an attempted or completed rape as a child and/or adult (18).
- About 14.8% of women and 2.8% of men in the United States are victims of rape; an additional 2.1% of women and 0.9% of men are victims of attempted rape (18).
- More than 52% of rape/sexual assault victims are females younger than 25 years (19).

The National Violence Against Women Survey found that "rape in America is a tragedy of youth" because the majority of rapes occur during childhood and adolescence (18).

- Of first or only rapes experienced by women, 21.6% occurred before the victim was 12 years old.
- Of all rapes, 20.8% were committed against girls between the ages of 15 and 16.

## Underserved Populations

Special attention and programs must address the needs of victims who have been overlooked in the past. The programs must include screening, diagnosis, treatment, evaluations, and psychological as well as case service assistance, which take into consideration the special needs of each group.

### The Elderly

Older people are often the target of sexual assault. Females with impaired functioning are particularly at risk. Health care professionals who are not aware of the signs may fail to respond to the problem. The elderly are sometimes assaulted in health care facilities, where they are unable to resist or escape their predators. Care and attention must be given to this special population.

### Disabled People

A person with a disability has a physical or mental impairment that substantially limits one or more major life activities, has a record of such impairment, or is regarded as having such impairment (20). Special programs with skilled and trained staff must be available throughout the continuum of care (including the criminal justice system) to meet the needs of individuals with impairments, whether medically based or the result of mental illness. More than 49 million Americans have disabilities, with a vast array of impairments. Persons with disabilities are devalued when programs and systems are not fashioned with their special needs in mind. Basic information regarding the hearing impaired, deaf people, and individuals with speech impairments (such as their preferred means of communicating) must be considered. Victims with visual impairment or blindness may not be able to visually identify their assailant or describe from sight the events of their victimization; nevertheless, through heightened other senses, the victim will be able to provide extensive information. Every device and effort should be used to ensure that these victims have access to resources that address their needs. Sexual assault victims with mental disabilities, mental retardation, or mental illness require special protocols for criminal justice participation and aftercare.

### Gay Men, Lesbians, Bisexuals, and Transgendered People

The gay, lesbian, bisexual, and transgendered (GLBT) community is an "invisible minority" because its members do not look different from others in their respective ethnic groups. About 2% of Americans—about 5 million people—are gay (20). Gay and lesbian victims of sexual assault tend to refrain from reporting their victimization because they fear the response will be insensitive and inadequate. Some victims do not wish to disclose their sexual orientation because they fear that such disclosures will jeopardize their jobs, family relations, and other vital aspects of their lives.

### Victims of Domestic Violence

In relationships in which violence is a common and recurring process, sexual assault is considered an appendix of the violence. Forced rape is seldom reported and is often used by the spouse rapist as punishment, retaliation, or a bargaining tool in custody issues. Sexual assault is tied to patterns of abusive behaviors associated with domestic violence. This type of forced sex is tied to the belief still held by some that a woman is obligated to submit to her husband on demand.

### Non–English-Speaking, Ethnic Minority, and Foreign-Born Victims

When considering the aftercare of victims from culturally diverse backgrounds, myriad issues emerge. Language and culture are primary in setting up protocols for response. Victims of sexual assault will view the rape dynamic from its occurrence throughout the aftermath based on their cultural experience. They must be assisted in special ways that eliminate barriers to information and available services tailored to their needs.

### Refugees and Resettlement Victims of Sexual Assault

Many women have been displaced from their countries for political or other reasons, such as war and natural disaster. They may be resettled to refugee camps, where they are sometimes forced into prostitution, forced to trade sex for food for their children, and/or brutalized by systematic rape. Victims who have experienced gang rape and repeated rapes often fail to report the crimes and blame themselves based on relegated submissive roles and on religious and cultural mores.

### The Aftermath of Sexual Assault

Forensics is the silent witness . . . it does not speak for or against the victim. It merely speaks the truth.

*Detective Jeffrey Miller, Forensic Expert, Fairfax, Virginia*

The rape victim deserves the best evidentiary examination possible through a program designed for the gathering, collection and documentation of that evidence for the court system.

*Sue Brown, Sexual Assault Nursing Examiner, Fairfax, Virginia*

In sexual assault cases, the victim's body is the primary "crime scene," and the forensic medical examination is an extremely important part of evidence collection (8). Emergency medical care, especially the collection of evidence through a forensic examination, is critical both for the victim and for protection of evidence for the prosecution. Trained medical professionals must meet the rape victim's medical and emotional needs and they must collect evidence to be used in a legal proceeding. When victims are made a part of this process as a stockholder, their cooperation increases and the procedures are not as difficult and prolonged. The local protocol, which may include agreements and cooperation among participating agencies, should be explained to victims. They need information about the process—what, how, why, and when—with simple direct explanations that can be understood even in the midst of conflict.

A comprehensive medical protocol to be used in the aftermath of rape includes the following components:

- Evidentiary examination (the patient has the right to refuse an examination for this purpose)
- Police report
- Gynecologic examination
- Consent for the taking of photographs
- Minors and parental notification
- Directions for taking medication to prevent pregnancy; side effects of drugs
- Referrals to anonymous human immunodeficiency virus (HIV) antibody testing facilities
- Counseling referrals
- Information regarding victim services for information regarding legislation, court proceedings, and civil suits

### Sexual Assault Response Team

Sexual assault response team (SART) is a designated group of professionals available to respond on demand when a sexual assault has occurred. The team consists of a law enforcement officer, a sexual assault advocate, a nurse examiner, a SANE, and a physician when necessary.

### *Collection of Forensic Evidence*

Examination of a rape victim includes the following:

- An internal examination
- Pubic hair combings
- Nail scrapings
- Saliva samples
- Medical history
- Medical care and treatment of injuries
- Diagnosis and treatment of sexually transmitted diseases
- Pregnancy test
- Collection of clothing

### Recommendations for Health Care Providers

1. Create a sensitive environment where patients are encouraged to express feelings, concerns, and needs related to the assault.
2. Be responsive to questions and concerns regarding procedures and treatment and involve patients in decision making regarding follow-up care and notification of family members.
3. Comply with the global challenge recommendation in *New Directions from the Field: Victims' Rights and Services for the 21st Century* (7) to institute victimology as curriculum in medical schools, nursing schools, and schools of social work.
4. Ensure that policies, procedures, and protocols are in place to deal with identification, medical histories of victims, treatment of victims, reporting, and follow-up evaluation.
5. Ensure that culturally appropriate information is available to victims of sexual assault. Victims should be able to read and understand medical information, which will help in their recovery process. In addition, when language is a barrier, ensure that interpreters are available to help in dispensing services.

6. Engage in campaigns to heighten public awareness regarding sexual assault as a preventive measure as well as to garner support for victims.
7. If forensic evidence has been collected, ensure that expert testimony is available for court cases.
8. Create programs that train personnel as a SANE, sexual assault nurse clinician, (SANC), or sexual assault/forensic examiner (SAFE) to offer sensitive outreach to adult and child victims of sexual assault in a nonthreatening environment. These programs employ highly trained and skilled medical professionals who are contacted immediately by law enforcement to respond to victims. They are present in the emergency department to address the injuries, initiate the process of evidence collection for prosecution, and provide special counseling to victims to allay their fears of infection and pregnancy. Medical professionals are the only agents qualified to make careful diagnosis, dispense treatment, and prescribe medications for victims of sexual assault. Additional help from other agents is satellite to the physical and mental issues set in motion by an emergency response to the problem.

The National Victim Assistance Academy (21) offers a "Promising Practices" segment that outlines innovative programs and approaches to working with victims. A few of these exceptional programs are described below:

- Medical care programs addressing the needs of recent rape victims. An initial medical examination immediately after a rape is recommended to assess the victim for sexually transmitted diseases (STDs) and for provision of prophylactic treatment. Rape victims should be seen for follow-up medical examination to assess any new infections that may be related to the assault, to counsel victims about STDs and hepatitis B, and to treat existing diseases. Guidelines from the Centers for Disease Control recommend follow-up care at 2 weeks after the assault for repeat STD testing and additional blood testing for syphilis and HIV, which can be repeated at 6, 12, and 24 weeks.

Despite these guidelines, most medical care is supported financially by the state or by partial payment from sources such as Crime Victims Compensation. However, since most rape victims do not report the assault to police, they cannot take advantage of subsidies for medical treatment of acute injuries.

- Some programs offer follow-up medical care for victims (19, 22). The Medical University of South Carolina provides medical care to women regardless of whether or not they have reported an assault to police. In addition, follow-up care is provided at 6 weeks and 6 months after the assault. Such care includes reassessment and treatment of STDs and long-term follow-up blood testing for HIV and hepatitis B.
- Another multidisciplinary aspect of the program at the Medical University of South Carolina is the development of a brief video-based intervention to help prepare women for the medical examination and to provide education and instruction designed to reduce post-rape symptoms of posttraumatic stress syndrome, substance abuse, panic, and depression. The program is coordinated with a local rape treatment center.
- Most women who report a rape are seen for medical care within hours of the assault. Thus, the medical community has an opportunity to give early intervention that could prevent some of the negative mental health consequences of rape. Rather than reducing anxiety, the medical examination contains many cues that might actually increase a rape victim's distress. Previous data indicated that women's initial distress is a strong predictor of long-term distress. Therefore, an intervention that could reduce distress at the time of the medical examination might help women in their recovery (21).

## DOMESTIC VIOLENCE

What's love got to do with it?

*Tina Turner*

The human heart is a strange mystery.

*Alexandre Dumas*

### Consider

Angela, a state department employee, and Tom, an insurance claims adjuster, were married for 3 months before the indicators of violence became apparent. Angela recalls that what she once considered Tom's love was in fact a mean, sinister obsession with every aspect of her life. He monitored her phone calls, her mail, and her relations with co-workers and family. He demanded control of her income and portioned out a limited allowance for incidentals only. He required special meals and formal eating arrangements. Tom always explained his actions as manifestations of his love, protection, and concern for Angela. He called himself a perfectionist who had found the perfect wife for the perfect family and life. He explained that his aggression was intended to guard and protect their perfect life.

By the end of their first year of marriage, Angela had become the victim of Tom's physical, verbal, sexual, and emotional abuse. The first attack was swift and harsh. Tom confronted Angela when she arrived home after working late on a Friday night. As she exited the car, Tom struck her with such force that she fell to the ground, scraping her face and fracturing her right cheekbone and several bones in her right foot. She was knocked unconscious and remembers awaking to Tom's concerned face as he applied ice to her bloody and rapidly swelling face, forehead, and hands. She was baffled and confused. Tom was remorseful and loving. He vowed never to hurt her again. He begged for forgiveness and promised that his newly acquired habit of drinking every night would stop. Angela was subsequently treated at the emergency department of a local hospital. Tom explained her "fall" as a nasty accident. That initial incident ushered in the start of 8 years of beatings, sexual abuse, drinking bouts, rages, fear, embarrassment, shame, stalking, threats, and attempts by Angela to conceal the effects of abuse, as well as many attempts to escape the condition. After the birth of two children and three miscarriages (caused by severe beatings), Angela finally, with the support of the criminal justice system and legal, health, and mental health service agencies, received safe passage to a new life.

[About 16% of pregnant women are abused. Several complications of pregnancy—including low birth weight, insufficient weight gain, substance abuse, inadequate prenatal care, and premature delivery—have also been associated with abuse (23). Connections between abuse during pregnancy and miscarriages are strongly suspected (24).]

Angela found asylum from years of pain and the threat of death from a husband determined to possess her on his own terms. She endured broken limbs; severe injuries to her eardrums, ribs, nose, fingers, and throat; frequent black eyes and broken teeth; and a spinal cord injury. She had also been forced to participate in painful and humiliating sexual acts. Conviction for his crimes against Angela and her eventual escape did not come swiftly or easily. It took years, starting with Angela's process of leaving a destructive relationship. Time after time she left and sought help through family and friends. Each time she tried to leave him, Tom was able to convince her that life would be different and he would change.

Over the years, the beatings became more severe and the psychological/emotional abuse became more intense. The children were exposed to Tom's drinking bouts and irrational behavior, and Angela feared for their physical safety as well as her own. After regaining consciousness following one of Tom's choking episodes, Angela finally resolved that he would never change and that she had to escape or die. Years of being locked in a violent and destructive relationship resulted in Angela's engaging in whatever Tom wanted or needed, including criminal activities such as fraud and theft. She describes her self-loathing and shame in having engaged in certain behavior. Her physician, who documented his findings and followed through with his suspicions regarding the reason for her frequent injuries, asked Angela the right questions. It was this informed physician who identified and recognized that Angela was the victim of recurring violence in her home. The same physician was responsible for recognizing and reporting the emotional and psychological abuse

of Angela's two children. The end of Angela's ordeal with Tom came as a result of medical intervention, not the workings of the criminal justice system. Her cries for help to law enforcement were minimized, overlooked, and in several cases denied. When police were called in, they encouraged the couple to work it out. When she attempted to obtain orders of protection, the system denied them based on the assumption that they were not needed to stem the situation. Tom has long since served his brief term in jail for assault. Angela has relocated and seemingly moved on with her life. Her children have grown into teenagers without the presence of their father in the home. To her knowledge, Tom is unaware of their location. For Angela, the years of violence still dominate her life. She confesses that she is never free from her fear that Tom will find her and kill her.

The intense concerns of victims of domestic violence were summarized by Brown (13):

- Physical safety of self and children
- Fear of the abuser locating them
- Concern about how they will survive
- Not having a safe place to stay away from the abuser
- Not having money, a job, or work skills
- Having no transportation

Additional problems emerge as aspects of secondary victimization:

- Lack of protection from law enforcement agencies
- Lack of services available to help with transition
- Lack of training, money, and information about how to increase work skills
- Stigmatization by being labeled a "spouse abuse victim"

### Definition of Domestic Violence

All aspects of abuse (physical, sexual, and controlling behavior, including emotional degradation) are important to the resultant effects on women's health and opportunities for interventions in the health care system.

*Jacquelyn C. Campbell* (25)

### Consider

Angela's story is a typical example of the cycle of violence. Confusion, imbalance of power, isolation, appeasement, secrecy, separations/reunions, as well as alcohol and drug use all reflect this complex and insidious practice of violence. Domestic violence is defined as a systematic pattern of abusive behaviors, occurring over a period of time, that may become more frequent and severe and are carried out for the purpose of control, domination, and/or coercion. Such behaviors may include verbal abuse and threats; physical, psychological, and sexual abuse; and destruction of property and pets. The batterer frequently accomplishes the abuses in an environment of his own creation that ultimately traps the victim in a state of fear, isolation, deprivation, and confusion.

Domestic violence episodes are not random acts of violence or incidents of mere loss of temper. Rather, such episodes are part of a complex, continuing pattern of behavior, of which the violence is but one dynamic (4). A general definition of domestic violence is any assault, battery, sexual assault, sexual battery, or any criminal offense resulting in personal injury or death of one family or household member by another, who is or was residing in the same dwelling unit. Generally speaking, "family or household member" means spouse, former spouse, persons related by blood or by marriage, persons who are presently residing together, as if a family, or who have resided together in the past, as if a family, and persons who have a child in common regardless of whether they have been married or have resided together at any time.

We are knowledgeable about the cycle of violence, we know about power and control. We understand the drama and tragedy of abuse. We even have a long list of why women stay in abusive relationships, but what we fail to talk about is the power of love often inherent in those destructive relationships. Love being battered and tortured . . . no way. Love and long for the battering partner to change his behavior, absolutely. Most women are initially shocked and confused by the battering behavior perpetrated by the men they love and trust. Such violence usually appears after a bond of commitment develops. The victim is caught unaware and is soon caught in a web, with the belief that the batterer's behavior will change. Domestic violence victims generally return to their violent situations six to eight times before finally leaving the relationship. They usually return because they do not want to separate their children from their father, because they love their partners, and they have no options for other living choices. During the process of leaving, the victim is never in greater danger than when the batterer recognizes that the leaving is final. During this period, he may increase his attacks, stalk the victim, vandalize, assault, rape, kidnap her and/or the children, and threaten and even attempt to kill them. Separating and returning only reinforces the batterer's violence, and he becomes convinced that his aggression accomplishes the goal of keeping his partner under control.

Working with battered women is especially difficult, requiring great patience on the part of listening parties. Women who are victims of domestic violence typically establish a history with law enforcement, child protective services, and the courts. When women have been in a violent situation for a long time and it is perceived that they are reluctant to leave, they need help from sensitive sources who understand that leaving is a process. Just as the cycle of violence progresses as a process, so does the eventual leave taking. It sometimes takes years before the woman is able to finally accomplish this goal. Battered women are sometimes assumed to be weak and ineffectual, but the opposite is true. There is strength in the ability to withstand and endure the amount of abuse that is inflicted in violent relationships.

Battered women can develop symptoms of post-traumatic stress disorder (PTSD) (26). PTSD is defined as a cluster of symptoms that almost anyone subjected to trauma outside the range of usual human experience would develop. These include but are not limited to intrusive recollection of the trauma(s), psychic numbing of emotions, flashbacks, appetite and/or sleep disturbance, hypervigilance, exaggerated startle response, disturbance concentration, unpredictable irritability or anger, anxiety, and depression. Victims of domestic violence may also experience symptoms of learned helplessness; passivity; indecisiveness; and chronic physical illnesses that range from frequent colds, flus, and allergies to chronic urinary, vaginal, and gastrointestinal problems. In the most serious cases, ulcers and eating disorders have also been related to abuse (27). According to research conducted by Kilpatrick, "victims of violent crime may suffer undiagnosed PTSD for many years, at great cost to their health and the healthcare system."

### Children Who Witness Violence

Children who witness violence in their homes are affected by the experience in various ways. The immediate negative effects appear to translate into low self-esteem, behavioral problems, reduced social ability, depression, and anxiety (28). Children who experience violence in the home as victims or observers are at risk for continuing the cycle of violence in their lives as adults (29). Men and women who report being hit by their parents are more likely to hit their own children (30).

### A Measure of the Problem

- In 1996, women experienced an estimated 840,000 rapes, sexual assaults, robberies, aggravated assaults, and simple victimization at the hands of an intimate.
- Intimate violence is primarily a crime against women. In 1996, females were the victims of three of every four murders of intimates and about 85% of the victims of nonlethal intimate violence (1).
- Data from the National Violence Against Women Survey (18), the first national study on stalking, sponsored jointly by the National Institute of Justice and the Centers for Disease Control and Prevention, confirm previous reports that violence against women is predominantly intimate-partner violence. Of the women who reported being raped and/or physically assaulted since the age of 18, three fourths were victimized by a current or former husband, cohabiting partner, date, or boyfriend.
- Women are significantly more likely than men to report being raped or physically assaulted by a current or former intimate partner,

whether the time frame considered was the person's lifetime or the 12 months preceding the survey. Moreover, when raped or physically assaulted by a current or former intimate partner, women are significantly more likely than men to sustain injuries (18).
- Women of all races are about equally vulnerable to violence by an intimate partner (17).
- Women between the ages of 19 and 29 and women in families with incomes below $10,000 are more likely than other women to be victims of violence by an intimate partner (17).
- Among victims of violence committed by an intimate partner, the victimization rate of women separated from their husbands is about three times higher than that of divorced women and about 25 times higher than that of married women (17).
- Females were more likely to be victimized at a private home (their own or that of a neighbor, friend, or relative) than in any other place. Males were most likely to be victimized in public places such as businesses, parking lots, and open spaces (17).
- About 4 in 10 inmates serving time in jail for intimate violence had a criminal justice status—on probation or parole or under a restraining order—at the time of the violent attack on the intimate (17).
- About one in four convicted violent offenders confined in local jails had committed their crime against an intimate; about 7% of state prisoners serving time for violence had an intimate victim (17).

### Recommendations for Health Care Providers

Be aware of the dynamics of domestic violence; be clear that no one should ever have to submit to violence. Domestic assaults can involve pushing, shoving, kicking, grabbing, throwing things at the victim, strangulation, beatings, punching, and emotional/verbal abuse, including threats of violence.

Be familiar with local and national resources for victims. For example:

- Children's Hospital in Boston was the nation's first program to offer advocacy and support to abused mothers at the same time that the hospital offered protection to abused children. AWAKE (Advocacy for Women and Kids in Emergencies) was formed to broaden child abuse programming to include intervention on behalf of battered women and to coordinate services that were often offered separately, and in conflict, to women and to children (21).

- The American Academy of Facial Plastic and Reconstructive Surgery, in partnership with the National Coalition Against Domestic Violence, the umbrella group for the majority of domestic violence shelters across the nation, provides free medical services to victims of domestic abuse (21).

Design a set of questions that will help detect possible violence in the home. Be specific and ask directly about violence. The following set of questions was compiled by Salber and Taliaferro (31):

1. You have a number of bruises. How did they happen?
2. What happens when your spouse loses his temper?
3. Are you in a relationship in which you are being hurt?
4. Has your partner ever harmed or threatened to harm someone or something you love?
5. Does your spouse use drugs or alcohol? How does your spouse behave toward you when he is drinking or using drugs?
6. Do you have children? Are they living in a safe environment?

It is imperative to ask these questions when the patient has been separated from anyone who has accompanied her to the appointment. She will most likely refrain from any admissions or discussions until she feels the information can be imparted to an empathetic listener.

Physicians specifically should look for evidence of domestic violence. In *The Physician's Guide to Domestic Violence,* Salber and Taliaferro (31) suggest that some clues to the presence of domestic violence can be ascertained from the history and physical examination:

- The reported history of the incident is not consistent with the kind of injury.

- There is a time delay between injuries and presentation.
- The patient has a history of being "accident prone."
- The patient has attempted suicide or experienced depression.
- The patient has had repeated psychosomatic complaints

Further actions to be taken by health care professionals are as follows:

1. Develop multidisciplinary approaches to working with domestic violence victims. Ensure that medical personnel join coalitions, boards, and committees whose task is to provide service to domestic violence victims.
2. Develop threat assessment protocols to ensure the safety of victims.
3. Provide emergency department security for victims of domestic violence.
4. Develop a protocol for questioning patients when domestic abuse is suspected.
5. Ensure continuity of services to victims through coordination with all agents of the care continuum.
6. Document the patient's condition in medical records.
7. Educate patients about domestic violence.
8. Participate in public health campaigns to educate the public about domestic violence based on research.
9. Optimize technology to inform victims about the medical aspects of domestic violence.
10. Develop a multicultural approach to dealing with victims of domestic violence in an attempt to help overcome ethnic, cultural, and religious barriers to help and healing.
11. Provide educational resources for health care personnel:

- The Family Violence Intervention Model for Dental Professionals Projects, funded by the Office for Victims of Crime, has developed comprehensive curricula and educational videos for dentists and dental ancillary staff that provide information about the dynamics of family violence and appropriate interventions by dental providers (21).

- The American College of Obstetricians and Gynecologists has produced a slide lecture about the health care needs of domestic violence victims. Target audiences include ob-gyn residents; third-year medical students; first- and second-year medical students in courses such as "Introduction to Clinical Medicine"; and other health care providers, including emergency department personnel, dentists, nurse midwives, nurse practitioners, and mental health providers (7).

## STALKING

Stalking is recognized as criminal victimization rather than simply nuisance behavior. Stalking is unwanted pursuit, following, contacting, or harassment. It occurs when an individual pursues a relationship that is unwanted by the object of the stalking behavior. Stalking is a close relative of domestic violence. Stalkers are likely to follow their targets, monitor their activities, bombard them with telephone calls, and spy on them using binoculars, telescopes, microphones, and cameras to achieve their end, which is to exert control and create fear. They will use any means to connect with their victims. Stalking behavior is obsessive, can escalate in intensity, and can be extremely dangerous because it inflicts emotional distress, injury, and, in some instances, death. Before 1990, when the first antistalking statute was established, stalking was not considered illegal. The exploration of this strange and insidious crime is new, and data are developing on a daily basis about its psychological nature.

A 1998 National Institute of Justice survey of stalking victims provided the first glimpse into the kinds of tactics stalkers most often employ in the commission of their crimes (18). Victims report being subjected to the following tactics:

- Being followed or spied on from outside their home or place of work (82%)
- Receiving unwanted phone calls (61%)
- Receiving unwanted letters or items (30%)
- Having property vandalized (30%)
- Having pet threatened or killed (9%)

The number and nature of these behaviors, and the context in which they occur, communicate a threat. It is this element of threat to the safety of another that makes their conduct a crime. Most legal definitions of stalking specifically address the presence of an element of threat (18).

### Categories of Stalking

1. Simple obsession stalking represents 60% of all stalking cases, including those arising from previous personal relationships (e.g., those between husbands/wives, girlfriends, domestic partners). Many simple obsession cases are actually extensions of a previous pattern of domestic violence and psychological abuse. The exercise of power and control over their victims gives stalkers a sense of power and self-esteem that they otherwise lack. These individuals often relentlessly pursue and are fixated upon the object of their affection. They imagine that their feelings are reciprocated. The psychological disorder defined as erotomania is associated with this type of obsessive preoccupation with another, very often a celebrity figure, who becomes the object of the stalking behavior. Erotomaniacs are delusional and virtually all of them suffer from mental disorders—often schizophrenia.
2. Vengeance/terrorism stalking is fundamentally different from the other types of stalking. Vengeance stalkers do not seek a personal relationship with their targets. Rather, they attempt to elicit a particular response or a change of behavior from their victims. Although vengeance is their primary motive, these stalkers seek to punish their victims for some wrong they perceive the victim has visited upon them.
3. Love obsession stalking involves stalkers who seek to establish a personal relationship with the object of their obsession—contrary to the wishes of their victims. Love obsession stalkers tend to have low self-esteem and often target victims they perceive to have exceptional qualities and high social standing. These stalkers seek to raise their own self-esteem by

associating with those whom they hold in high regard (7).

Victims who are pursued and harassed by stalkers experience a wide range of reactions, including loss of sleep, weight loss, depression, anxiety, and difficulty in concentrating. Stalking victims represent a category that deserves not only study but also programs that offer safety and relief from this menacing criminal behavior.

## ELDERLY CRIME VICTIMS

Winter is on my head, but eternal Spring is in my heart: I breathe at this hour the fragrance of the lilacs and violets, as at twenty years ago. The nearer I approach the end the plainer I hear around me the immortal symphonies of the heavenly chorus that waits to welcome me.

*Unknown*

Old age is often thought of as a time of loss and separation. Physical abilities, eyesight, hearing, agility, memory, and health can become diminished or lost. Loss also occurs through the death of friends, the abandonment of activities, and physical limitations. Pipher (32) likened being elderly to living in another country, where the terrain and the language are different, a country that provides little escape from violence and crime. Old age brings almost a natural reliance on support from others in new and different ways. Roles become reversed: children become parents, and parents become childlike in their need for protection and care.

Victimization of the elderly includes sexual assault, domestic violence, physical assault, homicide, burglary, and fraud. Elderly victims are particularly vulnerable in their limited ability to endure the aftermath of the crime if they do indeed survive the crime event. Their vulnerability is not only the result of physical and mental considerations but also the result of living in a time and place where beliefs and values were vastly different from those of present day.

People born early in the 20th century were taught to keep their feelings to themselves. For example, most World War II veterans do not talk about their wartime experiences. They were shell shocked and did not necessarily understand their own psychological states. They also thought that their friends and families would not want to hear the truth (32). The importance placed on privacy and independence by elderly people as well as their attitudes toward gender roles and sexual relations is sometimes evident in their response to victimization. Sexual assault victims in particular are extremely reluctant to report the assault, and most express strong reluctance about family members being made aware of the nature of the assault. They need help in understanding the ramifications of the crime and in accepting the help that is available.

Victims of fraud admit shame and humiliation at being "taken in" at their age by unscrupulous criminals. When marriages/relationships between elders become violent for the first time, the victim is fearful of both the violence and the discovery of the violence by their children or other intervening agents. That fear is often predicated on retaliation by the abuser, loss of support, or loss of the relationship with the abuser. When the abuser is the child of the elderly victim, the parent may feel shame and guilt at having raised an abusive child. An elderly relative of a homicide victim can be greatly affected by the crime. The typical reactions to death by homicide are magnified for the elderly. Their attempts to comprehend the criminal justice process, media attention on the crime, limited support systems, and resulting physical, emotional, behavioral, and cognitive reactions combine to create an overwhelming circumstance for the elderly relative of a homicide victim.

The elderly population has more exposure to the medical profession than do younger patients. Theirs is a world of frequent medical considerations, balancing doctor appointments and securing prescriptions. Members of the elderly population tend to regard physicians highly and may not likely admit to abuse for fear of judgment. On the other hand, some patients may be willing to disclose based on trust. Whatever the circumstances, abuse must be differentiated from the normal aging process. For example, the elderly are naturally more likely to lose their balance and fall; more likely to suffer skeletal fractures and bleed; and more likely to experience poor vision, mental confusion, bruising, and stiffness. These conditions can also be indications of abuse. The health care provider is crucial in the recognition of abuse and therefore can make a significant difference in the quality of life for elderly victims of crime.

## A Measure of the Problem

Until recently, little attention was given to specific crimes against the elderly. In 1996, the first National Elder Abuse Incidence Study was conducted by the National Center on Elder Abuse of the U.S. Department of Health and Human Services. The study showed that during 1996 at least one-half million older persons in domestic settings were abused or neglected or experienced self-neglect and that for every reported incident of elder abuse, neglect, or self-neglect, approximately five are unreported (33). The nation's oldest elders (80 years and older) are abused and neglected at a two to three times their proportion of the elderly population (33).

## Consider

Ruth, a 79-year-old retired teacher, was recovering from a stroke that left her partially paralyzed. After making excellent progress and regaining some normal functioning of her legs and speech, Ruth was released from the hospital and moved in with her daughter, Jane. Jane, a registered nurse, was skilled in balancing her career with the care of her mother. She engaged a number of family members, friends, and home companions to help with Ruth's care. After years of independent living, driving her own vehicle, and managing her own affairs, Ruth was now totally reliant on Jane. But she was spirited and anxious to recover, and Jane's roster of helpers worked well. Frank, Ruth's nephew, volunteered to sit with her on Tuesday nights while Jane attended choir rehearsal. During those evenings, Frank began to sexually assault Ruth. It started with inappropriate touching under the guise of helping her get in and out of bed. He put sleeping pills in her nightly drink. After she was asleep, he removed her clothing and engaged in fondling and masturbation. When Jane returned home, her mother was always sleeping soundly. Jane assumed that all was well and

proclaimed the offending nephew as her best sitter.

Three months later, Jane became aware of the abuse. Ruth became withdrawn and depressed. In contrast to her early enthusiasm to regain her physical functioning, she now had little to no interest in her therapy. She was tearful and frightened when Jane was away from the house, and she became hysterical when Jane was preparing to leave on Tuesday nights. At the same time, Jane was becoming concerned about the deep sleeping episodes, which transpired only after Frank's watch. Jane questioned Ruth about Frank's visits and discovered that Ruth had some awareness of his activities but was afraid to address the issue with her daughter. She was able to tell Jane that she was not entirely asleep on occasion and was aware that Frank was touching her body and himself. Ruth also expressed how concerned she was that Frank's behavior be kept a secret. Jane promptly dismissed Frank without explanation. Ruth's excessive sleeping ceased. Jane did not confront Frank directly; however, she did consult Adult Protective Services and Victim Services regarding her discoveries. The situation ended only with Frank's banishment from the family; Jane was not willing to follow through with any real investigation of the behavior. She has become an advocate for the elderly and tells her story to help others become aware of the exploitation and victimization of the elderly.

## The Aftermath of Domestic Violence Against the Elderly

All too often, as with crimes against children, crimes against the elderly are underreported and, even when there are convictions, sentences are light. Elderly victims have extreme difficulty in recovering from the disruptiveness of a crime. When the crime involves a family member, the burden is magnified by the betrayal. Elderly victims sometimes have limited mobility and require special transportation. Their financial resources are also limited, which influences their ability to recover from the ravages of victimization. Most elderly people spend a great deal of time in their homes, which is where they are most often victimized by exploitation, caregiver abuse, or sexual assault. Elderly victims do not always have the opportunity to engage in the criminal justice process because of their diminished capacities.

Brown (13) summarized some of the concerns held by elderly people who have become increasingly dependent on others and who are threatened with or have become victims of abuse:

- Fear of retaliation (applies to abuse by a relative or an institution)
- Fear of relocation
- Fear of senility
- Fear of death
- Fear of becoming a burden
- Embarrassment about being abused by a relative/child
- Fear of having to go to court
- Fear of institutionalization
- Fear of further abuse or death
- Fear of having food or medication withheld

## Forms of Domestic Violence Against the Elderly

The following definitions of abuse, exploitation, and neglect pertain to elders living in domestic settings (where the majority of crimes against the elder transpire):

*Physical abuse* is the use of force that may result in bodily injury, physical pain, or impairment. Physical abuse may include such acts as striking (with or without an object), hitting, beating, pushing, shoving, shaking, slapping, kicking, pinching, and burning. The inappropriate use of drugs and physical restraints, force feeding, and physical punishment of any kind are also examples of physical abuse.

Signs and symptoms of physical abuse include the following:

- Bruises, black eyes, welts, lacerations, and rope marks
- Bone and skull fractures
- Open wounds, cuts, punctures, and untreated injuries; injuries in various stages of healing
- Sprains, dislocations, and internal injuries
- Broken eyeglasses, physical signs of punishment, and signs of being restrained
- Laboratory findings of medication overdose or underutilization of prescribed drugs

- An elder's report of being hit, slapped, kicked, or mistreated
- An elder's sudden change in behavior
- The caregiver's refusal to allow visitors to see an elder

*Sexual abuse* is nonconsensual sexual contact of any kind. Sexual contact with a person incapable of giving consent also is considered sexual abuse. It includes unwanted touching, all types of sexual assault or battery such as rape and sodomy, coerced nudity, and sexually explicit photographing.

Signs and symptoms of sexual abuse include the following:

- Bruises around the breasts or genital area
- Unexplained venereal disease or genital infections
- Unexplained vaginal or anal bleeding
- Torn, stained, or bloody underclothing
- An elder's report of being sexually assaulted or raped

*Emotional or psychological abuse* refers to the infliction of anguish, pain, or distress through verbal or nonverbal acts. Emotional/psychological abuse includes verbal insults, threats, intimidation, humiliations, and harassment. Other examples are treating an older person like an infant; isolating an elderly person from his or her family, friends, or regular activities; giving an older person the "silent treatment"; and enforcing social isolation.

Signs and symptoms of emotional/psychological abuse may manifest in the following ways in an elderly person:

- Being emotionally upset or agitated
- Being extremely withdrawn, noncommunicative, or nonresponsive
- Exhibiting unusual behavior associated with dementia, such as sucking, biting, and rocking
- Reporting verbal or emotional mistreatment

*Neglect* refers to the refusal or failure to fulfill any part of a person's obligation or duties to the elder. Neglect may also involve a person who has fiduciary responsibility to provide care for an elder (e.g., not paying for necessary home care services). Neglect typically means the refusal or failure to provide an elderly person with necessities such as food, water, clothing, shelter, personal hygiene, medicine, comfort, and safety.

The following are signs and symptoms of neglect:

- Dehydration, malnutrition, untreated bedsores, and poor personal hygiene
- Unattended or untreated health problems
- Hazardous or unsafe living conditions/arrangements (e.g., improper wiring, no heat, no running water)
- Unsanitary and unclean living conditions (e.g., dirt, fleas, lice, soiled bedding, fecal/urine smell, inadequate clothing)
- An elder's report of being mistreated

*Financial or material exploitation* refers to the illegal or improper use of an elder's funds, property, or assets. Examples include cashing an elderly person's checks without authorization or permission, forging an older person's signature, misusing or stealing an older person's money or possessions, coercing or deceiving an older person into signing any document (e.g., a contract or will), and improper use of guardianship or power of attorney.

### Elderly Victims of Domestic Violence

Much of what is known about the older battered woman is anecdotal or drawn from practical wisdom. There are several patterns of domestic violence among the elderly:

- "Spouse abuse grown old": the victims have been abused for most of their adult lives
- "Late onset" cases: the abuse begins late in life by partners who had not previously been abusive. This type of abuse seems to be associated with age-related conditions or stresses, including retirement, dependency, changing patterns in relationships, or sexual dysfunction.
- Entering abusive relationships late in life: the abuser is frequently the victim's second or third spouse or intimate partner. In many instances, financial gain through financial abuse accompanies the physical abuse.
- Situations in which elderly women who were battered earlier in their lives by their husbands

(or who abused their children) are battered by their sons and daughters (7).

Many situations of abuse are unreported as a result of elderly victims' being unable to ask for help or having no one to tell because of isolation. Health care providers are the gateway to ending the neglect and abuse of our oldest citizens.

### Recommendations for Health Care Providers

1. Make the identification of elder abuse and neglect a priority. Work with other community agents to ensure that communication and understanding are paramount in terms of the health and safety of the elderly. Participate in partnerships, coalitions, and boards to facilitate support, understanding, and knowledge regarding issues and concerns related to the elderly. Become familiar with TRIAD, Association for the Advancement of Retired Persons (AARP), Adult Protective Services, Area Agency on Aging, and other organizations that exist to assist the elderly.
2. Provide public education regarding guidelines for detecting symptoms of abuse and neglect as well as diagnosis, treatment, referral, and reporting for health and safety purposes.
3. Create specialized units to establish protocols for early detection of abuse in order to ensure patient safety as well as aid in the active investigation and prosecution of the abuser.
4. Provide scientific and medical evidence to help in the prosecution of the perpetrators of crimes against the elderly.
5. Ensure that health care professionals are knowledgeable about local and national resources for services for the elderly.
6. Establish reciprocal referral systems among victim service providers, social service counselors, mental health professionals, and criminal justice agents.
7. Establish training on the cultural diversity of elderly victims; stress the importance of awareness of ethnic and cultural differences.

8. Ensure that the elderly are assessed routinely for indications of abuse and neglect and that any sign or symptoms are documented in their medical records.

9. Provide continuing education about the consequences of victimization for the health care providers in the community who come into contact with elderly victims.

10. The health care community should provide specific training for victim service providers about the important role they can play in assisting victims.

## CHILD VICTIMS

Just when I think I've outdistanced "it" the runner catches up again and comes alongside me to let me know that it has enough wind to keep on running and can overtake me anytime it wants to. It takes the time to rest and recharge, but I just keep on running.

*An adult who was sexually abused as a child*

You are a child of the universe no less than the trees and the stars; you have a right to be here.

*Max Ehrmann, Desiderata, 1927*

Perhaps our nation's greatest scourge is the victimization of our most vulnerable population. Children are sexually abused, beaten, and murdered by their own family members at an alarming rate each year. When children are subjected to emotional abuse and neglect, experience the trauma associated with domestic violence, and deal with physical and sexual assault, they are forced to engage in a difficult, complex psychological aftermath. The same disturbing reactions of humiliation, shame, anger, low self-esteem, blame, and confusion as experienced by adult victims become a part of the child victim's world. Children should not have to cope with the magnitude of such emotions, particularly related as they become to sexual issues. Little girls and boys are not supposed to have venereal diseases. They are not supposed to satisfy the crazed need of a demented mind. Children should not have to endure the pain of blows, kicks, choking, and burns. They should never have to be hungry or dirty or maltreated in any context. Children are not supposed to grapple

with devastating long-term effects, which continue to haunt their dreams.

The maltreatment of children has its origins in the historical premise that children were the property of their parents. As property, children could be sold into bondage, abused, married off at any age and to anyone the parents selected, abandoned, or murdered. There were no legal repercussions to offending parents. Sadly, this type of thinking and behavior remains in some cultures. However, all states have laws that require certain persons (teachers, doctors, social workers, police officers, and others) to report suspected abuse or neglect of children and youth under the age of 18 years.

### Prevalence of Child Abuse/Neglect

In 1996, there were 969,018 cases of substantiated abuse or neglect reported from 47 states (34). It is estimated that:

- 116,500 children were sexually abused (34)
- 232,560 children were physically abused (34)
- 58,150 children were emotionally abused (34)
- 29,070 children were medically neglected (34)
- 155,050 children endured some other form of maltreatment (34)
- 52% of child abuse and neglect victims were girls, and 48% were boys (34)
- An estimated 2,000 children died in 1995 as a result of abuse or neglect (35).
- Children younger than 3 years account for 75% of the annual deaths resulting from abuse or neglect (34).
- Almost 50% of the children who die from maltreatment in the United States are already known to child protection services (34).

### Forms of Child Abuse

The National Victim Assistance Academy defined the following types of child victimization (21):

*Physical abuse* is most often classified as a nonaccidental injury to a child under the age of 18 by a parent or caregiver. This type of abuse occurs when a parent willfully injures or allows a child to be injured, tortured, or maimed out of cruelty or excessive punishment.

Mental health professionals recognize *emotional abuse* and *emotional neglect* as two forms of emotional maltreatment of children. The former consists of a chronic pattern of behavior in which the child typically is belittled, denied love to promote specific behavior, marginalized from siblings, or subjected to extreme and inappropriate punishments. The latter is characterized by the failure to provide a child with appropriate support, attention, and affection. Occurring alone and coupled with other forms of abuse, emotional maltreatment can impair the psychological growth and the emotional development of the child.

*Acquaintance perpetrators,* such as family friends, neighbors, teachers, coaches, religious leaders, and peers, normally will win the confidence of the child through affiliation with the family or community. They tend to prey on children with low self-esteem and children who are unsupervised. Perpetrators who command positions of respect due to positions in community affairs, such as church, civic, and business affiliations, are more likely to intimidate or threaten the child once sexual abuse has occurred. There has been a marked increase in the number of juvenile perpetrators committing sexual abuse.

*Sexual abuse* is the exploitation of a child or adolescent for another person's sexual and psychological gratification. Family members, trusted friends, acquaintances, child-related community program personnel, day care workers, and other paid caregivers as well as strangers are known perpetrators. Child sexual abuse ranges from such acts as oral and genital stimulation and penetration to voyeurism and the involvement of a child in prostitution or the production of pornography.

*Intrafamilial sexual abuse* is committed most often by an individual known to the child. The abuser can be a blood relative who is part of the nuclear family or a surrogate parent such as a live-in companion or stepparent. Older siblings are frequently responsible for child sexual abuse. The family will likely be dysfunctional in other areas. It may have been destabilized by alcohol and substance abuse or severe spousal discord with a history of physical violence.

*Stranger sexual abuse,* frequently referred to as pedophilia (although the term describes any individual who has a sexual preference for children), is by far the most publicized form of child sexual abuse but constitutes only 10% of all reported cases. There is no evidence that perpetrators choose child victims based on race, but there is increased victimization of children of lower socioeconomic groups.

*On-line sexual predators,* a new breed of child abuser, have entered the picture as a result of children's increased and often unsupervised recreational use of the Internet. Investigations of computer sex offenders demonstrate that on-line sexual predators roam chat rooms and post sexually explicit material on the Internet to make contact with young children and teenagers. Victimization may be indirect and limited to showing a child pornographic sites to initiating sexually overt conversation in a chat room, by e-mail, or by instant messages.

## Consider

Kelley is 40 now, but she can still hear Uncle Bruce pleading to her when she was 8 years old. He was left in charge of Kelley and her baby sister Katy when their parents made occasional trips away from home. Uncle Bruce was single and only 21 years old, but to Kelley he seemed ancient. It started with Uncle Bruce bouncing her on his knee and tickling her until she nearly wet her pants. It was so much fun, and even her parents enjoyed watching Uncle Bruce entertain Kelley. One day while bouncing on Bruce's knee, Kelley felt his hands touch her between her legs. She wasn't sure she had felt that sudden shift in his attention to her body, but when the touch returned she knew. She also knew there was something different, dark, but pleasant about the touch. It was compelling and then it stopped as abruptly as it started. Uncle Bruce left and Kelley didn't see him for a while, but when he returned Kelley was anxious to start the games and curious about the strange touch. It came again, but this time it was more directed and rhythmic. Uncle Bruce was stroking her between her legs and telling her how wonderful it was and how he thought she was the most beautiful little girl in the world. Although the abuse ended when Kelley reached 13, the secret is still alive.

## The Aftermath of Child Abuse

The concerns of abused children have been summarized by Brown (13):

- Inability to trust others
- Removal from home or removal of offender
- Guilt, shame, and stigma
- Disclosure
- Loss of family/friends
- Healing from physical/sexual injuries
- Misunderstanding of what is happening emotionally
- Helplessness, lack of control

When adults betray children by shepherding them into negative behavior, the children suffer long-term reactions to the experience. Guilt and shame coupled with humiliation are feelings that seem to accompany this type of victimization. The child can be overwhelmed by feelings of anger, generally self-directed. In addition, sexually abused children may sexually abuse younger children. When there is no avenue for disclosure of the abuse, children are forced to compartmentalize the event. Sometimes they become preoccupied with sexual activities and engage in sexual acting out. Young children who become victims of sexual abuse are vulnerable and have little or no knowledge about STDs. They may recognize that the sexual behavior is inappropriate but have difficulty in processing the magnitude of the episode. The sexual arousal can be pleasant yet embedded in a blanket of ill feelings that cling, confuse, and harm. Sexually abused children may experience nightmares, hostile behavior, changes in eating habits, and change in school performance, including radical improvement in grades (overachieving) (13). Medical systems must be positioned to recognize the symptoms of child sexual assault.

## Recommendations for Health Care Providers

The following recommendations are from *New Directions from the Field: Victims' Rights and Services for the 21st Century* (7). Representing the collective thinking of programs throughout the nation, these recommendations are offered here in broad terms to serve as a guide for instituting programs and protocols for action.

1. Communities should establish children's advocacy centers to provide child-friendly locations where abused children can receive the services they need to heal and to provide information for the evaluation and investigation of their cases. To ensure the highest quality of intervention, training should be provided to professionals on conducting forensic interviews, to medical professionals on conducting child abuse examinations, and to mental health professionals on employing abuse-specific treatment approaches.
2. Children who witness violence should be provided the same level of victim assistance and special protections within the criminal and juvenile systems as child victims.
3. To ensure child abuse cases are recognized and reported as early as possible, training in the identification of signs of abuse as well as the impact of child victimization should be provided to all professionals who come into contact with child victims.
4. There should be improved governmental response to the problem of missing, abducted, and sexually exploited children.
5. All jurisdictions should establish or support "court school" programs to educate child victims and witnesses about the court process.
6. States should enact legislation to open access to criminal history records, and they should adopt regulations and policies necessary to meet the requirements of the National Child Protection Act.
7. Early intervention programs, such as Head Start and Healthy Start, should be implemented nationwide. The staff of these programs must be trained in how to recognize the signs of child abuse, how to report abuse to appropriate authorities, and how to provide referrals for victims and their families.
8. Specially trained lawyers and court-appointed special advocates should be provided to children in all civil child protection and other abuse-related proceedings.

9. All states should consider alternatives to live in-court testimony for children younger than 18 years.
10. Federal and state governments should support the significant additional research that is needed to document effective treatments for child victims, especially victims of child sexual and physical abuse and children who witness violence.

## Recommendations Specific to the Health Care Community

1. All professional schools that educate future health care professionals, including schools of medicine, nursing, social work, rehabilitation, hospital administration, and public health, should incorporate victim issues into their curricula.
2. All patients should be assessed routinely for indications of domestic abuse or other history of violence. Any signs or symptoms of abuse should be documented in their medical records.
3. Hospitals should establish training programs and protocols for all hospital personnel about the rights and needs of victims of crime.
4. Medical facilities, including hospitals and rehabilitation and trauma centers, should serve as gateways to assist victims of crime. Response staff should be available in these settings to provide on-site crisis counseling and follow-up with patients and to serve as links to in-house and community resources.
5. Victims of sexual assault should be given emergency medical care, forensic examinations, and testing for HIV and STDs at no out-of-pocket cost and in a supportive setting. More hospitals should consider establishing SANE programs to respond sensitively to the needs of sexual assault victims.
6. Cultural competency guidelines should be developed to help health care providers improve screening and intervention services for victims from diverse backgrounds.
7. Medical personnel should be knowledgeable about statutory privacy protections and have policies that ensure that statutory privacy protections are applied to medical records, abuse reporting forms, and medico-legal evidence. They should respect the confidentiality and privacy needs of all victims of crime and assist them in dealing with unwanted media attention, especially in cases of sexual assault and assaults on children.
8. Counseling and prevention programs and/or a referral system to such programs should be established in medical facilities that treat violence-related injury, including gunshot victims, to address the broad spectrum of needs of these victims.
9. Protocols for appropriate security and safety procedures should be developed to assist hospital personnel in responding to gang, family, and other violence that might result in staff victimization.
10. Pediatricians, emergency physicians, family practitioners, internists, and other health care professionals treating young children should be educated about the effects on children of witnessing domestic violence and violence in the community.
11. Technology should be utilized to improve medical services for crime victims, especially in underserved and rural areas.
12. All health care professionals should be educated about sensitive techniques for notification of death.
13. Statutes and policies should be adopted to prevent insurance companies from discriminating against victims of crime by denying and/or canceling coverage or by charging higher premiums for such coverage.
14. Victims with catastrophic physical injuries, including survivors of assaults and crashes caused by drunk drivers, should receive specialized neuropsychological evaluation in health care facilities.

Major challenges have been placed before our response systems through recommendations from the field, as outlined in *New Directions from the Field: Victims' Rights and Services for the 21st Century* (7). This excellent compilation of data collected in the field of victim service provision over a 20-year period offers five global challenges from the field of victim assistance to our total response systems:

1. To enact and enforce consistent, fundamental rights for crime victims in federal, state, juvenile, military, and tribal justice systems and administrative proceedings
2. To provide crime victims with access to comprehensive, high-quality services regardless of the nature of their victimization, age, race, religion, gender, ethnicity, sexual orientation, capability, or geographic location
3. To integrate crime victims' issues into all levels of the nation's educational system to ensure that justice and allied professionals and other service providers receive comprehensive training on victims' issues as part of their academic education and continuing training in the field
4. To support, improve, and replicate promising practices in victims' rights and services built on sound research-advanced technology and multidisciplinary partnerships
5. To ensure that the voices of victims of crime play a central role in the nation's response to violence and those victimized by crime

Implicit in each of the challenges is the need for the health care community to emerge as the front-line player.

## REFERENCES

1. Gilligan J. *Violence: reflections on a national epidemic.* New York: Vintage Books, 1997:19.
2. Herman JL. *Trauma and recovery.* New York: Basic Books, 1992.
3. Matsakis A. *I can't get over it: a handbook for trauma survivors.* Oakland, CA: Harbinger Publications, 1996:17.
4. Schornstein S. *Domestic violence and health care: what every professional needs to know.* Thousand Oaks, CA: Sage Publications, 1997.
5. Corey G. *Theory and practice of counseling and psychotherapy.* Belmount, CA: Brooks/Cole, 1991:110.
6. Office for Victims of Crime, National Victim Assistance Academy. *Child victimization,* chapter 10 (10-2). Washington, DC: U.S. Department of Justice, 1999.
7. Office for Victims of Crime. *New directions from the field: victims' rights and services for the 21st century.* Washington, DC: U.S. Department of Justice, 1999.
8. Kilpatrick DG, Resnick HS, Saunders BE, Best CL. Rape, other violence against women, and posttraumatic stress disorder: critical issues in assessing the adversity–stress–psychopathology relationship. In: Dohrenwend BP, ed. *Adversity, stress, and psychopathology.* New York: Oxford University Press, 1998:161–176.
9. Gilligan J. *Violence: reflections on a national epidemic.* New York: Vintage Books, 1997.
10. Douglas J, Olshaker M. *The anatomy of motive.* New York: Scribner, 1999.
11. Raine NV. *After silence: rape and my journey back.* New York: Crown Publishers, 1998.
12. Burgess AW, Holmstrom LL. Rape trauma syndrome. *Am J Psychiatry* 1974;131(9):981–986.
13. Brown SL. *Counseling victims of violence.* Alexandria, VA: American Association for Counseling and Development, 1991.
14. Russell DEH. *Rape in a marriage.* Indianapolis: Indiana University Press, 1990.
15. Campbell JC. Women's responses to sexual abuse in intimate relationships. *Health Care Women Int* 1989; 10:335–346.
16. Carosella C. *Who's afraid of the dark? A forum of truth, support, and assurance for those affected by rape.* New York: HarperCollins, 1995.
17. Ringel C. *Criminal Victimization in 1996, Changes 1995–1996 with trends 1993–1996.* Washington, DC: U.S. Department of Justice, Bureau of Justice Statistics, 1997.
18. Tjaden P, Thoennes N. Prevalence, incidence, and consequences of violence against women: findings from the National Violence Against Women Survey. *Research in Brief.* Washington, DC: U.S. Department of Justice, National Institute of Justice, November 1998.
19. Perkins C. *Age patterns of victims of serious crimes.* Washington, DC: U.S. Department of Justice, Bureau of Justice Statistics, September 1997.
20. Ruffino NC. *Managing diversity: people skills for a multicultural workplace.* Thomson Executive Press, 1995.
21. National Victim Assistance Academy. Office for Victims of Crime, U.S. Department of Justice, in conjunction with Victim's Assistance Legal Organization, California State University—Fresno, National Crime Victim's Research and Treatment Center, University of New Haven, Washburn University, 1999.
22. Holmes MM, Resnick HW, Frampton D. Follow-up of sexual assault victims. *Am J Obstet Gynecol* 1998; 79:336–342.
23. Parker B, McFarlane J, Soeken K. Abuse during pregnancy: effects on maternal complications and birth weight in adult and teenage women. *Obstet Gynecol* 1994;84(3):323–328.
24. Campbell JC, Pugh LC, Campbell D, Visscher M. The influence of abuse on pregnancy intention. *Women's Health Issues* 1995;5(4):214–223.
25. Campbell JC, Humphreys J. *Nursing care of survivors of family violence.* St. Louis: Mosby, 1993.
26. American Psychiatric Association. *Diagnostic and statistical manual of mental disorders: DSM-IV.* Washington, DC: 1994.
27. Snipe B, Hall EJ. *I am not your victim.* Thousand Oaks, CA: Sage Publications, 1996.
28. Carlson B. Adolescent observers of marital violence. *J Fam Viol* 1990;5:285–299.
29. Stark E, Flitcraft A. Woman-battering, child abuse and social heredity: what is the relationship? In: Johnson N, ed. *Marital violence.* London: Routledge and Kegan, 1985.
30. Cappell C, Heiner RB. The intergenerational transmission of family aggression. *J Family Violence* 1990;5: 135–152.

31. Salber PR, Taliaferro E. *The physician's guide to domestic violence.*Volcano, CA: Volcano Press, 1995.
32. Pipher M. *Another country: navigating the emotional terrain of our elders.* New York: Penguin Putnam, 1999.
33. National Center on Elder Abuse. *Incidence study: final report.* Washington, DC: U.S. Department of Health and Human Services, Administration of Children and Families, and Administration on Aging, 1998.
34. National Center on Child Abuse and Neglect. *Child maltreatment 1996: reports from the States for the National Child Abuse and Neglect Data System.* Washington, DC: U.S. Department of Health and Human Services, 1998.
35. National Center on Child Abuse and Neglect. Child maltreatment 1995: reports from the States for the National Child Abuse and Neglect Data System. Washington, DC: U.S. Department of Health and Human Services, 1997.

# 3

# Interviewing Techniques

## John S. O'Brien II

## FORENSIC MEDICAL INTERVIEWING

Medical interviewing serves as the cornerstone for the performance of medical evaluations and the formulation of treatment plans. The patient's medical history serves as the background and context within which the presenting clinical complaints have arisen. When undertaken in a thorough and comprehensive fashion, the history provides a rich source of clinical information that can be of major assistance in the diagnosis and treatment of medical, surgical, and psychiatric conditions. The medical interview and history, correlated with findings on examination, assist with the diagnostic process and often serve as the primary factor in the formulation of directions for further clinical work-up. This combined information is also useful for following a patient's clinical response to treatment.

The format of medical interviewing and general medical history taking is directly applicable to evaluations occurring in emergency departments and in forensic contexts. The overall format includes documentation of the patient's clinical complaint, usually in his or her own language, followed by a history of present illness, a review of medical history, family and social history, and a review of systems. An overview of general medical interviewing and history taking appears in Table 3-1. This structure is always useful as the basic outline for case assessment, documentation, and case presentation in emergency departments and all other clinical/medical settings. It serves as a structured approach to data gathering, focusing on a chief complaint for the purposes of diagnosis and

treatment. It is also useful for documentation in medico-legal contexts. In the clinical/medical context, clear, structured documentation is useful to carry out the essential function of medical records—serving as a communications device that summarizes clinically relevant information for subsequent caregivers to permit these individuals, who may not have direct contact with one another, to collaborate efficiently and effectively. In a medico-legal context, structured, thorough documentation is useful for documentation of clinical presentation, diagnosis, and management; demonstration explicitly or implicitly of the rationale underlying clinical conclusions and diagnoses; and recording of therapeutic interventions undertaken in response to the clinical conclusions and diagnoses as well as the patient's response to them.

Medical interviewing or history taking in an emergency department is essentially the same as general medical interviewing and history taking, except that it is more focused on the chief complaint and the patient's immediate needs for evaluation and treatment. Documentation tends to focus primarily on pertinent positives and negatives, both historically and on examination. The interview and documentation are oriented around evaluation of the patient's urgent clinical needs and the initiation of lifesaving and/or immediate appropriate treatment. An additional purpose is triage of patients for referral for outpatient follow-up or subspecialty evaluation and further treatment. Clinical/medical documentation in the emergency department is essential for communication about the patient's chief complaint, pertinent history, and clinical presentation

**TABLE 3-1.** *Medical interviewing and history taking*

1. General medical interviewing—history taking
2. Chief or presenting complaint—"patient's own words"
3. History of present illness
4. Medical history
   a. Medical
   b. Surgical
   c. Psychiatric
   d. Substance abuse
   e. Trauma
5. Family history
   a. Medical
   b. Surgical
   c. Psychiatric
   d. Substance abuse
6. Social history
   a. Life circumstances
   b. Habits, e.g., drugs or alcohol (see medical history)
7. Risk exposure
   a. Interpersonal
   b. Vocational
   c. Avocational/recreational
8. Review of systems

to subsequent clinicians for the purpose of facilitating further evaluation and management. These clinicians either function as part of the emergency care team or provide care for the patient following treatment and release from the emergency department. Medico-legally, the emergency department record is a useful retrospective source of information that summarizes the patient's history and clinical presentation, the diagnoses or conclusions drawn about the patient, and the treatment initiated or triage undertaken for further evaluation and follow-up. Retrospective medico-legal assessment of the record often focuses on the conclusions drawn, the treatment provided, and the rationale for both, and seeks to legally establish "facts" based on what is documented in the record. It also allows assessment of the appropriateness of clinical conclusions drawn and of subsequent treatment sought by the patient after emergency department evaluation.

Forensic medical interviewing/history taking is essentially the same as general medical interviewing/history taking. It also includes consideration of clinical and legal issues defined by the context in which the interview or history is taken

and the nature of the legal issues being considered. Such interviewing and history taking has a variety of purposes, such as evaluation of the patient's clinical presentation; arrival at diagnosis or explanation of the presentation and making of recommendations for treatment; establishment of a record of the evaluation and the conclusions drawn as future evidence that may be useful in a legal proceeding; and preservation of observations and findings for future reference in legal contexts.

Perhaps the most significant difference between forensic medical interviewing/history taking and general medical or emergency medical interviewing/history taking is the attention to documentation that is necessary. The documentation must be as objective and detailed as possible, including observations of and conversations with the patient. It should be primarily data oriented and include only those conclusions or explanations that are based soundly on the data collected both historically and clinically. Forensic medical records should also be written in a way that avoids rendering legal conclusions or definitive opinions that are the province of a legal fact finder. The clinician should thoroughly document the patient's history, general observations of the patient, and results of the clinical examination. The clinician can draw clinical conclusions and can express an opinion that those conclusions are consistent with a particular cause, without arriving at a conclusion with factual certainty. This approach allows for the cause to be determined factually in a legal context later, following consideration of all the evidence, which often is not known or understood by the clinician at the time of the evaluation. The clinician may also make appropriate referrals for follow-up treatment and other support services based on clinical conclusions consistent with a particular cause, without arriving at a definitive conclusion about the cause of the patient's clinical presentation.

Treating patients in emergency departments often involves evaluation of clinical complaints that have medico-legal significance, either at the time of presentation or later. Most patients who present as victims of violence or abuse have immediate medico-legal involvement, and patients who were injured in accidents may be involved in subsequent litigation focusing on the injuries they sustained. Therefore, a large proportion of cases seen in emergency departments may ultimately have medico-legal significance. Preparation of the emergency department record with an awareness of its medico-legal significance may be extremely helpful to the patient, who may later be involved in litigation, and to the clinician, who may be called on to testify retrospectively and who may need to rely on the record as the primary source of information for the purposes of testimony. Frequently, this testimony is requested after a significant time has passed since the emergency department visit.

Although there may appear to be tension between the necessity to evaluate, treat, and triage patients in an emergency department and to document that process efficiently, and the necessity to generate a comprehensive and informative medical record for medico-legal purposes, the two necessities are not incompatible. The approach to documentation must be flexible enough to permit the addition of more extensive information when it is both clinically and medico-legally indicated. In this manner, the patient's narrative and/or the clinician's observations of the patient's demeanor and behavior, or other potentially relevant medico-legal information, can be included in the emergency department documentation to assist a fact finder in assessing the clinical presentation and determining its cause in subsequent legal proceedings.

Underlying the process of performing clinical interviews and obtaining medical histories are interview techniques oriented to eliciting information from the patient for the purposes of diagnosis, treatment, and medico-legal documentation. Generally, medical interviewing techniques commence with open-ended or broad questioning and proceed to more focused or narrower questioning. The clinician attempts to elicit the patient's history in the patient's own narrative, which is very useful in the clinical evaluation of the presenting complaint and especially helpful in forensic contexts. Some patients are not communicative, for a variety of reasons, and the clinical history must be obtained from collateral sources.

Those sources should be documented in the record in terms of both identity and content. If a patient is not communicative about his or her own history, the record should reflect that fact and should contain observations of the patient and an assessment of any clinical reasons for the inability to communicate. Furthermore, if the patient is conscious and alert but not communicative, collateral history is most appropriately obtained outside the patient's presence and documented as such to reduce the possibility that any subsequent communication by the patient was prompted or suggested by the collateral source. This is especially necessary if the patient is an awake but reticent or mute young child who may be developmentally susceptible to prompting, which can result in an inaccurate history.

A mental status examination or cognitive capacity screening examination should be done as part of the assessment of the potential clinical reasons for the patient's uncommunicativeness. These exams may also have clinical importance for assessment of the patient's clinical presentation, diagnosis, and initiation of further workup or appropriate treatment. When evaluating noncommunicative patients, observations of their behavior must be documented as thoroughly as possible. Such patients may never provide information regarding their history or circumstances, so that behavioral observations and clinical findings documented in the record may be all that will be available for clinical evaluation and treatment and for future use in medico-legal contexts.

Victims of violence and abuse represent a variable but significant percentage of the patients who present to physicians' offices and emergency departments for clinical evaluation. As many as 3 million children have been reported to state agencies as victims of child abuse or neglect in single calendar years, and roughly 200,000 new cases of child sexual abuse are predicted to occur each year (National Center on Child Abuse and Neglect [NCCAN]). Approximately 10% to 15% of cases of child abuse are first reported by medical care providers (1).

Victims of violence and abuse presenting to emergency departments can be divided into four categories by age and by virtue of whether or not they are directly and reliably communicative: child noncommunicative, child communicative, adult noncommunicative, adult communicative. For communicative individuals, both children and adults, interviewing and history taking are based largely on the patient's narrative. Very young children (younger than 4 or 5 years) represent a special population whose narratives may not be credible or reliable. The narratives of very young children should be recorded and documented; however, historical information may also need to be derived from collateral sources, outside the presence of the child, to evaluate more thoroughly the young child's presenting complaint. For noncommunicative patients, information must be obtained from collateral sources. These sources should be identified in the record, along with careful observations of the patient and thorough documentation of the results of mental status or cognitive capacity screening examination performed upon the patient to assess the basis for the noncommunicativeness.

## INTERVIEWING CHILDREN

Interviewing or obtaining a medical history from a communicative child relies largely on the patient's own description of his or her history and chief presenting complaints. A potentially significant issue when talking with a child is assessing credibility and reliability. Reference to the definition of child competency may be of benefit in this regard, although child competency definitions vary somewhat among jurisdictions as defined by statute and case law. Generally, competency consists of the ability to understand and answer questions intelligently and accurately, to provide truthful versions of an experience, and to understand the difference between right and wrong, and truth and falsehood. Studies of child credibility focus on the influence of childhood development, on the content of the information provided, on the relationship between the content and the context in which the event occurred, and on subsequent statements about the event (2). One measure of a child's credibility is the stability of information provided and its unchanging nature over time.

The stability of information must be placed into the psychological context of the child providing it (3). In a study of children receiving therapy for sexual abuse, 75% initially denied the abuse and 22% recanted previous disclosures, whereas other studies indicate that the majority of children maintain their claims of abuse and never deny them to officials once they are questioned (4). One clinically observed pattern of disclosure is that the child begins initially silent, but allegations emerge once an adult becomes suspicious and questions the child. Upon questioning, the child may at first deny the allegations, but he or she subsequently discloses because of weariness of the abuse or fear that something worse may happen. However, often children will not disclose because of shame, fear, or embarrassment or because they do not want to get in trouble (5).

There appears to be a general agreement that children younger than 3 years cannot be competent witnesses and that there is significant variability of competency among children between the ages of 3 and 5 years (6). The older the child, the more likely he or she will be to discuss child abuse and be a reliable informant. Children older than 4 years make more disclosures of abuse than nondisclosures or inconclusive disclosures in comparison with 2- and 3-year-olds. Some studies suggest that allegation-blind interviewing techniques, requiring more patience and attentiveness to the child and fostering the development of better rapport, facilitated disclosure by the child (7). These techniques also appear to yield higher disclosure rates of abuse by children to interviewers unknown to them.

When interviewing a communicative child, it is best to begin with open-ended questions such as, "Why are you here today?" This type of questioning is not suggestive and thus allows the child to provide his or her own information instead of responding to prompts (1). However, some children do not respond to open-ended questioning. Younger children provide less information spontaneously during free recall or in response to open-ended prompts. At some point, directed questioning usually becomes necessary to elicit information about body touching, the circumstances of the abuse, and the identity of the abuser (8). Sternberg and colleagues showed that open-ended questions yielded longer and richer responses from child witnesses than direct, leading, or suggestive questions. An explanation for this difference is that open-ended questions probe recall memory, whereas focused questions probe recognition memory, which is more likely to elicit erroneous responses. Open-ended questions also yield more relevant and detailed information from children who have reported multiple incidents of abuse than from children who reported only one act of abuse (9). Some studies suggest that open-ended questions used in the introductory or report building phase of the evaluation help the child become comfortable with the interviewer and with the interviewer's expectations of the child (10).

It may be necessary to pose two types of specific questions to children: questions that request particular information and questions that require only yes/no answers to confirm or disconfirm information posed to the child (11). Questions intended to elicit particular information do not suggest a predetermined answer, whereas yes/no questions provide the child with adult-generated information with which the child must agree or disagree. Questions requesting particular information are preferable, except for very young children, most of whom do not yet have the syntactic ability to form appropriate responses (11).

Some studies have examined the influence of leading and misleading questions on the accuracy of child reports about an event. For all age groups, responses to leading questions were very accurate, but responses to misleading questions were less accurate (and extremely inaccurate from very young children) (12). Older children are more resistant to misleading questions. Younger children tend to agree with misleading questions, possibly because of their desire to comply with the authority figure asking the question. Furthermore, children presented with misleading information are more suggestible when the information is provided by a stranger. Children not presented with misleading questions are more likely to disclose both accurate and inaccurate information to their parents as opposed to strangers. Children tend to be more suggestible when they perceive the interviewer to be

authoritarian, intimidating, or unfriendly. They tend to comply with the interviewer when their knowledge of the event is limited, assuming the interviewer to be more knowledgeable (13). At a threshold age of about $4\frac{1}{2}$ years, childhood suggestibility decreases. Developmental advances in the ability of children to understand conflicting mental representations are accompanied by age-related declines in suggestibility among 3- to 5-year-olds. However, there appears to be some disagreement about the reasons for changes in reliability of reporting between ages 3 and 5 years: some investigators point to developmental linguistic capability (14), whereas others attribute unreliability to feelings of discomfort about an emotional or painful situation, and not to limited vocabulary or linguistic ability (15).

In general, the literature supports interviewing children in a minimally suggestible manner and in a setting that is comfortable and informal. Furthermore, it appears that allegation-blind interviewers fare better in terms of establishing rapport with children and minimizing the likelihood of leading or misleading with information obtained from collateral sources. There may, therefore, be clinical and forensic benefit to interviewing the communicative child first and then obtaining collateral information afterward, again preferably outside the presence of the child. A child's suggestibility may also be reduced if the interviewer clarifies expectations and emphasizes the importance of telling the truth and admitting confusion over guessing. Furthermore, telling a child that repeated questions do not imply that the initial response was incorrect may minimize the child's tendency to change an answer (13).

Evaluating noncommunicative children presents significant challenges to the emergency department physician. Documentation of collateral information and observations about the child during the physical examination are essential. Assessment of the reasons for the lack of communicativeness is clinically, and maybe forensically, appropriate and necessary. Mental retardation should be documented, as should the results of a cognitive capacity screening and/or mental status examination, if conducted. Intellectually or cognitively deficient children who may be victims of violence or abuse can be evaluated if they are not regarded as incompetent in a legal sense, and documentation of any history provided by them should be undertaken (16). A patient's silence during the interview may be completely unrelated to any mental disease or defect. A child may be attempting to collect his or her thoughts or decide whether or not to trust the interviewer. A child may fall silent because of the interviewer's insensitivity (17). Children with specific impairments of speech or hearing may require an evaluation utilizing nonverbal interview techniques, such as playing, drawing, or painting. Such approaches are usually the province of specialists trained in evaluating children with those deficiencies. Severely depressed children may not speak during interviews; however, they may become communicative later, after effective treatment has been initiated (18). If a child is exhibiting elective mutism, there is no universally successful method for eliciting verbal responses; the record may have to reflect observations of the child's appearance, demeanor, and behavior, as well as the results of his or her examination, as well as document the child's mutism and the fact that all of the history was obtained from collateral sources. Referral of the patient to a specialist trained in child interviewing may be necessary to conduct as thorough an examination as possible and avoid inappropriate and unproductive utilization of emergency department personnel.

Documentation of the evaluation of a noncommunicative child in an emergency department should include observations of the child and any clinically relevant information regarding the lack of communication along with the physical examination. Collateral information obtained outside the child's presence should be documented and observations made regarding the interaction of the child with the collateral source. The collateral source can be called on to comfort the child or facilitate conversation between the clinician and the child if the child is communicative in the presence of the other person, but care should be taken to avoid leading or prompting the child on the part of the physician or the collateral source, and documentation should reflect the presence of the source and any observable effect that it has on the child.

## INTERVIEWING ADULTS

Adult victims of violence can also be communicative or noncommunicative. A communicative adult is evaluated using his or her own narrative and relying on techniques that elicit a general medical history. The information should be documented, with consideration given to the medico-legal importance of the record generated. Open-ended interview techniques are generally favored; however, reticence can create a barrier to the free flow of information, particularly in situations of spousal abuse or other forms of intrafamilial violence. These circumstances may prompt the patient to avoid discussion or misrepresent the history underlying physical injuries. The patient's behavior and demeanor should be documented and correlated with the reported history of injury and the actual physical findings. It may be necessary to point out discrepancies between the verbal representation and the clinical findings as a means of sympathetically eliciting greater disclosure. However, such efforts may be met with resistance and might not be successful. In those instances, merely documenting the discrepancies between the patient's account and the physical findings, and providing the patient with appropriate resources to discuss the possibility of familial violence may be all that is possible in an emergency department setting.

Some adults may appear to be communicative, but their communication is unreliable as a result of another clinical condition. Patients with delirium as a result of substance abuse or withdrawal and those with dementia may appear communicative but, on further questioning, are revealed to be incapable of providing accurate or useful information or clinical data. Again, the discrepancy between the patient's verbal report and any injuries or physical problems should be identified in the record, along with the clinician's observations of the individual and his or her performance on mental status or cognitive capacity screening examination. As with children, some noncommunicative adults whose mental status examination reveals depression may become more communicative after treatment for the underlying depression has been initiated.

More than 4 million Americans suffer from Alzheimer's disease, with variable but at times highly significant impairment in mental processing, comprehension, and communication. This group is at high risk for neglect and abuse. Some studies suggest that closed-ended questions are easier for this type of patient to answer (19), but other studies reveal no significant difference in the proportion of relevant responses between open, closed, and mixed types of questioning (20). As patients' cognitive capacity screening examination scores decrease, the number of questions necessary to elicit a response increases and the proportion of relevant responses to open-ended questions decreases (20). This highlights the need to further characterize the basis for impairment in communication with clinical examination and mental status and cognitive capacity screening examinations. The findings available from such examinations have diagnostic importance and also help the clinician choose an interview strategy that will be most likely to elicit reliable information. In the emergency department, documentation of observations of the patient, objective data regarding his or her cognitive capabilities, as well as findings on physical examination may be all that can be accomplished in the evaluation of patients suspected to have been victims of violence or abuse. These patients should be referred to appropriate agencies for further evaluation and follow-up.

## SUMMARY

Clinical interviewing and history taking is a skill applicable in all clinical settings. Approaching patients with a genuine sense of interest and in a manner indicating that they are being listened to is highly beneficial to the establishment of trust and rapport. The subsequent elicitation of information about the patient is an invaluable tool for the evaluation, diagnosis, and initial clinical management of patients and their subsequent referral for treatment. Victims of violence or abuse require the same care and attention as other patients but may need additional intervention to soothe emotional upset and to establish rapport and trust. The challenge for emergency department personnel is to undertake this process effectively in as time-efficient a manner as possible, but also in a manner that makes the patient feel as comfortable and as communicative as possible, given their age, emotional state, and any concurrent medical, mental, or neurocognitive conditions.

A significant percentage of emergency medical intervention may have medico-legal significance in the future. Integral to the forensic aspects of emergency medical practice are patient interviews, the elicitation of medical and event histories, and accurate and thorough documentation of that information and of behavioral observations and physical findings. Approaching the patient with an open mind, listening, documenting what is said, and observing the patient and documenting those observations are essential. Some patients present specific challenges. This chapter has suggested approaches to those patients to elicit as much reliable information as possible for the purposes of clinical assessment and forensic documentation. The goal is to generate a medical record that accurately and thoroughly reflects the patient's clinical presentation, emergency evaluation, and treatment for future reference by other clinicians, and documents a descriptive snapshot of the patient for future reference and consideration during fact finding in a legal context.

## REFERENCES

1. Monk M. Interviewing suspected victims of child maltreatment in the emergency department. *J Emerg Nurs* 1998 Feb;24(1):31–34.
2. von Klitzing K. Credibility examination of children and adolescents on the question of sexual abuse. *Acta Paedopsychiatry* 1990;53:181–190.
3. Jáskiewicz-Obydzinska T, Czerederecka A. Psychological evaluation of changes in testimony given by sexually abused juveniles. In: Davies G, Wilson C, Lloyd-Bostock S, et al., eds. *Psychology, law, and criminal justice: international developments in research and practice.* Berlin: Walter de Gruyter, 1995;160–169.
4. Bruck M, Ceci SJ. The suggestibility of children's memory. *Annu Rev Psychol* 1999;50:419–439.
5. Kellogg ND, Hoffman TJ. Child sexual revictimization by multiple perpetrators. *Child Abuse Negl* 1997 Oct; 21(10):953–964.
6. Lamb ME, Sternberg KJ, Esplin PW. Making children into competent witnesses: reaction to the amicus brief

in re Michaels. *Psychol Public Policy Law* 1995;1(2): 438–449.

7. Cantlon J, Payne G, Erbaugh C. Outcome-based practice: disclosure rates of child sexual abuse comparing allegation blind and allegation informed structured interviews. *Child Abuse Negl* 1996;20(11):1113–1120.

8. Faller KC. Interviewing children who may have been abused: a historical perspective and overview of controversies. *Child Maltreatment* 1996;1(2):83–95.

9. Sternberg KJ, Lamb ME, Hershkowitz I, et al. The relation between investigative utterance types and the informativeness of child witnesses. *J Appl Dev Psychol* 1996;17:439–451.

10. Jones DPH. The influence of introductory style on children's ability to relay information in forensic interviews [Editorial]. *Child Abuse Negl* 1997;21(11):1131–1132.

11. Peterson C, Biggs M. Interviewing children about trauma: problems with "specific" questions. *J Trauma Stress* 1997;10(2):279–290.

12. Greenstock J, Pipe M-E. Interviewing children about past events: the influence of peer support and misleading questions. *Child Abuse Negl* 1996;20(1): 69–80.

13. Reed LD. Findings from research on children's suggestibility and implications for conducting child interviews. *Child Maltreatment* 1996;1(2):105–120.

14. Aldridge M, Wood J. Talking about feelings: young children's ability to express emotions. *Child Abuse Negl* 1997;21(12):1221–1233.

15. Harris PL, Jones DPH. Commentary on "Talking about feelings" (Aldridge and Wood, 1997). *Child Abuse Negl* 1997;21(12):1217–1220.

16. Quinn KM. Competency to be a witness: a major child forensic issue. *Bull Am Acad Psychiatry Law* 1986;14 (4):311–321.

17. Bates B. *A guide to physical examination and history taking,* 5th ed. Philadelphia: JB Lippincott, 1991.

18. Barker P. *Clinical interviews with children and adolescents.* New York: WW Norton, 1990.

19. Tappen RM. Alzheimer's disease: communication techniques to facilitate perioperative care. *AORN J* 1991; 54(6):1279–1286.

20. Tappen RM, Williams-Burgess C, Edelstein J, et al. Communicating with individuals with Alzheimer's disease: examination of recommended strategies. *Arch Psychiatr Nurs* 1997;11(5):249–256.

# 4

# Forensic Emergency Medicine

William S. Smock

Forensic emergency medicine is the application of forensic medical knowledge and appropriate techniques to living patients in the emergency department. Nowadays, most trauma patients seen in emergency room settings are victims. They are not victims of happenstance or accident, but of malice and intent at the hands of assailants. This phenomenon reflects a major change in our society's interactional dynamics. Given that this is the new reality of our patient population, physicians must practice medicine—in particular trauma medicine—in a new way, with attention to details heretofore overlooked. What was once considered confounding clutter that gets in the way of patient care (such as clothing and surface dirt) takes on a whole new significance when recognized for what it really is—evidence.

Traditionally, the emergency physician has been trained in the provision of emergency medical care without regard for forensic issues. In the process of providing patient care, critical evidence can be lost, discarded, or inadvertently washed away (1–10). Patients then lose access to information that can be of critical significance when criminal or civil proceedings arise secondary to their injuries.

## ACKNOWLEDGING THE VOID

The earliest references in the U.S. medical literature to the practice of forensic medicine on living patients in our country decry its absence (1,11). These articles were written by the forensic pathologists and pioneers in clinical forensic medicine, John Smialek, M.D. and the late William Eckert, M.D. In 1986, Cyril Wecht, M.D., J.D., former president of the American College of Legal Medicine, stated that:

> It's a great shame and a source of much puzzlement why a group similar to police surgeons hasn't developed here. Even within our adversarial judicial system and with our guaranteed civil rights—which are much greater than in many of the countries where forensic clinicians are commonly found—I believe those persons with both medical and forensic training could remove much of the guesswork, speculation and hypotheses from the disposition of accident or assault cases involving living persons (10).

## FILLING THE VOID

The first postgraduate training program for emergency physicians dealing with clinical forensic medicine was a 2-day seminar in Chicago in 1990, sponsored by the Illinois Chapter of the American College of Emergency Physicians. This program was suspended after its first year. An annual postgraduate clinical forensic medicine training seminar was subsequently established in Louisville in 1994 by the Kentucky Chapter of the American College of Emergency Physicians. This program continued through 1998.

The Department of Emergency Medicine at the University of Louisville School of Medicine and the Kentucky Medical Examiner's Office established the first formal clinical forensic medicine training program for residents in the United States in 1991 (3,4,9,12). Two years later, the first fellowship in clinical forensic medicine was created, also in Louisville. Concomitantly, the first formal clinical forensic medicine consultation service in the United States was established (3,4,9).

## UTILITY OF FORENSIC EMERGENCY MEDICINE

The emergency physician, by design and default, evaluates and treats victims with gunshot and stab wounds, and victims of physical assault, sexual abuse and assault, domestic violence, and motor vehicle–related trauma. All of these patients have injuries or conditions that have criminal or civil forensic medical implications and the prospect or specter of courtroom sequelae (2). A patient's emergency medical evaluation must be detailed and documentation comprehensive. Comprehensive documentation ideally contains all three components: narrative, diagrammatic, and photographic. The failure to document a number of clinical findings comprehensively may have far-ranging consequences for a patient, an accused suspect, and, potentially, the treating physician (1,2,5,6,8,9, 14–17). Carmona and Prince reported in a review of 100 charts of emergency department patients who presented to a level 1 trauma center in California that there was poor, improper, or inadequate documentation in 70% of cases (2). In 38% of these cases, potential evidence was improperly secured, improperly documented, or inadvertently discarded (2).

The forensically *untrained* emergency physician may easily overlook and inadvertently destroy evidence, both gross and trace, in the course of providing patient care. He may misinterpret physical injuries and evidence and form an inaccurate opinion as to their cause (1–8,10,13, 15–17). Such opinions, when recorded in the patient's emergency department chart, may pose a considerable problem for the patient, the court, and the emergency physician if circumstances progress to legal proceedings at a later date.

If the forensically untrained physician can make mistakes that may haunt him and others in court, the trained one may be able to preclude the courtroom consequence entirely. One example of such avoidance is seen in a case involving a 20-year-old black man who presented to a level 1 trauma center with a perforating gunshot

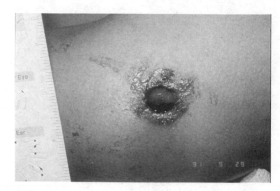

**FIG. 4-1.** The presence of soot and seared wound margins is indicative of a loose contact wound. The patient stated that he was shot from a distance of 40 feet. The physical evidence does not support the history given by the patient.

wound to the left shoulder (4). The patient stated that he had been shot from a distance of 30 feet and that he knew the assailant's name. When the police arrived in the emergency department, the patient requested that the assailant be arrested immediately, as he felt his life was in danger. Examination of the wounds revealed the presence of soot surrounding the larger anterior wound, as well as soot on the patient's shirt (Fig. 4-1). The examining emergency physician was aware that the presence of soot was indicative of a close range of fire and that the physical evidence did not support the history given. When the patient was confronted with this information, he recanted his story and admitted that the wounds were self-inflicted in an attempt to "set up" the accused (4). The ability of the emergency physician to determine that the wound was consistent with having been inflicted at a close range prevented the accused from being arrested for a crime he did not commit. Traditionally, such wounds have been cleaned and debrided, removing all evidence in the process, including evidence that would distinguish entrance from exit and range of fire.

## FORENSIC ASPECTS OF GUNSHOT WOUND MANAGEMENT

Emergency physicians treat in excess of 250,000 victims of gunshot wounds each year. Because they evaluate gunshot wounds before therapeutic or surgical intervention obscure the wound's appearance, they are in an ideal position to evaluate and document it. Documentation of gunshot wounds in the medical record by the treating physician should include the number, location, size, shape, and characteristics of the wound(s). A precise description of a gunshot wound requires a basic understanding of wound ballistics and a familiarity with relevant forensic terminology.

## WOUND BALLISTICS

Wound ballistics is the study of the effect(s) that penetrating projectiles have on the body (18–23,37,38). Several factors determine a bullet's potential for wounding (18–21,24–26). They are the bullet's velocity and weight, deformations/fragmentation upon impact with tissue, and the characteristics and location of the impacted tissue itself (18–23,25–26). The mechanism by which the bullet wounds is the transference of its kinetic energy to the relatively stationary tissue it impacts. The severity of the wound inflicted is directly related to the amount of kinetic energy transferred to the tissue rather than the total amount of kinetic energy possessed by the bullet itself (19–21). Bullets traveling at higher velocities have more kinetic energy and theoretically higher wounding potential; however, the physician should not assume that injuries associated

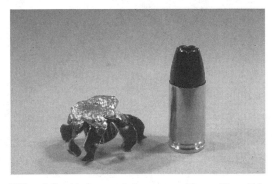

**FIG. 4-3.** Hollow-point ammunition, like this 9-mm "Black Talon" bullet, has the capacity to significantly increase its surface area upon impact with tissue.

with high-velocity projectiles (like those propelled by a rifle) are necessarily more severe than those associated with low-velocity projectiles (Fig. 4-2). Wound severity is dictated by the interplay of several variables and not the bullet's velocity alone.

Crushing is the principal mechanism by which bullets from handguns impart damage to tissue. A bullet traveling through tissue generates two cavities. The first is a temporary one, lasting only 5 to 10 milliseconds from its generation until its collapse. The second is the permanent one, the crushed tissue we observe. The size of the cavity remaining (i.e., the wound) varies with the size, shape, and configuration of the bullet. A hollow point bullet that mushrooms upon impact can increase its diameter by as much as 2.5-fold (Fig. 4-3). This hollow-point bullet's capacity to change its shape will increase the area of tissue crush it generates by 6.25 times that of a nondeformed bullet of a similar caliber (21).

## FORENSIC TERMINOLOGY ASSOCIATED WITH GUNSHOT WOUNDS

The majority of misinterpretations of gunshot wounds made by physicians are ones involving the distinction between entrance and exit wounds. The errors are invariably based on the fallacious assumption that an exit wound will be larger than its corresponding entrance wound.

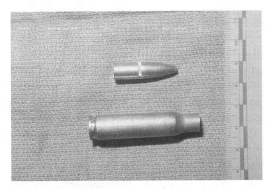

**FIG. 4-2.** A wound from a .308 caliber high-velocity rifle round. High-velocity rounds have the potential to transfer large amounts of energy to body tissue.

The first study to compare the interpretations of emergency physicians, trauma surgeons, and neurosurgeons at a level 1 trauma center with those of a forensic pathologist determined that fatal gunshot wounds were correctly interpreted in only 47.8% of cases.

There are five factors that determine the size of gunshot wounds, both entrance and exit: the size, shape, configuration, and velocity of the bullet as it contacts tissue, and the physical characteristics of the impacted tissue itself.

### Entrance Wounds

Range of fire is the distance between the gun muzzle and the victim. There are five categories of range of fire. Each has an entrance wound whose characteristics are unique to it. The entrance wounds bear the name of the range of fire from which they are inflicted: indeterminate or distant range and graze wounds, intermediate or medium range, near-contact or close range, and contact wounds.

#### *Contact Wounds*

A contact wound is generated when the barrel or muzzle of the gun is in actual contact with the victim's skin or clothing. These wounds can be further divided into "tight contact," where the barrel is pushed hard against the skin, and "loose contact," where the barrel is incompletely or loosely held against the skin or clothing. Tight contact wounds can vary in appearance from a small hole with seared blackened edges (Fig. 4-4) to a gaping stellate wound (Fig. 4-5). The large stellate wound is caused by gases expanding under the skin and is often mistaken for an exit wound. The small tight contact entrance wound's blackened edges are caused by the discharge of hot gases and an actual flame.

In tight contact wounds, all materials—bullet, gases, soot, incompletely burned pieces of gunpowder, and metal fragments—are forced into the wound. When the wound occurs over thin or bony tissue, the hot gases cause the skin to expand to such an extent that the skin stretches and tears (Fig. 4-6). These tears generally have a triangular configuration, with the base of the

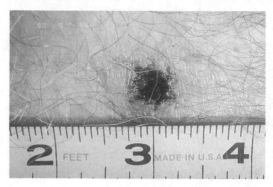

**FIG. 4-4.** A tight contact wound from a .22 caliber handgun. The wound margins are seared and soot covered. Small, triangular-shaped tears are the result of tissue expansion from the injection of gases into the wound.

triangle overlying the entrance wound. Tears are usually associated with ammunition of .32 caliber or greater, or magnum loads (Fig. 4-7A–C).

However, stellate tears are not pathognomonic for contact wounds. Some exit wounds appear stellate, as do wounds associated with ricochet or tumbling bullets (Fig. 4-8A, B). Tangential wounds frequently appear stellate, also. One way to distinguish the wounds that mimic the tight contact wound from the tight contact wound itself is the absence of soot and powder within and around the wound.

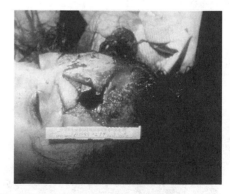

**FIG. 4-5.** A large stellate laceration from a contact wound with a .357 magnum handgun. The triangular shaped lacerations are the result of the injection of gases. Emergency physicians should not base an opinion of entrance versus exit on the size of the wound.

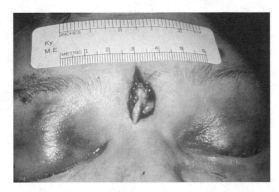

**FIG. 4-6.** Seared wound margins and a triangular-shaped laceration from a tight contact wound with a .38 caliber revolver. That patient's husband stated that the wound was self-inflicted from a distance of approximately 14 in. On the basis of statements made to the treating physicians, which were inconsistent with the physical properties of the wound, the husband was charged with murder.

In some tight contact wounds, a contusion that mirrors the muzzle can be seen. This pattern contusion results when the hot gases cause the skin to expand back against the muzzle tip (Fig. 4-9A, B; see Colorplate following page 144). Patterns like these are helpful when establishing the type of weapon used (revolver vs. semiautomatic) and should be documented before debridement or surgery.

Soot is a black, dusty by-product of combustion and will be observed within and around a contact wound in which the gun's muzzle is loosely contacting (incompletely contacting) or angled, relative to the skin (Fig. 4-10). The angle between the muzzle and the skin dictates the soot pattern observed. A perpendicular, loose, or near-contact wound causes searing of the skin surrounding the wound as well as the deposition of soot. A tangential, loose, or near-contact wound results in

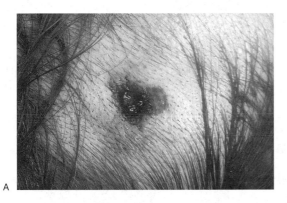

A

**FIG. 4-7. A:** A tight contact wound from a .25 caliber handgun. The wound displays soot, seared margins and a muzzle contusion at the 3 o'clock position. The muzzle contusion resulted from the forceful displacement of skin against the gun muzzle. **B:** Tight contact wound with a muzzle contusion from a .38 caliber handgun. **C:** Large stellate lacerations from a tight contact wound with a .380 semiautomatic handgun. The large wound is the result of tissue expansion from the injection of gas into the tissue.

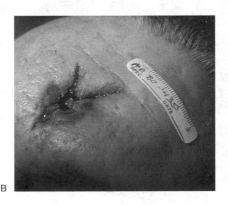

B

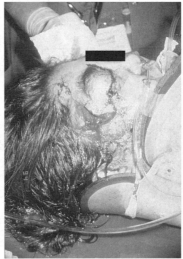

C

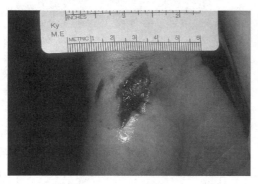

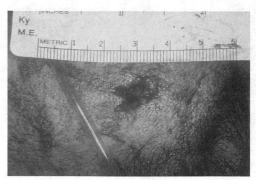

**FIG. 4-8. A:** Exit wounds may also have a stellate appearance. The lack of soot and searing of the wound margins can differentiate stellate-appearing exit wounds from contact wounds. **B:** Stellate exit wound from a .380 semi-automatic handgun.

searing and soot deposition that are elongated in shape, marking the path the bullet took at entry.

### *Close-Range Wounds*

Close range is defined as the maximum range at which soot is deposited on the wound or clothing (Fig. 4-11A–C). This muzzle-to-target distance is usually less than 6 in. Soot has been noted on victims whose skin-to-muzzle distance was 12 in., but this is very rare (20–22). Beyond 6 in., the soot usually falls away and does not reach the target. The concentration of the soot varies inversely with the muzzle-to-target distance and is influenced by the type of gunpow-

der and ammunition used, the barrel length, and the caliber and type of weapon used. A precise range of fire, such as 1 cm versus 10 cm, cannot be determined from a soot pattern.

If the patient is stable and therapeutic manipulation of the wound can be delayed, the soot pattern should be described in detail and photographed before it is removed. Forensic crime laboratories can determine the range of fire of an assault by test-firing the offending weapon at a target at various distances until they succeed in reproducing the soot pattern observed on the patient. Of course, they must use ammunition similar to that which caused the wound.

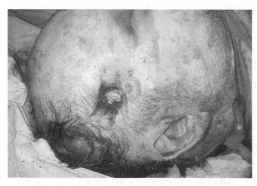

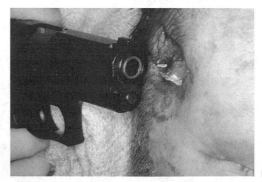

**FIG. 4-9. A:** A "muzzle contusion" or "muzzle abrasion" overlying the right temple associated with a tight contact wound. Close examination of contact wounds may reveal clues as to the type of handgun used (i.e., semi-automatic vs. revolver). **B:** Forceful expansion of the skin overlying the right temple resulted in a muzzle contusion from the barrel of a 9-mm semi-automatic handgun.

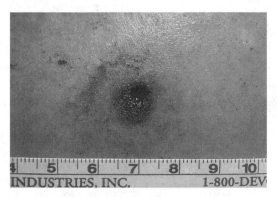

**FIG. 4-10.** Soot deposition is associated with both loose contact and close-range gunshot wounds. This asymmetrical soot pattern is produced when the handgun barrel-to-skin angle is less than 90 degrees when the weapon is discharged.

### Intermediate-Range Wounds

"Tattooing" or "stippling" is caused by contact with partially burned and wholly unburned pieces of gunpowder. They appear as punctate abrasions and are pathognomonic for intermediate-range gunshot wounds (Fig. 4-12A–C; see Colorplate following page 144). Therefore, the medium- or intermediate-range wound is one that is sufficiently close to cause tattooing.

Tattooing is generally seen in wound-to-muzzle distances of 60 cm or less, but has been reported as close as 1 cm and as far away as 1 m. The pattern and density of the tattooing are dictated by the muzzle-to-skin distance, the length of the gun's barrel, the type of ammunition used, the type of gunpowder used, and the presence of intermediate objects (such as clothing and hair).

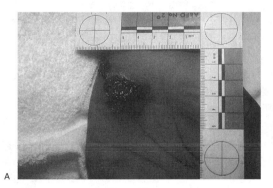

A

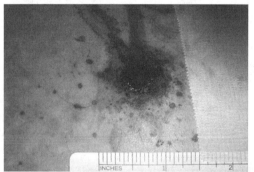

B

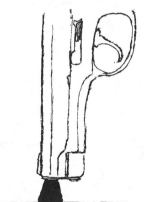

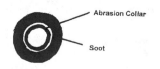

C

**FIG. 4-11. A:** Visible carbonaceous material or soot will be deposited on wounds when the barrel of the handgun is discharged within 6 in. The presence of soot defines a wound as "close range." **B:** Soot associated with the discharge of a 9-mm semi-automatic pistol from a distance of 1 in. **C:** Deposition of soot associated with the wound in Fig. 4-11B.

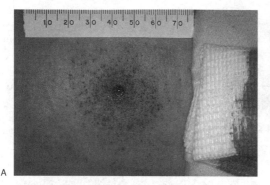

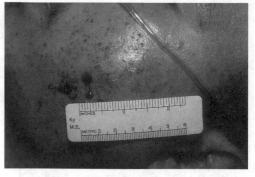

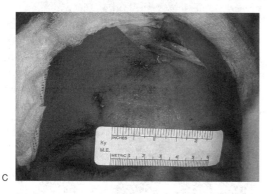

**FIG. 4-12. A:** "Tattooing" is the result of partially burned or unburned gunpowder impacting skin. The "tattoos" are punctate abrasions and are associated with an intermediate-range gunshot wound. Tattooing has been seen with wounds as close as 1 cm and as far away as 1 m. **B:** This patient stated that he was shot with a .22 caliber handgun at a distance of 12 in. His cheek exhibited punctate abrasions or "tattooing" associated with intermediate-range gunshot wounds. **C:** Forehead "tattooing" from an intermediate-range gunshot wound. The patient reported he was shot with a .38 caliber revolver from a distance of 18 in.

### Long-Range Wounds

The long-range or distant wound is inflicted from a range sufficiently far that only the bullet makes contact with the clothing and skin. No tattooing or soot is observed. As the bullet penetrates the skin, the skin is indented resulting in the creation of an "abrasion collar," also called "abrasion margin," "abrasion rim," and "abrasion ring" (Fig. 4-13A, B). The collar is an abraded area of tissue that surrounds an entry wound and is caused by friction between the bullet and the epithelium, not by thermal changes associated with a hot projectile. The abrasion

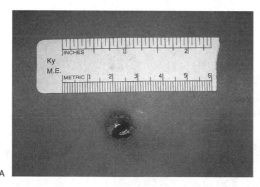

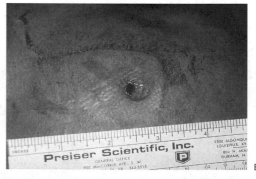

**FIG. 4-13. A:** An abrasion collar is the result of friction between a bullet and the skin. Abrasion collars are associated with gunshot wounds of entrance. **B:** An abrasion collar may also be called an "abrasion rim" or "abrasion ring." The width will vary with the angle of the bullet's impact.

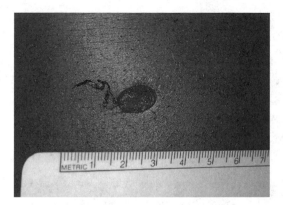

**FIG. 4-14.** An entrance wound associated with a high-velocity handgun round (.357 magnum). The abrasion collar can only be seen when the tissue is everted.

collar's width will vary with the angle of impact (Fig. 4-12C). Almost all entrance wounds have abrasion collars. Some high-velocity rounds will produce very small abrasion collars which can only be seen with examination of the tissue (Fig. 4-14). Because of the inelasticity of the tissue in these areas, entrance wounds on the palms of hands and soles of feet usually appear slit-like and lack abrasion collars (21).

## Exit Wounds

Exit wounds are the result of a bullet pushing and stretching the skin from the inside out. The skin edges generally are everted, with sharp but irregular margins. True abrasion collars, soot, and tattooing are not associated with exit wounds.

Emergency physicians should remember that exit wounds can assume a variety of shapes and configurations and are not necessarily consistently larger than the entrance wounds that preceded them (Figs. 4-15A–C). The exit wound's size is dictated principally by the amount of energy that the bullet still possesses as it exits the skin. Other factors that affect wound size are the bullet's size and configuration. A bullet's configuration will change from its usual nose-first attitude on entering the skin to a tumbling and

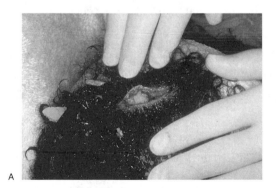

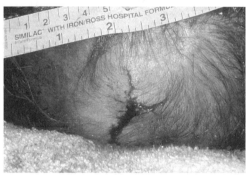

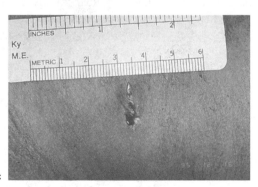

**FIG. 4-15. A:** An exit wound at the vertex of the skull associated with an intraoral entrance wound. Forceful extrusion of bone at the wound site resulted in enlargement of this exit wound. **B:** A triangular-shaped exit wound with irregular wound margins. Exit wounds may be larger or smaller than their associated entrance wounds. **C:** A slit-like exit wound on the lateral neck. The size of the exit wound is dependent on multiple variables including bullet velocity and tissue elasticity.

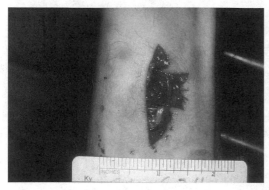

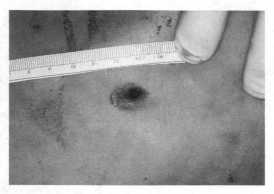

**FIG. 4-16.** A stellate-shaped exit wound of the forearm from a .22 caliber-long rifle bullet. The wound size and shape are the result of bone extrusion. The lack of soot and seared skin distinguishes this wound from a contact wound.

**FIG. 4-17.** A shored exit wound. The "false" abrasion collar occurs when the exiting projectile pushes the skin against a supporting object. This shored exit wound resulted from a .357 magnum projectile exiting the patient's back when he was against a brick wall.

yawing one after impact with tissue. A bullet with sufficient energy that exits the skin in a sideways configuration, or one that has increased its surface area by mushrooming, will have an exit wound larger than its corresponding entrance wound (Fig. 4-16) (18,20,21).

### Atypical Exit Wounds

A "shored-exit" wound is one with a *false* abrasion collar. If the skin is forcibly pressed against or supported by a firm object or surface at the moment the bullet exits, the skin can be squeezed between the exiting bullet and the supporting surface (Fig. 4-17) (22,23). Examples of supporting structures include floors, walls, doors, chairs, and mattresses, as well as less flexible articles of clothing, such as belts or jewelry.

On rare occasions, soot may be present at an atypical exit wound site (24). If an entrance wound is located sufficiently close to it, soot may be propelled through the short wound track and appear faintly on the exit wound's surface.

### Entrance versus Exit

Emergency physicians, health professionals, and law enforcement officials will make grievous errors in documentation and the determination of entrance versus exit wounds if the diagnosis is based solely on the size of the wound (2,4,5,8,13,16). If an emergency physician receives adequate forensic training and has familiarity with the proper forensic terminology, then distinction of entrance from exit wounds will not be difficult. When in doubt, the emergency physician should refrain from placing statements regarding "entrance" and "exit" in the medical record. At such times, the patient and physician will be better served if the wound is measured, photographed, and accurately described using appropriate forensic terminology and tissue sent to the forensic pathologist for microscopic analysis.

### EVIDENCE

In the evaluation and treatment of patients who are victims of a gunshot wound, assault, or trauma, the emergency physician usually has the opportunity to preserve and collect short-lived evidence, but first he must recognize it as such. Carmona and Prince have reported that trauma physicians "usually have little or no training in the forensic aspects of trauma care and therefore necessary evidence may often be overlooked, lost, inadvertently discarded or its admissibility denied because of improper handling or documentation" (2).

In the case of gunshot wounds, the victim's clothing may yield information about the range

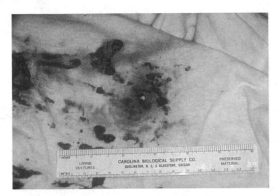

**FIG. 4-18.** Soot deposition is associated with a close range of fire. Examination of the patient's clothing by the emergency physician will assist in the determination of entrance versus exit wounds and the range of fire. Each article of clothing should be packaged separately in paper bags to avoid the transfer of residues between articles.

of fire and help distinguish entrance from exit wounds (Figs. 4-18, 4-19, 4-20A–E) (1,7,20–22, 25). Clothing fibers will deform in the direction of the passing projectile. Gunpowder residues and soot will deposit on clothing, just as they do on skin. Some of the residue will be invisible to the naked eye but can be detected using standard forensic laboratory staining techniques.

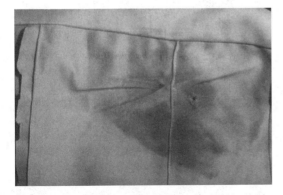

**FIG. 4-19.** Invisible vaporized lead residues can be visualized with colorimetric testing by the forensic crime laboratory. All clothing associated with victims of gunshot wounds should be preserved for crime lab testing, even if no visible residues are appreciated.

Bullet wipe is a lead and/or lubricant residue left on clothing through which a bullet has passed (Fig. 4-21). When articles of clothing are removed from a wounded patient, they should be packaged separately (to avoid cross-contamination) and placed in a paper bag (to minimize the risk that static electricity will lift fragile evidence off their surface).

A gunshot residue (GSR) test may determine whether a victim or suspect has fired a weapon (21,26–34). The GSR test checks for the presence of invisible residues from the primer: barium nitrate, antimony sulfide, and lead peroxide. The sensitivity of the test decreases with the passage of time, and law enforcement agents may not have access to a patient during the "golden hour" (21). Factors that affect the sensitivity include washing the skin with alcohol or povidone-iodine (Betadine), placing tape on the skin, rubbing the hands against clothing, and placing plastic bags over the patient's hands, which may cause moisture to develop on the skin. If a GSR test is to be performed or if soot is noted on the patient's hand, paper bags should be placed over the hands early in the treatment of the patient (Fig. 4-22A, B).

When a weapon is discharged, it imprints multiple unique microscopic marks on the side of a bullet (20,21). The bullet's markings result from its contact with the tool marks or "rifling" in the gun's barrel (Figs. 4-23 and 4-24A, B). The emergency physician must try not to compromise these markings when removing a bullet from a patient (22). Bullets should be handled with gloves. Surgical instruments, like hemostats or pickups, should be covered with gauze to ensure the preservation of these microscopic "fingerprint" marks (Figs. 4-25 and 4-26).

Radiographs may be used to help locate retained projectiles and may be of evidentiary value when determining the number of projectiles and the direction of fire (20–22,25). However, they should not be exposed less than 72 in. from a bullet. Closer exposure will distort the image of the projectile and cause it to appear larger than it is. Emergency physicians should not render opinions on a projectile's caliber.

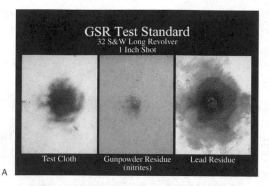

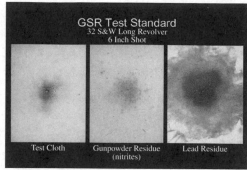

A

B

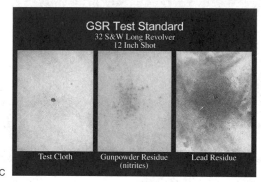

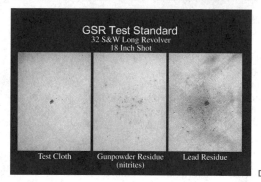

C

D

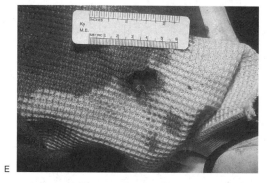

E

**FIG. 4-20.** Gunshot residue testing of a .32 cal-iber handgun on cloth. The forensic crime lab-oratory will examine clothing for evidence of visible and invisible gunshot residues, includ-ing carbonaceous soot from the burning of gunpowder, nitrates from unburned gunpowder, and vaporized lead residue. Nitrates and lead residues are only visible with the application of specialized forensic testing. **A:** At the 1-in. range, there are heavy concentrations of soot, nitrates, and lead residues deposited on the test cloth. **B:** At the 6-in. range, there is mini-mal soot with heavy concentrations of nitrates and lead residues. **C:** At the 12-in. range, there is no soot and heavy concentrations of nitrates and lead residues are present. **D:** At the 18-in. range, there are no visible residues. The con-centrations of nitrates and lead residues are significantly reduced. **E:** At the 24-in. range, no residues are deposited on the test cloth.

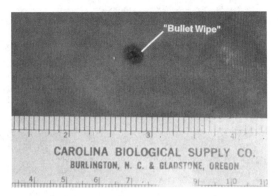

**FIG. 4-21.** "Bullet wipe" on clothing is the deposition of lead and lubricants by the projectile as it penetrates. This residue is best appreciated on white clothing but may be detected on dark clothing utilizing forensic testing for lead residues.

## FORENSIC ASSESSMENT OF BLUNT TRAUMATIC PATTERN INJURIES

A pattern injury is one that is recognized by the imprint left on the skin by the offending object. Blunt traumatic pattern injuries include pattern abrasions, pattern lacerations, and, most commonly, pattern contusions. Pattern injuries are reproducible and are "mirror images" of the weapon, whether hand, gun muzzle tip, baseball bat, belt, and so forth, that inflicted them.

## Pattern Abrasions

An abrasion is defined as an injury that rubs or scratches away the superficial layers of the epidermis. Common examples of pattern abrasions include bite marks, ligature marks, fingernail marks, and carpet imprints (Fig. 4-27A–C).

## Pattern Lacerations

A laceration is a tear in the skin, produced by blunt force trauma. The edges of a laceration will exhibit tissue breaking and appear torn or abraded. This is in contrast to the sharply deformed edges of an incised wound.

## Pattern Contusions

The pattern contusion is the most common pattern injury produced by the application of blunt force. Blood in the tissue underlying the striking object is forcibly displaced to the sides, resulting in an epithelial print that essentially traces the outline of the weapon used. For example, a blow from a linear object leaves a contusion that is characterized by a set of parallel lines separated by an area of central clearing (Fig. 4-28A–G).

When circular contusions are observed, the emergency physician should be highly suspicious

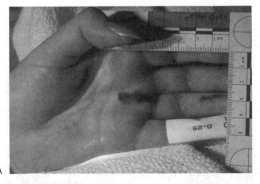
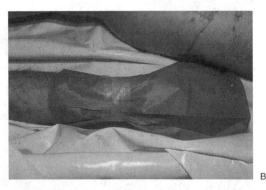

A                                                                                                           B

**FIG. 4-22. A:** Examination of the hands may reveal the presence of visible gunshot residues. The presence of soot indicates that the patient's hand was within 6 in. of the weapon when it was discharged. This patient held a .32 caliber revolver in her left hand during her suicide. **B:** Placement of paper bags over the hands of a gunshot wound victim helps preserve the presence of any gunshot or primer residues. *Never* cover the hands with plastic bags. Placement of plastic bags will result in the accumulation of moisture and result in the degradation and contamination of evidence.

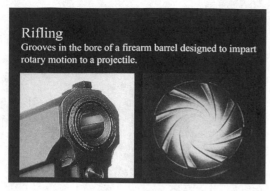

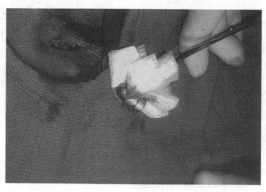

**FIG. 4-23.** Bullets will have microscopic marks or "rifling impressions" imparted to them as they travel down the gun barrel. The impressions are a mirror image of the marks left in the gun barrel during its manufacture. Like a fingerprint, the barrel etchings are unique to each barrel.

**FIG. 4-25.** To avoid damage from surgical instruments to the bullet's microscopic impressions, hemostats and pickups should be covered with gauze. Any metal-to-metal contact will destroy these microscopic marks and make the job of the forensic scientist more difficult.

of abuse or battery. Circular contusions 1.0 to 1.5 cm in diameter are characteristic pattern contusions left by excessive fingertip pressure (Fig. 4-29A–C; see Colorplate following page 144). An easily overlooked anatomic location where fingertip pressure contusions are often found is the medial aspect of the upper arm (Fig. 4-30).

### Bite Marks

The pattern injury that is the most useful in identifying the actual individual responsible for inflicting an injury is the bite mark (Fig. 4-31). The bite mark may be seen as a pattern contusion, a pattern abrasion, or a combination of the two. Bite marks vary greatly in the quality of their identifiable features, depending on the anatomic location of the bite and the motion of the teeth relative to the skin. Some bite marks may not even be recognizable as such.

When an acute bite mark is identified, the emergency physician must guard against destroying residual evidence. The skin surface

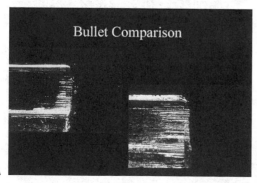

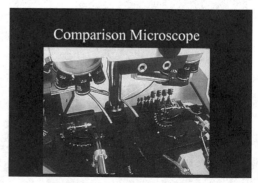

**FIG. 4-24. A:** The microscopic impressions are a unique fingerprint of the gun's barrel and can be examined with a comparison microscope. Care must be taken in the collection of bullets to avoid metal-to-metal contact from surgical instruments, such as hemostats, or damage from the dropping of projectiles into surgical pans. **B:** The comparison microscope is utilized to compare bullets collected from a patient with a known bullet standard.

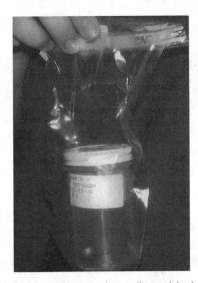

**FIG. 4-26.** Bullets must be collected in breathable containers (paper boxes or envelopes). Placement of bullets in airtight containers will result in contamination and degradation of the evidence from the collection of moisture and the proliferation of bacteria.

should be swabbed with a sterile cotton-tipped applicator moistened with sterile water or normal saline. This procedure may succeed in collecting some of the assailant's buccal cells. The cells can be analyzed for DNA and blood group antigen. Blood group antigen is only detectable for a short time. This test should be sent to a crime laboratory as quickly as possible.

Ideally, a forensic odontologist will be available to evaluate a bite mark if an accurate identification is to be made from the injury. Only a forensic odontologist should render an opinion that includes or excludes a suspect.

## Dating Contusions

The emergency physician may be asked to render an opinion regarding the age of a contusion. This topic has received much debate in the forensic community. A number of variables

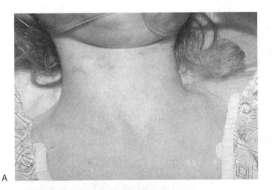

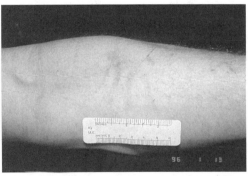

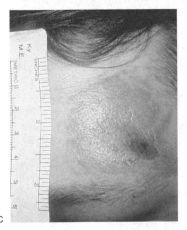

**FIG. 4-27. A:** Ligature abrasions are associated with hanging and strangulation. This patient sustained a ligature mark from a near-fatal strangulation at the hands of her husband. **B:** Fingernail abrasions are generally linear and parallel. These abrasions are frequently seen in domestic and sexual assaults. Tissue and hair can be found under the fingernails of the assailant. **C:** An imprint of carpet weave was transferred to the patient's forehead when her head was slammed to the floor by her boyfriend. This pattern injury is most frequently seen in victims of domestic violence.

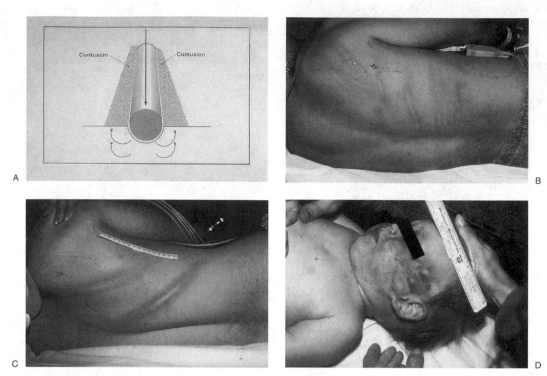

**FIG. 4-28. A:** Impact with a rounded-liner object will displace the blood directly beneath the blow laterally. This will result in a characteristic contusion that has an area of central clearing bounded by parallel linear contusions. **B:** Multiple pattern contusions with central clearing with surrounding linear contusions. These injuries resulted from repeated blows from a police baton. This pattern is associated with forceful blows and should be well-documented by the treating physician. **C:** These pattern contusions resulted from two forceful blows from a pool cue. The area of central clearing was subjected to the most pounds per square inch during the blow. **D:** A blow from an open hand imparted this pattern contusion on the cheek of a 1-year-old. The areas of central clearing surrounded by linear contusions mirror the extended fingers of the hand.

come into play where contusion development is concerned. The amount of blunt force applied to the skin, the vascularity of the tissue, the fragility of the blood vessels, the tissue density, and the amount of blood that escapes into the surrounding tissue. All affect contusion formation and configuration (35, 36). As a result, no reproducible standard for the dating of a contusion is possible based on its color or size. There are ongoing scientific studies evaluating contusions from the standpoint of hemoglobin degradation. But for now, emergency physicians should not attempt to date a contusion on the basis of physical examination alone.

## FORENSIC ASSESSMENT OF SHARP FORCE TRAUMA

There are two types of sharp force injuries: incised and stabbed. The incised wound is one generated by a drawing motion and is therefore longer than it is deep. The stab wound is a puncture-type wound and is, as a result, deeper than it is wide. The wound margins of sharp force injuries are clean and lack the abraded edges of injuries generated by blunt force trauma.

Information of a forensic nature can be gleaned from the examination of a stab wound. Certain characteristics of a knife's blade, whether single- or double-edged, can be determined from

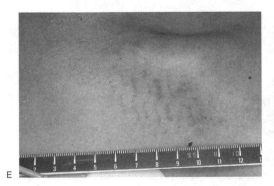

E

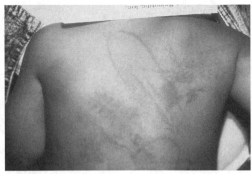

F

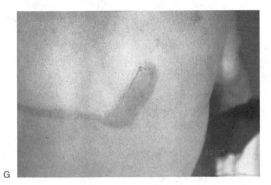

G

**FIG. 4-28.** *(Continued.)* **E:** The imprint from the sole of a tennis shoe was imparted to the skin overlying the clavicle during an assault. This pattern contusion was matched to the sole of the accused suspect's tennis shoe. **F:** Blows from a single belt can inflict different pattern contusions depending on the configuration of the belt when it strikes the skin. A looped linear pattern occurs when the belt hits on edge. When the broad surface of the belt impacts the skin, a mirror image of the belt's weave is imprinted. **G:** A pattern contusion was imprinted on this patient's back from a blow with a golf putter. Impact from a flat object does not permit the lateral displacement of the blood beneath the blow as is seen with blows from a rounded-linear object. This male victim of domestic violence sought treatment when he developed shortness of breath from underlying rib fractures.

visual inspection (Figs. 4-32A, B). Additional characteristics, such as whether the knife was serrated or sharp, can be determined if the blade was drawn across the skin during its insertion or withdrawal (Fig. 4-33). Serrated blades do not always leave these characteristic marks. In cases where the knife has been inserted to the proximal portion of the blade, a contusion may result from contact with the hilt (Fig. 4-34). When the emergency department physician encounters more than one missed wound on a patient, self-inflicted injuries must be suspected (Fig. 4-35A–C).

## SUMMARY AND CONCLUSION

It is a brave new world. The practice of medicine must evolve to meet the needs and accommodate the reality of our society. Perhaps more so in emergency medicine than in any other specialty, physicians are confronted by the fallout from a society stressed by rapid change, easy access to inexpensive weapons, and the soul-numbing bombardment of images of violence.

As before, and always, our highest calling is saving lives. It is the nature of the wounds from which we are saving patients that is changing. The medical management isn't so very different, and yet new skills are required of us. Emergency physicians today must have a working knowledge of wound mechanics and pattern injuries. We must know how weapons wound and watch with an ever-vigilant eye for injuries indicative of abuse and battery. Forensics belongs in the emergency room now out of necessity and out of an ethical obligation to fulfill a critical role in safeguarding patients.

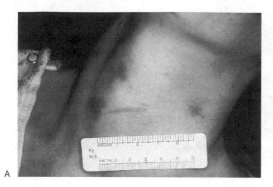

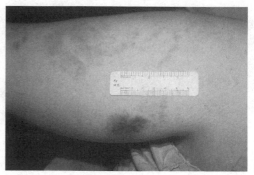

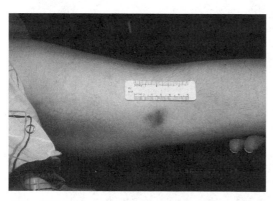

FIG. 4-29. A: Fingertip and web space contusions are present over the anterior neck of this victim of domestic violence. Fingertip contusions are generally rounded and measure 1.0–1.5 cm in diameter. Web space contusions are associated with strangulation and are imparted when the skin between the thumb and forefinger are forcibly applied to the neck. B: "Grab marks" are associated with fingertip pressure. Examination of the inner surface of the patient's upper arm revealed the two types of grab marks. A fingertip contusion from a thumb is located on the lower aspect of the arm. The outline of a finger (central clearing surrounded by a horseshoe-shaped petechial hemorrhage) is located above the superior aspect of the arm. C: Horseshoe-shaped petechial hemorrhage with central clearing is associated with pressure applied by the pad of the finger. This victim of sexual assault displayed two horseshoe-shaped contusions with petechial hemorrhage with central clearing on the lateral aspect of her neck.

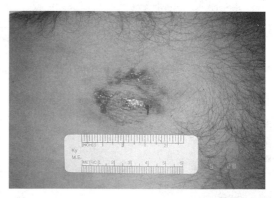

FIG. 4-30. Fingertip contusions may be subtle but are always associated with a significant amount of pressure applied to the epithelium. Close examination of the inner aspects of the upper arms and thighs of suspected domestic violence and sexual assault victims may reveal their presence.

FIG. 4-31. A human bite can provide a multitude of valuable forensic evidence. Swabbing of the bite with a sterile swab can provide DNA from deposited buccal cells and saliva for ABO blood typing. Bites from unknown assailants should be swabbed for evidence before medical care is initiated. The tooth pattern imparted to the skin can also be used to identify or exclude suspects.

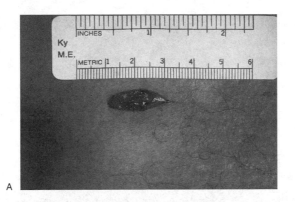

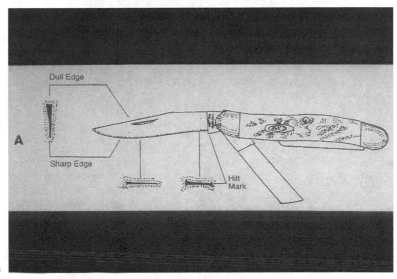

**FIG. 4-32. A:** A stab wound from a single-edged knife blade. In this picture, the dull portion of the blade is associated with the right wound margin of the wound and the sharp edge of the blade with the left wound margin. **B:** Diagram of a stab wound and the associated single-edged knife blade.

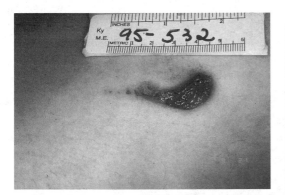

**FIG. 4-33.** A single-edged stab wound from a serrated knife blade. Abrasions from the blade's serrated edge are visible at the left margin of the wound. These abrasions can result from either the insertion or withdrawal of the knife blade.

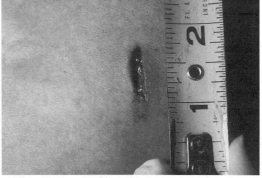

**FIG. 4-34.** A single-edged stab wound with a small "hilt mark" at the superior wound margin. The hilt mark occurs when the hilt of the blade (see Fig. 4-32B) forcefully contacts the skin.

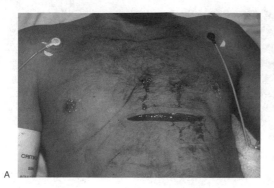

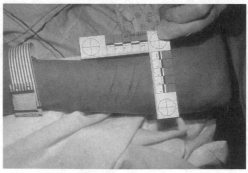

A

B

C

**FIG. 4-35. A:** This patient sustained 39 superficial incised wounds to his anterior thorax, reportedly inflicted by his wife. Upon pointed questioning, the patient admitted that the wounds were self-inflicted. Self-infliction behavior must be ruled out in any patient with more than one incised wound. **B:** Self-inflicted incised wounds to the wrist in a suicidal patient. The physician must reserve the use of the term "laceration" for wounds associated with blunt force trauma. **C:** A patient with four superficial incised abdominal wounds reported to police that he was assaulted with a box cutter during a robbery. Review of his medical record indicated a similar incident, with the same weapon, 3 years earlier. After pointed questioning, the patient admitted that the wounds from both "robberies" were self-inflicted. The patient was referred for psychiatric evaluation. Any patient with more than one incised wound must be evaluated for self-destructive behavior.

## ACKNOWLEDGMENT

I wish to thank Mr. Scott Doyle of the Kentucky State Police Crime Laboratory for his assistance and photographs.

## REFERENCES

1. Smialek JE. Forensic medicine in the emergency department. *Emerg Med Clin North Am* 1983;1(3):1685.
2. Carmona R, Prince K. Trauma and forensic medicine. *J Trauma* 1989;29(9):1222.
3. Smock WS, Nichols GR, Fuller PM. Development and implementation of the first clinical forensic medicine training program. *J Forensic Sci* 1993;38(4):835.
4. Smock WS. Development of a clinical forensic medicine curriculum for emergency physicians in the USA. *J Clin Forensic Med* 1994;1(1):27.
5. Smock WS, Ross CS, Hamilton FN. Clinical forensic medicine: how ED physicians can help with the sleuthing. *Emerg Legal Briefings* 1994;5(1):1.
6. Eckert WG, Bell JS, Stein RJ, et al. Clinical forensic medicine. *Am J Forensic Med Pathol* 1986;7(3): 182.
7. Mittleman RE, Goldberg HS, Waksman DM. Preserving evidence in the emergency department. *Am J Nurs* 1983;83:1652.
8. Godley DR, Smith TK. Some medicolegal aspects of gunshot wounds. *J Trauma* 1977;17(11):866.
9. Ryan MT. Clinical forensic medicine. *Ann Emerg Med* 2000;36(3):271.
10. Goldsmith MF. US forensic pathologists on a new case: examination of living patients. *JAMA* 1986;256(13): 1685.
11. Eckert W. Forensic sciences: the clinical or living aspects. *Inform* 1983;16:3.
12. Busuttil A, Smock WS. Training in clinical forensic medicine in Kentucky. *Police Surgeon* 1990;14:26.
13. Collins KA, Lantz PE. Interpretation of fatal, multiple, and exiting gunshot wounds by trauma specialists. *J Forensic Sci* 1994;39(1):94.
14. McLeer SV, Anwar RA, Herman S, Maquiling K. Education is not enough: a systems failure in protecting battered women. *Ann Emerg Med* 1989;18:651.

15. Breo DL. JFK's death: the plain truth from the MD's who did the autopsy. *JAMA* 1992;267(20):2794.
16. Randall T. Clinicians' forensic interpretations of fatal gunshot wounds often miss the mark. *JAMA* 1993;69 (16):2058.
17. Fackler ML, Riddick L. Clinicians' inadequate descriptions of gunshot wounds obstruct justice: clinical journals refuse to expose the problem. In: McCormick-Armstrong, ed. *Proceedings of the American Academy of Forensic Sciences,* vol. 2. Colorado Springs, 1996: 150.
18. DiMaio VJM, Spitz WU. Variations in wounding due to unusual firearms and recently available ammunition. *J Forensic Sci* 1972;17:377.
19. Fackler ML. Wound ballistics: a review of common misconceptions. *JAMA* 1988;259(18):2730.
20. Fatteh A. *Medicolegal investigation of gunshot wounds.* Philadelphia: JB Lippincott, 1976;88–89.
21. DiMaio VJM. *Gunshot wounds,* 2nd ed. Boca Raton: CRC Press, 1999:74–75, 86, 92.
22. Spitz WU. *Medicolegal investigation of death,* 3rd ed. Springfield, IL: Charles C Thomas, 1976:324, 345, 348.
23. Dixon DS. Characteristics of shored exit wounds. *J Forensic Sci* 1981;26(4):691.
24. Adelson L. A microscopic study of dermal gunshot wounds. *Am J Clin Pathol* 1961;35(5):393.
25. Dixon DS. Gunshot wounds: forensic implications in a surgical practice. In: Ordog GH, ed. *Management of gunshot wounds.* New York: Elsevier, 1988:168.
26. Andrasko K, Maehly AC. Detection of gunshot residues on hands by scanning electron microscopy. *J Forensic Sci* 1977;22(2):279.
27. Matricardi VR, Kilty JW. Detection of gunshot particles from the hands of a shooter by SEM. *J Forensic Sci* 1977;22(4):725.
28. Wolten GM, Nesbitt RS, Calloway AR, et al. Particle analysis for the detection of gunshot residue. I: Scanning electron microscopy/energy dispersive x-ray characterization of hand deposits from firing. *J Forensic Sci* 1979;24(4):409.
29. Wolten GM, Nesbitt RS, Calloway AR, et al. Particle analysis for the detection of gunshot residue. II: Occupational and environmental particles. *J Forensic Sci* 1979;24(2):423.
30. Wolten GM, Nesbitt RS, Calloway AR, et al. Particle analysis for the detection of gunshot residue. III: The case record. *J Forensic Sci* 1979;24(4):864.
31. Tillman J. Automated gunshot residue particle search and characterization. *J Forensic Sci* 1987;32(1):62.
32. Kee TG, Beck C. Casework assessment of an automated scanning electron microscope/microanalysis system for the detection of firearms discharge particles. *J Forensic Sci Soc* 1987;27(5):321.
33. Zeichner A, Levin N. Casework experience of GSR detection in Israel, on samples from hands, hair, and clothing using an autosearch SEM/EDX system. *J Forensic Sci* 1995;40(6):1082.
34. Gialamas DM, et al. Officers, their weapons and their hands: an empirical study of GSR on the hands of non-shooting police officers. *J Forensic Sci* 1995;40(6):1086.
35. Adelson L. *The pathology of homicide.* Springfield, IL: Charles C Thomas, 1974:384–385.
36. Wilson EF. Estimation of the age of cutaneous contusions in child abuse. *Pediatrics* 1977;60(5):750.

# 5

# Forensic Examination of Victims and Perpetrators of Sexual Assault

Georgina A. Groleau and M. Christine Jackson

Although the nation's crime rate is declining—a 7% decrease was reported in 1997 (1)—the rates of rape and sexual assault remain steady. According to the 1997 *Uniform Crime Report,* approximately 350,000 women are reported raped each year in the United States (2). The 1998 National Institute of Justice and Centers for Disease Control survey on the national violence against women documented that an estimated 302,100 women and 92,700 men are forcibly raped each year in the United States (3).

These statistics underestimate the number of sexual assault victims per year. In 1996, the National Crime Victimization Survey revealed that more than two thirds of rape/sexual assaults committed in the nation remain unreported (4). Women are not convinced that reporting the sexual assault will lead to conviction of the perpetrator. In fact, many women believe that their trauma after a sexual assault will be exacerbated if they take legal action. The 1993 Senate Judiciary Report Response to Rape stated that 84% of reported rapes do not result in conviction. Of the 16% of perpetrators convicted, half will be sentenced to less than 1 year in prison and 4% are not incarcerated at all (5). The sense of not being able to obtain justice from the legal system is one of many consequences of rape for women. Others include rape-related posttraumatic stress syndrome, depression, eating disorders, substance abuse, and suicide (6–9). The tangible, out-of-pocket cost of sexual assault (excluding child sexual abuse) is estimated at $3.3 billion per year (10). For each rapist who is not convicted there are usually subsequent victims because rapists tend to be repeat offenders (11). A rapist who has been caught has, on average, 14 previous victims (12). Appropriate conviction and incarceration of a rapist is justice served for the current victim and all prior victims; in addition, the rapist's future victims are spared.

When evaluating a victim of sexual abuse, the emergency physician must meet strict medical and legal standards. A preestablished systematic approach enables the busy emergency physician to complete an adult sexual assault examination adequately. Proper collection of evidence provides medical care for the victim as well as hope for legal recourse against the perpetrator.

## SEXUAL ASSAULT AND LEGAL ISSUES

Physicians who perform sexual assault evidentiary examinations must be familiar with the related legal aspects. They must know the definition of rape and sexual assault as well as the legal time limits on patient presentation after the assault for conducting the evidentiary examination. The rights of the victim must be understood and ensured prior to obtaining consent for and proceeding with an evidentiary examination. To ensure the legal validity of evidence, a chain of custody must be maintained. Failure to maintain this chain means that the forensic evidence collected can be thrown out of court. Since many cases rotate around the forensic evidence, maintaining chain of custody can make or break a case.

## DEFINITION OF RAPE

*Rape* is an act of forced vulvar penetration by a penis, object, or body part without the consent of a woman, during which ejaculation may or may not occur (13). The term *sexual assault* used in some states broadens the coverage of unwanted sexual acts to include rape, sexual abuse, and sexual misconduct involving either gender. Sexual assault also includes any sexual contact of one person with another without appropriate legal consent. The examiner needs to be familiar with the local jurisdiction's definitions of rape and nonconsensual sexual acts (see Appendix).

## TIME LIMITS

The usual legal time limit for collection of evidence is 72 hours from the time of the assault. Victims of sexual assault presenting within 72 hours should be assigned priority in triage along with other serious emergencies, as the evidentiary examination must be conducted without delay to minimize loss or deterioration of evidence. If more than 72 hours has passed since the assault, a complete physical examination still should be conducted to examine for injuries to the body and the genitalia. Depending on the sexual assault protocol of the local authorities, a modified evidential examination may be indicated. Based on spermatozoa survival data, there may be value in collecting cervical samples even when the patient presents more than 72 hours after the assault (14:108).

## CONSENT

To protect the rights and interests of both the patient and the hospital, an appropriate signed written consent must be obtained before beginning the examination, treatment, and evidence collection. The consent form for the evidentiary examination is in the standard sexual assault kit. Consent means that the patient understands that the evidence will be collected, preserved, and released to law enforcement authorities. Consent for the evidentiary examination also includes consent for obtaining photographs of physical trauma to be used as evidence in a court of law (some jurisdictions have a separate consent form for photographs). Signed written consent for the sexual assault evidentiary examination does not replace general consent for routine diagnostic and medical procedures that is standard with emergency treatment and in accordance with hospital policy.

If the patient consents to examination, treatment, and evidence collection, the local law enforcement agency needs to be notified. The agency will render a complaint number and send an investigative officer to the hospital to file a report. Even if the patient does not want to make a police report or have an evidentiary examination, the local enforcement agency needs to be notified to implement local procedures. Rape of minors and certain adults who are mentally challenged or disabled requires mandatory reporting; however, laws regarding mandatory reporting of adult victims vary from state to state.

When obtaining written, signed consent for a sexual assault examination and evidence collection, the physician must inform the patient of his or her rights. The patient has a right to refuse an examination that entails evidence collection, even if presenting within 72 hours of the assault. The patient needs to be made aware that evidence deteriorates over time and may be unobtainable if it is not collected and preserved promptly. The physician must explain that body fluids and swabs collected may lead to the identification of the offender, especially in light of DNA "fingerprinting" techniques. The patient must also be informed that consent for the evidence collection examination, once given, can be withdrawn at any time for all or part of the examination. The patient has the right to refuse the collection of reference specimens, such as hair strands and blood for profiling and alcohol determination. The patient must also be told that if he or she refuses the collection of reference samples at the time of the examination or at a later date, the crime laboratory cannot conduct a comparative analysis of the evidence in question.

Patients have the right to know if they are responsible for the cost of the examination. If an evidentiary examination is performed, the local government is responsible for the cost of the examination; otherwise, the cost of the examination and treatment is the patient's responsibility. (One exception to this is the State of Iowa, which covers the cost even if a report is not made.) Testing and treating for sexually transmitted diseases (STDs) and pregnancy will also be provided without charge. As appropriate, referral information for anonymous or confidential free HIV counseling and testing should be given to the victim if she or he chooses to not have the baseline HIV testing done at the time of the initial examination.

To maintain the chain of custody, there needs to be careful and proper handling and transfer of the collected evidence with documentation to verify who collected the evidence, who picked up and transported the evidence, and that the evidence was always guarded appropriately. This assists the courts by ensuring that no alteration of the evidence or loss of evidence occurred prior to trial. All transfers of custody of evidence documentation must include the following information: the name of the person transferring custody, the name of the person receiving custody, and the date and time of transfer. Transfers should be kept to a minimum, ideally limited to two persons. The collected evidence is turned over to law enforcement officers by the examiner after the examination has been completed and the reference samples, swabs, and the slides have been dried completely. If it is not possible to turn over the forensic evidence to law enforcement officers after collection, the evidence needs to be stored in a locked area accessible only to designated individuals. Any time evidence exchanges hands, that exchange must be documented. A recent retrospective study of sexual assault evaluations performed by emergency physicians or ob-gyn residents in an urban emergency department revealed that the chain of custody was documented properly in only 6% of cases (15).

## ADULT FEMALE SEXUAL ASSAULT VICTIM

### Patient Intake

When a woman who has been sexually assaulted comes to an emergency department within 72 hours of the assault, she should be triaged quickly, including assessment of stability, and then escorted rapidly to a private area for the interview and examination (Fig. 5-1). The examination should be conducted without delay to minimize the loss or deterioration of evidence. A trained support person should be assigned to each victim. If the patient is taken directly to an examining room and asked to put on a hospital gown, then clothing must be collected properly at that time. The police need to be notified upon the victim's arrival and a legal complaint number for the victim's case must be obtained from the law enforcement agency.

The process of the examination must be explained to the victim, which is best done by the examiner. After the victim has been informed of her rights and agrees to the examination, written consent for the exam needs to be obtained before proceeding. The examiner then obtains the history in a warm, professional manner, realizing the emotional challenge the victim faces when recounting the details of the assault.

### Victim Interview

All recorded information is admissible in court. The physician should document the following information:

- The name, age, and race of the victim
- The date, time, location and/or physical surroundings of the assault
- The patient's personal hygiene since the assault.
- The name(s), number, and race(s) of the perpetrator(s), if known
- The use of weapons, physical force, restraints, injuries, forced drug use, and verbal and/or nonverbal threats
- The threats, types of force, or other methods used by the perpetrators(s) and the area(s) of the body affected
- The sexual acts committed by the perpetrator(s)
- Details regarding attempt to penetrate or actual penetration of the vagina or rectum by penis, finger, or other object
- The occurrence of fellatio and any resultant injuries
- The frequency and the sequence of the sexual acts

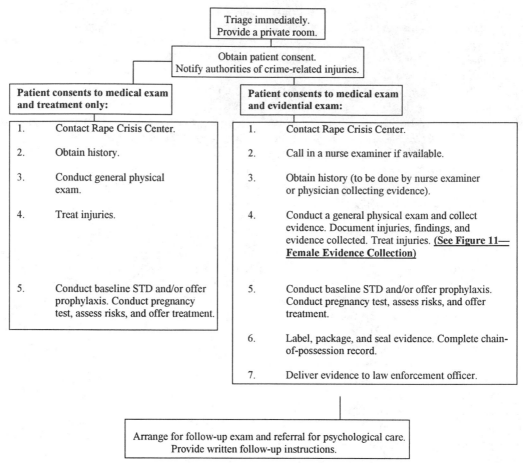

**FIG. 5-1.** Female sexual assault examination.

- The positions used during the sexual assaults
- Whether the assailant ejaculated and the location
- Which perpetrator committed which act, if there was more than one assailant
- Whether kissing, biting, or licking occurred and the site(s) involved

A careful history must be taken, as some victims may be reluctant to describe all the acts committed, particularly anal penetration (Fig. 5-2). The patient should be asked if she remembers injuring the assailant during the assault (e.g., by scratching or biting).

Any physical injuries, sites of bleeding, and/or pain described by the victim must be recorded as well as the area(s) of the body affected. Injuries occurring prior to and independent of the assault should be identified (e.g., fractured arm, lacerations, or bruising), with clarification of all findings. If the assault occurred within 72 hours of the examination, the victim's personal hygiene activities since the assault should be noted because this information affects the laboratory analysis of evidence. The physician should ask the patient if she has bathed, douched, urinated, or defecated since the assault. Information regarding the date of the patient's last menstrual period should be obtained to determine whether she is menstruating at the time of the examination, to evaluate the possibility of pregnancy, and to consider postcoital options. If the patient had consenting intercourse within the

**Victim Information**

General appearance_____

Demeanor_____

Last menstrual period_____

Recent surgeries, trauma, diagnostic procedures, or medical treatments (in the past 60

days)_____

Last consensual intercourse_____

**Assault Information**

Date of assault_____

Time of assault_____

Location of assault_____

**Victim's Personal Hygiene**

| | | |
|---|---|---|
| Bathed since assault | yes | no |
| Douched since assault | yes | no |
| Urinated since assault | yes | no |
| Defecated since assault | yes | no |
| Changed clothing since assault | yes | no |

**Perpetrator(s)**

Name of perpetrator(s)_____

Number of perpetrators_____

Race of perpetrator(s)_____

**Use of Force**

| | | |
|---|---|---|
| Use of weapon | yes | no |
| If yes, what?_____ | | |
| Physical force | yes | no |
| If yes, what?_____ | | |
| Restraints | yes | no |
| If yes, what?_____ | | |
| If yes, where?_____ | | |
| Verbal threats | yes | no |
| If yes, explain_____ | | |
| Non-verbal threats | yes | no |
| If yes, explain_____ | | |
| Other types of force used? | yes | no |
| If yes, explain_____ | | |

Wounds inflicted on assailant?                    yes              no

If yes, where?_____

**FIG. 5-2.** History checklist. *(Continued on next page.)*

past 72 hours, the approximate date and time should be recorded. This information is required by the crime lab because it can affect analysis of evidence.

Other information, such as use of medications, allergies, and general medical history, should be documented on the standard emergency department chart. The patient should be asked about drug or alcohol use within the previous 72 hours. Positive toxicologic test results for alcohol or drugs are not uncommon (16), and the examiner should not allow the results to place the victim's history in question. Information about anal-genital injuries sustained during the past 60 days as well

**Alcohol/Drug Use**

| | | | |
|---|---|---|---|
| Alcohol use | yes | no | |
|     If yes, amount?_____ | | | |
|     If yes: | forced use | consensual use | both |
| Drug use | yes | no | |
|     If yes, what?_____Route?_____ | | | |
|     If yes: | forced use | consensual use | both |

**Sexual Acts**

| | | | | |
|---|---|---|---|---|
| Oral penetration | yes | no | attempted | unknown |
| Vaginal penetration | | | | |
|     Penis | yes | no | attempted | unknown |
|     Finger | yes | no | attempted | unknown |
|     Foreign object | yes | no | attempted | unknown |
| Rectal penetration | | | | |
|     Penis | yes | no | attempted | unknown |
|     Finger | yes | no | attempted | unknown |
|     Foreign object | yes | no | attempted | unknown |

Frequency and sequence of the above acts/positions_____

_____

| | | | |
|---|---|---|---|
| Ejaculated | yes | no | unknown |
|     If yes, where?_____ | | | |
| Difficulty maintaining an erection? | yes | no | |
| Kissing/licking | yes | no | unknown |
|     If yes, where?_____ | | | |
| Biting | yes | no | unknown |
|     If yes, where?_____ | | | |

Use diagrams to document foreign material, excretions, trauma, physical injuries, and Wood's lamp findings.

**Evidence/Injuries**

| | | |
|---|---|---|
| Clothes torn | yes | no |
|     If yes, where?_____ | | |
| Clothes stained | yes | no |
|     If yes, where?_____ | | |
| Physical injuries | yes | no |
|     If yes, where?_____ | | |
| Fractures | yes | no |
|     If yes, where?_____ | | |
| Lacerations | yes | no |
|     If yes, where?_____ | | |

**FIG. 5-2.** *Continued.*

as surgeries, diagnostic procedures, or medical treatment performed within that period should be documented to prevent confusion of resultant lesions with injuries related to the sexual assault.

**Physical Examination**

The patterns of injury found with sexual assault result from the restraining methods of the perpetrator, the violent acts of the perpetrator, and the

Cuts      yes      no
     If yes, where?_____
Abrasions/ecchymosis      yes      no
     If yes, where?_____
Bite mark(s)      yes      no
     If yes, where?_____
     Size_____Shape_____
Foreign bodies found?      yes      no
     If yes, where?_____
     If yes, type?_____

**FIG. 5-2.** *Continued.*

resisting efforts of the victim. Despite evidence that sexual assault does not result in visibly detectable physical or genital injury in all cases, the criminal system still relies heavily on physical evidence of trauma to convict a perpetrator. The examiner needs to be knowledgeable of forensic medicine pertaining to sexual assault in order to detect physical injury, document trauma, and collect evidence appropriately, all of which are associated with a successful legal outcome (17,18).

On arrival, the sexual assault victim needs to be assessed for unstable vital signs. The clinician should determine if there has been a change in mental status or if there is a history of loss of consciousness. The patient should be examined to rule out any serious internal injuries (including tears of the rectouterine pouch). Complaints of moderate to severe pain should alert the examiner to possible serious injuries. A review of fatal sexual assaults revealed that the most common causes of death were mechanical asphyxiation, beating, lacerations, drowning, and gunshot wounds (19). Fatal injuries are sustained by 0.1% of women who are sexually assaulted (20). Five to ten percent of survivors of sexual assault sustain major nongenital injuries (20,21). Genital injuries requiring surgical intervention occur in approximately 1% of victims (21).

Once the trauma survey has been completed and the patient medically cleared, then the careful search for patterns of injury and evidence collection is initiated. Physical examination of the sexual assault victim focuses on the detection of physical (nongenital) injuries and genital injuries.

In addition to the standard trauma survey, the physician also needs to search carefully for evidence of physical injuries inflicted by the perpetrator during the assault. Studies conducted during the past two decades have found that 31% to 82% of sexual assault victims sustain physical injuries (16,17,22–28). The physical injuries most often involve the head, face, neck, and extremities (16,22,27). Although the incidence of injuries is significant for all ages and types of victims, women younger than 50 and nonpregnant women are more likely to be injured during sexual assault (16,27). The risk of sustaining physical injuries also increases if the assailant was a stranger (29,30). The lack of evident physical or genital trauma does not imply consent by the victim or the absence of rape (24).

Slapping, kicking, beating, and biting are methods the perpetrator employs to overcome the resistance of the victim. The entire body must be examined for areas of tenderness, soft-tissue swelling, abrasions, contusions, bruises, petechiae, bite marks, lacerations, fractures, and other evidence of violence. Areas of tenderness without bruising should be documented carefully. Bruises may develop 1 to 2 days later.

The back of the head is often banged against the ground during a sexual assault; therefore, soft-tissue swelling and lacerations may be evident. Another cause of scalp hematoma or soft-tissue swelling is violent pulling of the hair (31). If raccoon eyes or Battle's sign is present on examination, then the patient may have sustained a basilar skull fracture. If the patient lost consciousness at the scene, her Glasgow Coma Scale score should be determined.

Further evaluation for intracerebral trauma may be indicated. With blunt trauma to the head and face, associated injury to the cervical spine needs to be considered. Victims of sexual assault often sustain facial injuries, including mandibular fractures, nasal fractures, other facial fractures, broken or loose teeth, facial lacerations, and ocular trauma. The breasts should be examined for evidence of trauma, including contusions, lacerations, and bite marks. If the assailant pulls and twists the victim's clothing, then petechial hemorrhages or a line of punctate bruising may occur on the skin, commonly in the area of the bra strap or near the axilla (31).

The trunk and extremities need to be examined for evidence of trauma. The extremities should be inspected for evidence of the perpetrator overcoming the resistance of the victim. Fingernail abrasions or fingertip bruises on the wrists, ankles, and inner aspects of the arms and thighs are sustained when the perpetrator's hands restrain the victim. If the perpetrator forcibly twisted the wrists of the victim, erythema in that area may be noted (31). If the assailant overwhelms the victim and holds her in restraint, then bruises and abrasions may be seen over bony prominences.

Using the history as a guide, carefully examine the victim for evidence of bite marks. A typical human bite mark is a round or oval ring-shaped lesion with two opposing, often symmetrical U shapes with open spaces at the bottom. The intensity of force behind the bite will affect the pattern depth and characteristics (i.e., the pattern may have abrasions, contusions, or lacerations in the area of the teeth) (32) (Figs. 5-3 and 5-4, see Colorplate following page 144). The classic bite mark shape is not always present, so if a bite mark is suspected, then forensic evaluation of the lesion is indicated. In documenting the bite mark, the site, size, shape, color, and type of injury are included (e.g., contusion with ecchymosis, abrasion, laceration, incision, avulsion, petechial lesion). Findings such as smooth skin or indentation of the skin by the teeth should be noted. If the patient gives a history of being bitten in a certain area but tenderness is the only physical sign noted, the clinician must remember that bruising may develop later.

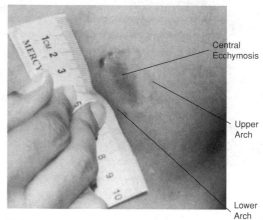

**FIG. 5-3.** Bite mark on the breast.

Different patterns of trauma are associated with an assailant's efforts to stop the victim from screaming. The methods include clamping the hand over the mouth, use of adhesive materials over the mouth, gagging, and strangulation. The mouth and lips must be inspected for evidence of trauma or residual adhesive material. Marks of brute force or strangulation should be sought. The presence of ligature marks, bruises, abrasions, or scratches on the neck should be noted. Gagging and strangulation both lead to asphyxia and may result in physical evidence, such as scattered petechial hemorrhages over the face and the eyelids. Subconjunctival hemorrhages and retinal hemorrhages may also result from attempted strangulation (31,33).

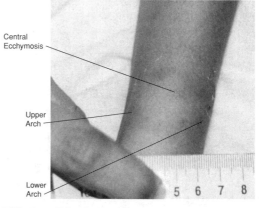

**FIG. 5-4.** Bite mark on the wrist.

The perpetrator may have used ligatures or tape (e.g., duct tape) to restrain the victim. The physical signs of restraint, usually on the ankles and/or wrists, vary and depend on the tightness and the length of time for which the victim was restrained. The patterned abrasion or bruise at the site of the restraint may differ, from tenderness only to slight erythema of the skin to a deeper skin lesion with distal edema (31).

Many assailants use threatening behavior with guns, knives, or other weapons to overcome the resistance of the victim. Research has shown that regardless of the victim's resistance efforts, the assailant's use of a weapon and/or force usually overcomes the victim (34). Cartwright et al. retrospectively reviewed 440 cases of sexual assault survivors to determine the factors that correlated with injury. The risk of physical injury was greatest if the assailant's weapon was a knife or club (79%) rather than a gun (34%). If no weapon was employed, the incidence of physical injury fell between that associated with use of a knife/club and a gun (29). The patient may or may not sustain an injury from the weapon itself. The weapon may be used as a threat and the physical trauma inflicted in a different manner. The patient's history will usually guide the physician toward detection of such injuries.

In certain circumstances, the victim may attempt to resist the assailant's attack and sustain injuries related to that effort. These injuries are typical for "fight" injuries. The victim may have contusions of the forearms or the legs, caused by self-defense movements. The hands, especially the knuckles, may reflect self-defense actions. There may be longitudinal abrasions on the trunk or limbs if the victim was dragged over a rough surface. The skin may have embedded dirt particles. The victim's fingernails may be broken if she scratched the assailant or defended herself during the attack. Her clothing may have been torn during attempts to resist the assault (31).

The amount of resistance offered by the victim is affected by many variables, one of which is the fear instilled by the assailant's verbal threats and/or threats with weapons. A victim held at gunpoint is less likely to resist the assailant's assault and therefore may lack injuries associated with such efforts. Although there is some consensus that resistance increases the chance of aborting rape, it is inconclusive if the victim's physical resistance alters her risk of being physically injured (20,34). Ulman et al. reviewed the cases of 274 women who were raped or avoided rape to identify factors associated with physical injury. The risk of physical injury correlated with the assailant's physical aggression and did not correlate with more forceful resistance by the victim (35).

The violent sexual acts of the assailant (e.g., forced vaginal intercourse, fellatio, sodomy) may or may not cause physical or anogenital injuries. A negative examination does not imply that sexual assault did not occur (24). However, because positive findings on examination are legally important in the prosecution of the perpetrator, the emergency medicine physician needs to do a careful examination and document all findings.

If during the interview the patient reveals that fellatio occurred as part of the sexual assault, her mouth and perioral area should be examined for evidence of trauma. The lips should be inspected for contusions, lacerations, and moist or dried collections of seminal fluid. Any evidence in the oral cavity of ecchymosis and/or petechiae, which are most commonly seen in the posterior pharynx or on the soft palate, should be noted. Erythema or hemorrhagic findings on the palate may be a result of the negative pressure associated with fellatio, direct trauma, and, in a few cases, candidiasis. Fellatio may also tear the frenulum under the tongue, cause other lacerations, and loosen teeth. However, in most cases there is a paucity of physical findings detected after forced fellatio, as usually fellatio does not produce clinical lesions or trauma (36).

The patient presenting after forced vaginal penetration needs a careful physical examination of the introitus and the vagina. This exam should be conducted even when the patient denies vaginal complaints after an assault. The external genitalia should be inspected for any evidence of foreign materials and collections of dried and/or moist secretions. Dried secretions may appear as areas of matted pubic hair. The external genitalia, fossa navicularis, posterior fourchette, and vestibule should be examined for

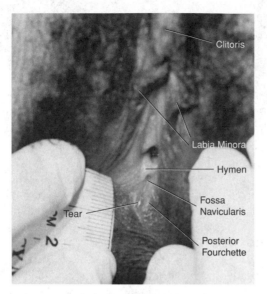

FIG. 5-5. Tear to posterior fourchette. Female Tanner 4 sexual assault patient.

evidence of trauma (Fig. 5-5, see Colorplate following page 144). A speculum examination of the vagina needs to be performed to observe for internal trauma. Vaginal pool secretions should be collected for the detection of spermatozoa, acid phosphatases, p30 (an antigen derived from the prostate epithelial cells and found in seminal plasma and urine from men, including those who have had a vasectomy) (14:117), and DNA testing. Cervical swabs should be obtained for cultures to detect sexually transmitted diseases. Any bleeding, abrasions, petechiae, ecchymosis, edema, contusions, hematomas, or lacerations sited on the external genitalia or internally should be noted. The most common areas of injury are the posterior fourchette, fossa navicularis, labia, and vagina (23,25,27,37,38).

Currently in the United States, a gross visual pelvic examination is still the standard when female sexual assault victims are evaluated in emergency departments. Studies have been conducted during the past 15 years to determine the incidence of genital trauma in sexual assault victims. Studies employing only a gross visual pelvic examination found the incidence of genital injuries to vary from 6% to 65%, with the majority falling between 10% and 30% (16,17,22–24, 26–28,37,38). Cartwright et al. found that elderly

victims of sexual assault (age 60 to 90 years) had a 52% incidence of genital trauma (28). Ramin et al. documented the incidence of genital trauma after sexual assault in postmenopausal women (women older than 50) using gross visual genital examination. The incidence of genital trauma more than doubled (43%) and was more often serious in postmenopausal victims. The most common sites of injury did not differ among victims younger or older than 50 (27). Satin et al. compared the incidence of trauma after sexual assault in pregnant versus nonpregnant women. Genital injury was more prevalent in nonpregnant victims (21% vs. 5%) (16).

Documentation of trauma sustained during sexual assault has improved with the introduction of toluidine blue dye and colposcopic examination with photography (Figs. 5-6 through 5-8, see Colorplate following page 144). Although these examinations are the preferred method, they are not yet standard for evaluating the sexual assault victim. Rather, they are currently used by centers established strictly to perform medical and forensic evaluations of victims of sexual assault or the suspects of the

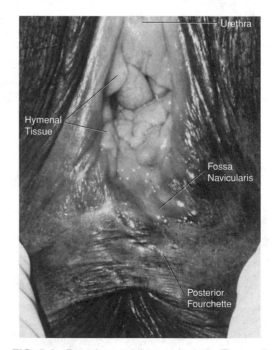

FIG. 5-6. Female sexual assault victim Tanner 5 before toluidine blue dye testing.

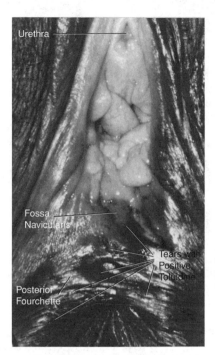

**FIG. 5-7.** Female sexual assault victim Tanner 5 after toluidine blue dye testing.

crime. In these centers, the main examiner is usually a nurse with specific training in the medical and forensic evaluation of the sexual assault victim (11). However, with increased recognition that the physician's role is to examine the sexual assault victim not only medically but also forensically, efforts have been made to incorporate forensic aspects of the sexual assault ex-

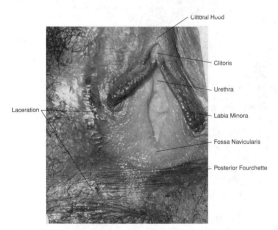

**FIG. 5-8.** Female sexual assault victim Tanner 5 after toluidine blue dye testing.

aminations into continuing medical educational programs and resident training curriculums.

Lauber and Souma introduced the use of a 1% aqueous solution of toluidine blue dye, a nuclear stain, to improve the identification of genital microlacerations during examination of rape victims. They found that microlacerations occurred in 40% of the victims of sexual assault and only 5% of patients with a history of recent consensual sexual intercourse (39). Normal vulvar skin does not contain nuclei and therefore does not bind the dye. The disruption of the normal vulvar skin by the trauma of sexual assault allows the dye to bind to nuclei in the deeper layers of the skin. Standard use of the dye during pelvic examination of a rape victim entails applying 1% aqueous solution of toluidine blue dye to the posterior fourchette area with gauze or by using cotton-tipped applicators (Table 5-1). After a few seconds, the dye is wiped away with lubricating jelly and 4/4 in. gauze squares or cotton balls, and the microlacerations are noted as linear areas of blue dye uptake. Diffuse uptake or no uptake of the toluidine blue dye is considered a negative examination. Because the dye is not absorbed systemically, it has a low-risk profile and thus can be used in pregnant women. The timing of the toluidine blue dye examination depends on the local sexual assault evidentiary examination protocol. In some areas, the protocol calls for the toluidine blue dye examination only after the anogenital examination has been performed and forensic samples have been collected. Other areas call for the dye examination to be performed before the speculum examination to exclude the possibility of trauma during insertion of the speculum.

McCauley et al. compared the incidence of genital microlacerations detected in sexual assault victims with gross visualization alone versus that with the addition of toluidine blue dye

**TABLE 5-1.** *Steps for the application of toluidine dye, 1% aqueous solution*

1. Apply to posterior fourchette or rectal area with a cotton-tipped applicator.
2. Let dry.
3. Remove with lubricating gel and 4 × 4 gauze.
4. Do not apply to mucosal surfaces
(Figs. 5-7 and 5-8, see Colorplate following page 144).

in the same patients. The detection of injuries increased substantially—from 4% to 58%—with toluidine blue dye testing. Their control group of patients had only 10% positive uptake with the toluidine blue dye testing, and the majority of those patients complained of dry and painful intercourse (40). The increased positive uptake of toluidine blue dye on testing in the sexual assault group suggests a lack of consent.

The ability to diagnose vaginal trauma after sexual assault is enhanced significantly by colposcopy. A colposcope is an instrument that allows up to 30 times binocular magnification with excellent lighting and has the capacity to take still photographs or video films without additional lighting or flash. It looks like a large microscope mounted on wheels. The main purpose of the colposcope in sexual assault evaluations is to improve the detection and documentation of injuries of the vaginal introitus, vagina, and cervix. The injuries can then be documented in the text of the chart, on diagrams of the female body, and by photographs of the injuries. The photographs can be reviewed later by medical experts for legal purposes.

Slaughter et al. added colposcopy to the standard sexual assault protocol to improve the detection of injuries sustained during sexual assault. They detected genital injuries with colposcopy in 87% of the victims presenting within 48 hours of assault (41). A subsequent study by Slaughter et al. revealed genital injuries in 68% of victims with the use of colposcopy. Again, the most common sites of injury were the posterior fourchette, fossa navicularis, hymen, and labia minora. Tears were noted most often on the posterior fourchette and the fossa navicularis, abrasions on the labia, and ecchymosis on the hymen (25). Lenahan et al. compared the differences in detection of genital injuries when using the standard gross visual genital examination versus the addition of colposcopy. The detection of injuries increased more than eightfold when colposcopy was added to gross visual examination in the same patients (26).

If the victim's history indicates that anal penetration has occurred, then the physical examination proceeds beyond the standard inspection of the anus and the perianal area to include

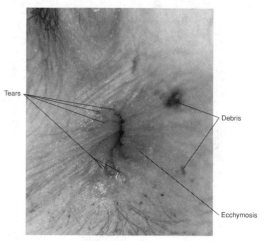

**FIG. 5-9.** Anal trauma in a female with a history of anal penetration.

a careful examination of the rectum (Figs. 5-9 and 5-10, see Colorplate following page 144). Injuries may include abrasions, ecchymoses, edema, contusions, petechiae, lacerations, and fissures. Moist or dried collections of secretions in the perianal area may be seen with gross visualization and with the assistance of a Wood's lamp or the Bluemaxx light. Semen tends to collect at the anal mucocutaneous juncture. The application of toluidine blue dye around the rectal area prior to the anoscopic examination

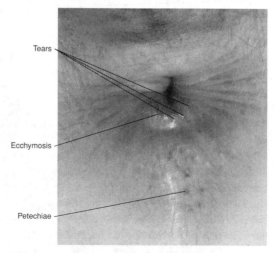

**FIG. 5-10.** Anal trauma in a female with history of anal penetration.

aids in the visualization of injuries. Anoscopy, and in some cases proctoscopy, is indicated when rectal trauma is suspected.

## Patient Support

Sexual assault may cause severe physical and psychological trauma. Victims have a wide range of possible demeanors. They may be calm and show little emotion, or they may be anxious and hysterical. All behaviors should be accepted by the staff as victims' means of coping with a violent experience. Victims should be encouraged to express their emotions, and the staff should acknowledge the traumatic nature of the experience.

The primary examiner and staff must demonstrate behavior that is both empathetic and nonjudgmental to help reduce the victim's acute psychological trauma. A sexual assault evaluation must not only address the medical and legal aspects of the assault but also include treatment for psychological trauma sustained by the victim. The psychological aspects of the assault should be addressed as soon as the victim arrives. Victims should be treated promptly and with respect to helping them regain self-esteem.

The complete sexual assault evaluation and examination is inherently a potentially degrading and humiliating experience for any patient. It is essential that it be carried out in a manner that is both competent and compassionate. Before the start of the examination, the victim should be asked if she would like an advocate to be present during the evidentiary examination. An advocate may be a nurse, a social worker, a person from a crisis intervention team, or a physician. The advocate not only gives emotional support to the victim, but also acts as a liaison with family and friends. Someone should stay with the victim at all times during the evaluation to ensure her sense of safety. The facility and staff should provide privacy for the victim during the entire examination. Only the primary examiner and the advocate should be present for the examination. If an advocate is not available, then one staff nurse should be assigned as the advocate for the entire evidentiary examination.

The primary examiner should introduce herself and explain her role. The patient should be asked how she wants to be addressed. Throughout the evidentiary examination, the clinician should explain the reasons for the questions that must be asked and the evidence collection process. Only questions pertinent to the evidentiary examination should be asked. Questions regarding the patient's reasons or motivations must be avoided. Before posing emotionally sensitive questions, the examiner should establish rapport with the patient. As the physical examination proceeds, the clinician should inform the patient of the findings. The patient can be involved in decisions regarding treatment, follow-up care, and notification of family or friends. She should be told about the benefit of counseling after sexual assault and given appropriate referral information. The staff must show confidence in the victim's ability to recover from such a violent crime.

After arrival at the emergency department, the victim should remain clothed until it is time to conduct the examination. After thorough documentation of the history, a complete evidential examination that meets the minimum standards must be conducted concurrently with the physical examination. The patient's general appearance and demeanor should be documented. Along with the vital signs, the patient's height, weight, and color of eyes and hair should be noted. The patient's clothing should be observed for rips, tears, stains, and other foreign materials, including fibers, hair, twigs, grass, soil, splinters, glass, blood, or seminal fluid. Before the patient's clothing is collected, it should be scanned for fluorescent exudates, and positive areas should be noted in the text. All clothing worn during and immediately after the assault should be collected, and the collection should be documented (Fig. 5-11). If the victim is not wearing the clothing worn at the time of the assault, then only the items that are in direct contact with the victim's genital area need to be collected. The police officer in charge should be informed to arrange for collection of the clothing worn at the time of the assault for forensic analysis at a later time.

The proper method of collecting the clothing is to have the patient stand on two sheets of clean paper on the floor, one sheet on top of the other. The disposable paper placed routinely on examination tables can be used for

All swabs and slides must be air dried before packaging. Code corresponding swabs and slides, e.g., oral
swab #1. oral slide #1
Expansion of #4, Figure 1

| CLINICAL SPECIMENS FOR LAB (TO GO TO HOSPITAL LAB) | | EVIDENCE FOR CRIME LAB (TO BE GIVEN TO LAW ENFORCEMENT) |
|---|---|---|
| | **4a.** Note condition of clothing on arrival. Collect outer and under clothing worn during or immediately after assault. Collect fingernail scrapings if indicated. Do colposcopic examination throughout as needed. **4b.** Conduct general physical exam. Scan entire body with Wood's lamp. Collect dried and moist secretions and foreign materials from body including head,hair, and scalp. Note and bite marks. Document findings. **(Figures 5-3 and 5-4,** see Colorplate following page 144) | **4a1.** Clothing (in separate bags) Fingernail scrapings, foreign material on clothing and body |
| **4c1.** *Neisseria Gonorrhoeae Culture (GC)* | **4c.** Examine oral cavity for injury. Document findings. If indicated by history, swab area around mouth. Collect 4 oral swabs. Take specimen for GC. | **4c2.** Four swabs from oral cavity |
| | **4d.** Examine external genitalia for injury. Scan with Wood's lamp. Collect dry and moist secretions and foreign materials. Document findings. Cut matted pubic hair. Comb pubic hair to collect foreign materials. **(Figure 5-5,** see Colorplate following page 144) | **4d2.** Any dried secretion, foreign material, matted pubic hair cuttings, pubic hair combings, and the comb. |
| **4e1.**GC and *Chlamydia* | **4e.** Examine vaginal and cervical areas for injury and foreign materials. Do Toluidine Dye applications **(Figures 5-6–5-8,** see Colorplate following page 144) Collect 4 swabs from vaginal pool, Prepare 1 wet mount slide and 2 dry mount slides. Examine wet mount for sperm. Document findings. Collect cervical swabs. Collect specimen for GC. Do speculum exam. | **4e2.** Foreign materials, four vaginal swabs, one wet mount slide, one dry mount slides. |
| **4f1.** GC, rectum | **4f.** Examine buttocks, perianal akin, and anal folds for injury. Collect dried and moist secretions and foreign materials. Document findings. If indicated by history or findings, collect 2 rectal swabs of rectal area. Conduct an anoscopic or proctoscopic exam if rectal Injury is suspected, and collect 2 swabs of internal rectal area, 1 dry mount. **(Figures 5-9 and 5-10,** see Colorplate following page 144) | **4f2.** Dried secretions foreign materials, and rectal swabs, wet mount slide, and dry mount slide |
| **4g1.** Syphilis and pregnancy | **4g.** Clinical Tests Pregnancy test-blood (red-topped tube) Syphilis serology (red-topped tube) | **4g2.**Alcohol and toxicology samples |
| | **4h.** Other evidence collected at the discretion of physician and law enforcement officer. Blood alcohol (red-topped tube)/toxicology # (grey-topped tube) Urine Toxicology screen # (urine specimen, # & 50ml) | **4h2.** Reference samples |
| **SEND CLINICAL SPECIMENS TO LAB.** | **4i.** Collect reference samples (these can be collected at a later date if patient refuses at time of exam): blood typing (yellow-topped tube) saliva specimen, 25 head hairs, 25 pubic hairs | **GIVE EVIDENCE TO LAW ENFORCEMENT OFFICER.** |

**FIG. 5-11.** Female evidence collection.

this process. The purpose of the bottom sheet of paper is to protect evidence from debris or dirt on the floor that can contaminate the clothing. The top sheet is submitted to the crime laboratory. The patient needs to remove her shoes prior to stepping on the paper for disrobing to avoid contamination of the loose trace evidence with nonevidential debris from the shoe soles. The shoes should be collected and packaged separately. The victim's clothing should not be shaken because microscopic evidence could be lost. Holes, rips, or stains in the victim's clothing must not be disturbed by cutting.

A head-to-toe skin surface survey must be conducted. The skin should be searched grossly for evidence of bleeding, lacerations, abrasions, bruises, erythema, edema, scratches, bite marks, burns, stains, moist secretions, dried secretions, and foreign materials. Then, with the lights darkened in the room, the entire body should be scanned with a long-wave ultraviolet light (Wood's lamp/Bluemaxx light), searching for fluorescent exudates. The ultraviolet light reveals evidence of dried or moist secretions, stains, fluorescent fibers, and subtle injuries (such as rope marks and contusions) not readily visible in white light. If findings are noted, their location, size, and appearance should be documented in the text and on the schematic figures of the female body. Photographs of the skin trauma should be taken. Photographs of bruises may be helpful in defining the object that inflicted the injury. With the proper technique, photographs of bite marks assist in identifying the perpetrator. If the bite mark has broken or perforated the skin, a cast of the bite mark by a forensic odontologist, if available, may be indicated. This evidence can be compared later with court-ordered impressions and wax bites from the suspect.

Bruises and bite marks may not be apparent immediately following an assault. A recommendation should be made to the police to arrange for a follow-up examination and additional photographs by the crime laboratory after the bruising has developed more fully. Photographs should be taken for 6 days at 24-hour intervals because bruises and bite marks become more evident with time.

Along with textual, diagrammatic, and photographic documentation, evidence (e.g., foreign materials, dried and moist secretions, and stains) on the patient's body should be properly collected. Foreign materials include fibers; hair; grass; dirt; and thicker stains of semen, saliva, or blood. A separate "miscellaneous" envelope should be used for each location on the body from which foreign material is collected. On the envelope write "debris" and describe the materials and the site of collection. The separate foreign material envelopes should be sealed and placed in the main miscellaneous evidence collection envelope. Findings should be recorded in the text, and the location of the foreign materials found on the body should be marked on the evidence diagram. For collection of foreign materials, a tweezer, a glass slide, or the dull side of a scalpel blade can be used to gently loosen or scrape the foreign substance onto the opened and flat miscellaneous paper collection envelope. Sometimes the use of a cotton-tipped swab moistened with sterile water can be helpful. The paper envelope should be refolded in a manner to retain the scraping and debris. If heavily crusted semen or blood is found on the pubic hair, the matted hairs bearing the specimen should be cut out and placed in a collection envelope, which is then labeled and sealed.

If the victim gives a history of scratching the assailant or if foreign material is observed under the nails, fingernail scrapings should be collected, as they may contain blood and/or tissue of the perpetrator or other evidence from the crime scene. The right- and left-hand collections are performed as separate procedures. The sexual assault examination kit provides the two fingernail scrapers and the collection envelopes required for the procedure (see Appendix). Each of the victim's hands should be held over an unfolded, flat collection paper envelope. Then scrapings are taken from under all five fingernails and the debris is allowed to fall into the collection envelope. The used scraper is placed in the center of the collection envelope, which is then refolded to retain the debris and the scraper. The two envelopes are identified as containing "right-hand fingernail scrapings" or "left-hand fingernail scrapings."

Evidence specimens of thin secretions and stains from blood, semen, and saliva need to be properly collected to improve the forensic yield when they are subjected to genetic typing tests, most importantly DNA testing. The method of collecting evidence from moist secretions or stains differs from collecting evidence involving dried secretions or stains. Both methods use swabs supplied in the sexual assault evidence kit. Each suspicious moist or dried secretion, stain, or fluorescent area needs to be approached as a separate procedure with separate swabs and labeled in detail. When blood stains are present, the stain pattern should be photographed before the evidence is collected. The area is swabbed, and injuries that might be associated with the blood should be noted. The two-swab technique is used for dried secretions or stain areas noted on the gross visualization examination and with the light scanning procedure (42). The first swab is moistened with sterile distilled water and then used to swab the evidence area. The wet swab is then air-dried for at least 1 hour either with a stream of cool air or on a drying rack. The second swab is left dry and used to swab the same site as the wet swab. Once the wet swab has dried, then both swabs from the one evidence site are packaged together in the original wrapper. The wrapper is labeled with the evidence collection site and placed in the main miscellaneous evidence collection envelope. If evidence is collected from a moist area of secretion or stain, a dry swab is used to avoid dilution of the evidence. The swab is allowed to air-dry for at least 1 hour and is then placed in a labeled envelope or tube, which is then sealed. If the area swabbed (moist or dried) was found with the use of Wood's lamp, "W.L." should be marked on the envelope. The findings are recorded, and the locations of the secretions or stains are noted in the text and on the diagram of the female body.

Dried semen stains have a characteristic shiny, mucoid appearance and tend to flake off the skin. Under an ultraviolet light, semen usually exhibits a blue–white or orange fluorescence and appears as smears, streaks, or splash marks. Since freshly dried semen may not fluoresce, each suspicious area should be swabbed, whether it fluoresces or not, with a separate swab. Not all fluorescent areas observed under ultraviolet light are indicative of seminal fluid; therefore, forensic confirmation of the findings is necessary. If the victim reports oral penetration, the area around the mouth and the oral cavity must be swabbed for evidence of seminal fluid. The area around the mouth is swabbed for evidence as would be done for other dried or moist secretions. If the assault occurred within 6 hours before the examination, two swabs

should be used to collect evidence from the oral cavity. Using both swabs simultaneously, the left inside cheek area and the left upper gum line are swabbed with gentle pressure. Two dry mount slides are then prepared—one from each swab—and labeled swab/slide no. 1 and swab/slide no. 2. The swabs are allowed to air-dry for at least 1 hour; then the slides are packaged in the miscellaneous collection envelopes, which are labeled and sealed. If the victim reports fellatio, a culture should be obtained for *Neisseria gonorrhoeae* after the evidence swabs have been collected.

Collection of the perpetrator's saliva and residual epithelial cells on bite mark wounds requires the two-swab technique for collection of dried secretions. The outside border of the bite mark should be swabbed toward the center of the bite mark, first with the wet swab, then the dry one. The greatest amount of saliva is usually deposited in the area of the bite mark caused by the lower teeth. The wet swab is allowed to air-dry for 1 hour. Then both swabs are submitted for forensic analysis of DNA.

Reference samples, including blood, serum, and head and pubic hair, are collected to determine whether or not specimens are foreign to the patient. They are also used for comparison with specimens from potential suspects. Plucking of hairs from the patient's head permits evaluation of hair length as well as variation of natural pigment or hair dyes from the root to the tip of the strand. The patient should be given the option of pulling out her own hair reference samples, as this gives her the feeling of having more control over the situation. The patient or the examiner should pull a minimum of 5 full-length hairs from each of the following scalp locations (total of 25 hairs): center, front, back, left side, and right side. The hairs should represent the variations in length and color. They are placed in a miscellaneous evidence envelope, which is labeled and sealed.

Reference samples of pubic hair can be collected simultaneously with the pubic hair evidence collection. A sheet of paper should be placed beneath the patient's buttocks. The pubic hair is combed forward from the mons pubis toward the vaginal area. A new unused comb should be used to remove any loose hairs or foreign materials that may have transferred from the assailant to the patient during the assault. The loose hairs, foreign materials, pubic hair, and comb are placed in the sheet of paper under the patient's buttocks, which is then folded with the contents inside. The folded paper and its contents are placed in a large labeled envelope, which is then sealed. Samples of the patient's pubic hairs are needed for comparison with the suspect's hairs. The patient or the examiner needs to pluck at least 25 hairs of various lengths and color from the pubic area. The hairs can be compared microscopically, and if hairs foreign to the victim are identified, they can be tested utilizing polymerase chain reaction (PCR) DNA.

A thorough and carefully documented anogenital examination follows. If the victim has bathed, showered, or douched since the assault, the examiner should still collect samples from the appropriate body orifices to attempt to preserve any trace evidence. To prevent loss of evidence from the genital area through wiping or washing, the patient should not void prior to the examination. If the patient must urinate, a specimen container should be provided and the urine sent to the hospital laboratory to be examined for motile or nonmotile sperm. The patient should place the tissue used for wiping in an envelope. The tissue is then dried, labeled, and submitted with the other evidence.

The external genitalia should be examined for any foreign material, bleeding, or evidence of trauma. Injuries may include abrasions, lacerations, ecchymoses, hematomas, edema, contusions, or petechiae. A common finding after recent coitus is erythema and superficial abrasion of the posterior fourchette. Most genital injuries from sexual assault involve the fossa navicularis and the posterior fourchette. Any extensive tears or bleeding should be evaluated and repaired surgically, if necessary, by a gynecologist. Any findings on gross visual examination should be documented on the diagram of the female body and in the text. The location of the anogenital findings should be documented by using the face of a clock and the patient in anatomic position as your reference (e.g., midline injuries at the entrance to the vagina over the posterior fourchette at the 6 o'clock position).

Any foreign materials and dried or moist secretions on the external genitalia should be collected as evidence. Any foreign bodies found in the vagina should be removed, photographed, and dried. For evidence collection, the two-swab technique is used for dry secretions and the one-swab technique for moist secretions. The area should be scanned with a long-wave ultraviolet light (Wood's lamp/Bluemaxx light), and any findings recorded in the text and on the diagram of the female body. On the diagram, place "W.L." next to the findings noted with a Wood's lamp or ultraviolet light.

Before the speculum examination, toluidine blue dye should be applied to the external perineal area and the findings recorded. The dye is applied with cotton-tipped applicators to the area of the posterior fourchette and, after several seconds, a lubricant or sterile water is applied to the area. The area is wiped gently with nonsterile pads until the blue dye is no longer seen on the pads. Then a dry cotton-tipped applicator is used to wipe away dye caught in the crevices of the posterior fourchette. Areas with retained royal blue dye uptake should be interpreted as having tested positive. The findings should be recorded and any abnormalities photographed. The area must be wiped completely dry to avoid entry of toluidine blue or lubricating jelly into the vagina and thus prevent contamination of forensic tests that follow. In some states and jurisdictions, the protocol calls for the collection of forensic specimens from the vaginal pool, cervical os, and anus prior to the use of toluidine blue dye to prevent contamination of specimens. This requirement conveys less concern about the possible, though unlikely, trauma that may be induced by insertion of the speculum. The method chosen will depend on local forensic protocols.

If the hymen is very redundant or thickened secondary to estrogen changes, the balloon technique can be used after all of the vaginal specimens have been collected. For this technique, the examiner inserts a Foley catheter into the vagina and then inflates the balloon with 5 to

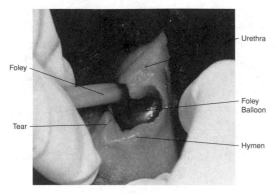

Foley

Tear

Urethra

Foley
Balloon

Hymen

**FIG. 5-12.** Use of a Foley balloon to show hymen tear on a 14-year-old sexual assault patient.

10 mL of water (Fig. 5-12, see Colorplate following page 144). The catheter is pulled out slowly until the hymen rests on the surface of the balloon, where it can be evaluated. The balloon is then deflated and the catheter removed (43).

The speculum examination is done to observe for trauma and to collect evidence from the vaginal and cervical area. A nonlubricated speculum moistened with warm water is used for this examination. Care should be taken in selecting the speculum size: Special consideration should be given if the woman is elderly, is an adolescent, or does not ordinarily have sexual relations with male partners. A speculum should not be used to examine a girl or woman who is less than Tanner 3. For Tanner 1 and 2, gentle traction on the labia majora along with good positioning is usually sufficient for visualization of the vagina and cervix and for obtaining evidence. If more visualization is needed because of bleeding, a tear, or other forensic findings, then a nasal speculum can be used.

Generally, swabs are collected from the vaginal pool before evidence is collected from the cervical os. Specimens from the cervix and cervical os should be collected and labeled separately. The number of swabs collected depends on local protocol and the contents of the particular state's sexual assault kit. For evidence collection, two swabs are held together as a unit and then inserted into the vaginal pool. The swabs are rotated to ensure uniform distribution of the sample on them. A swab from the first

swab unit is used to prepare a slide that the crime laboratory will examine for the presence of sperm. The slide is allowed to air-dry (without a cover slip) and is then immersed in 70% ethanol for a minimum of 30 seconds. The swabs and the slide should be labeled and placed in a labeled miscellaneous evidence envelope (e.g., vaginal swab no. 1, vaginal slide no. 1). The cervical os is swabbed using another two swabs as a unit. The swabs are labeled and allowed to air-dry. Then they are returned to the labeled miscellaneous evidence envelope.

After collection of the vaginal swabs, separate specimens may be collected for the detection of spermatozoa. If the clinician chooses to have a separate slide to look for spermatozoa at the hospital, one swab is used to prepare the wet mount slide using normal saline, which is examined immediately for motile or no-motile sperm. This slide should not be discarded! It should be heat preserved and placed in a separate miscellaneous evidence envelope (labeled). Nonmotile sperm can be detected for up to 3 days in samples from the vaginal pool and up to 5 to 7 days in the cervix after coitus. Sperm or ejaculate may be absent if the assailant used a condom, did not ejaculate, or had a vasectomy.

Colposcopy, if available, should be performed to confirm signs of minor injury to the genital area. The magnification setting on the colposcope should be recorded. Many colposcopes have photographic capability and, if findings are noted, they should be photographed. In addition, the findings should be documented in the text and on the diagram of the female body. At the conclusion of the genital examination, a specimen for gonorrhea culture should be collected from the endocervix as a baseline and other cultures for STDs should be obtained as indicated.

The anorectal area should be examined for signs of injury and foreign materials. The presence of seminal fluid, dried or moist secretions, fecal matter, bleeding, lubricants, and any other foreign materials should be noted. Injuries may include abrasions, lacerations, fissures (both fresh and healed), ecchymoses, edema, contusions, or petechiae. Injuries should be photographed at the time of their detection (e.g., before the use of swabs in the anorectal area). Dried secretions are collected using the two-swab technique and moist secretions using the single-swab technique. When present, semen tends to collect at the anal mucocutaneous juncture. Foreign material should be deposited in a separate, labeled envelope. The area is scanned with a long-wave ultraviolet light (Wood's lamp/Bluemaxx light). Any suspicious substance or fluorescent area should be swabbed. If indicated by patient history or physical findings, toluidine blue dye should be applied around the rectal area before an anoscopic examination is performed. Any abnormalities noted after application of the dye should be photographed. The anorectal findings are documented in the text and on the diagram of the female body. Any long-wave ultraviolet light findings (Wood's lamp/Bluemaxx light) are indicated as "W.L." If rectal injuries are suspected, the necessity of anoscopic or proctoscopic examination is considered. Ecchymoses, petechiae, focal edema, internal fissures, lacerations, and excoriations may be seen with anoscopy. Proctoscopy, with an appropriately sized instrument, is indicated when significant rectal trauma is suspected. If a colposcope is available, trauma should be identified and described in the text.

A minimum of two anorectal swabs should be obtained to type semen when present. For the anal swabs, two swabs are used as a unit from the miscellaneous evidence collection envelope to carefully collect evidence from the anal cavity. A slide is prepared without a cover slip and allowed to air-dry. The swabs and slide are labeled as the "anal swabs" and "anal swab slide" and placed in the miscellaneous evidence collection envelope.

The rectal swab evidence must be collected after anal swab evidence collection is complete. The first step in the collection of rectal swabs requires the area around the anus to be cleaned to prevent the transfer of semen that may be present on the perianal area to the rectum. The sphincter is dilated using a small, nonlubricated speculum moistened with warm water or by instructing the patient to use the lateral decumbent or prone knee-to-chest position. Sometimes gently placing a finger next to the sphincter and applying gentle pressure for about a minute will cause the

sphincter to relax. During collection of seminal fluid from the rectum, the swab should be introduced slowly and rotated 360 degrees. If needed, the swab can be moistened with sterile water; saline solution should not be used. Two slides are prepared from the rectal swabs. They are then air-dried and labeled. The slides and the original wrapper are marked as "rectal swab" and "rectal slide." They should be placed in the original wrapper and then in the miscellaneous evidence collection envelope along with the anal swab and slide. If the patient reports sodomy, a specimen should be collected for gonorrhea culture from the rectum as a baseline. Specimens for other STD cultures should be obtained as indicated.

Before completion of the evidence examination, a sample of venous blood must be obtained. A lavender-topped tube should be sent to the crime lab for the patient's reference DNA testing. Blood should be sent to the hospital laboratory for a pregnancy test, alcohol test, syphilis serology, and, if indicated by protocol, a hepatitis panel. Blood for baseline HIV testing may also be obtained, depending on the local hospital protocol, but the patient must sign a consent form specific to HIV testing. In addition to the blood work, a urine sample should be sent for a toxicologic screen. It is optimal to not obtain the urine sample until the evidentiary examination is concluded to prevent loss of evidence.

When performing a vaginal examination on a mentally challenged patient, extra time needs to be spent on obtaining the patient's cooperation. Some patients may require sedation.

## Medical Treatment

The sexual assault victim's injuries must be evaluated and treated. Patient stability is the priority. The forensic evidence collection examination should proceed only after significant injuries have been addressed. The treatment of wounds includes tetanus prophylaxis. The surgery or gynecology service should be consulted for moderate to severe physical or genital injuries.

During the sexual assault evaluation, the patient must be tested to rule out preexisting pregnancy. If the patient was not pregnant before the assault, then she needs to be counseled regarding the options for preventing pregnancy related to it. The risks and benefits of postcoital contraceptive medication should be explained. The patient must be informed that the prophylactic regimens are approximately 98% effective if started within 24 hours of being raped and are recommended only if the victim is seen and treated within 72 hours of the assault. There is a 1% to 2% failure rate with the prophylactic regimen in addition to potential teratogenic effects on the fetus. Nausea and vomiting may also be caused by prophylactic pregnancy medications but can be alleviated with the use of hydroxyzine (Vistaril pamoate), 25 mg by mouth, taken prior to prophylactic medication. A separate consent form should be obtained when giving a patient emergency contraceptive pills. Example contraceptive pill regimens are norgestrel/ethinyl estradiol (Ovral) (50 mg)—two pills taken immediately and two pills in 12 hours—and Lo/Ovral (or other low-dose hormone)—four pills taken immediately and four pills in 12 hours (44–46).

The sexual assault victim should be counseled about exposure to and prophylaxis for STDs. The risk of acquiring an STD as a result of sexual assault is unknown, as it is difficult to determine if the infection was present prior to the assault. Jenny et al. (47) studied STDs in victims of rape to focus on the incidence of newly acquired disease after the assault versus the incidence of preexisting disease. They concluded that for victims of rape the prevalence of preexisting STDs is higher than the incidence of acquiring an STD as a result of the assault. The most common preexisting STDs detected with screening (in descending order) were bacterial vaginosis and infection with *Trichomonas vaginalis, Chlamydia trachomatis,* cytomegalovirus, *Neisseria gonorrhoeae,* herpes simplex virus, *Treponema pallidum,* and HIV. The newly acquired diseases detected on return visit (in decreasing order) were bacterial vaginosis, trichomoniasis, and *N. gonorrhoeae* and *Chlamydia* infection (47). Other studies revealed a similar transmission rate for gonorrhea and syphilis after sexual assault: 2.5% to 13.3% and 0 to 2%, respectively (22,48–50). Although HIV-antibody seroconversion has been reported among persons with sexual assault as the only known risk factor, the risk for acquiring HIV infection through sexual assault is low. That risk is influenced by the risk factors of the assailant(s), type of sexual acts during the assault (e.g., oral, vaginal, or anal), and whether ejaculation occurred (51).

Other diseases and conditions associated with sexual activity, such as hepatitis B, head lice infestation, venereal warts, and nonspecific urethritis in males, should also be considered, especially during the follow-up visit.

Screening cultures should be obtained for *N. gonorrhoeae* and *C. trachomatis* from any site of penetration by the assailant(s). A wet mount and culture should be obtained to test for *T. vaginalis,* bacterial vaginosis, and yeast infection. The patient's serum should be collected to establish a baseline for syphilis, hepatitis B, and HIV infection. A separate consent form needs to be signed for HIV testing, and counseling should be provided before and after testing in accordance with local protocols.

Routine preventive therapy for the most common STDs should be administered at the time of the initial evaluation. Only 30% to 53% of sexual assault victims return for follow-up appointments (17,47), so the initial examination may be the only opportunity for STD prophylaxis. The 1998 CDC guidelines for the treatment of STDs recommend prophylactic treatment against hepatitis B, *Chlamydia, N. gonorrhoeae, Trichomonas,* and bacterial vaginosis. A postexposure hepatitis B vaccination (without hepatitis B immunoglobulin) at the time of the initial evaluation should adequately protect against hepatitis B. The recommended antimicrobial regimen is ceftriaxone (125 mg IM, single dose) plus metronidazole (2 g orally, single dose) plus azithromycin (1 g orally, single dose) or doxycycline (100 mg orally twice a day for 7 days) (51). Should there be a contraindication to this treatment regimen, then the most recent CDC guidelines for treatment for STDs should be consulted.

If the sexual assault victim is pregnant, doxycycline is contraindicated. The safety of azithromycin in the pregnant or lactating female has not been established. Therefore, for the pregnant victim of sexual assault, an alternative regimen to treat *Chlamydia* infection prophylactically would be erythromycin (500 mg orally 4 times a day for 7 days). If the patient is pregnant and allergic to cephalosporins, then spectinomycin (2 g IM, single dose) may be an alternative prophylaxis for *N. gonorrhoeae* (51).

Although the risk of acquiring HIV infection through sexual assault is low, concern about transmission remains because the consequences are grave. However, prophylaxis against HIV is not known to be effective following sexual assault and is generally not recommended (46,51). (The examiner should follow local protocols regarding prophylaxis treatment for HIV infection.) If prophylaxis for HIV infection is considered, the risks and benefits of treatment with anti-retroviral agents need to be explained to the patient. If the patient decides to take postexposure therapy for HIV, the guidelines for occupational mucous membrane exposure should be followed (51).

Sexual assault victims should be scheduled for follow-up in 14 days to ensure successful prophylaxis. A repeat test for syphilis and HIV infection should be obtained 6, 12, and 24 weeks after the assault, as the incubation period is longer than for the more common STDs. Follow-up doses of the hepatitis B vaccine should be given 1 or 2 months and 4 to 6 months after the initial dose (51).

The influence of drugs must be considered in each sexual assault case. The victim may have a change in mental status on presentation or have poor recollection of the assault because of the effects of illicit drugs, medications, or alcohol. In addition, the assailant may have given the victim a drug such as flunitrazepam (Rohypnol) or γ-hydroxybutyrate (GHB) to diminish the victim's resistance. Neither drug is legal in the United States. During the forensic examination, urine should be collected for toxicologic screen to detect these drugs. The urine must be collected within 72 hours of drug ingestion and tested immediately or frozen until the test is performed.

Rohypnol, a benzodiazepine, is prescribed in 80 countries around the world (excluding the United States and Canada) for the treatment of debilitating sleep disorders. Rohypnol is 10 times more potent than diazepam (Valium). Illegally obtained Rohypnol can be "slipped into a drink" by someone known or unknown to the victim. In the past, it was a small pill that usually went unnoticed in drinks because the pills were colorless, odorless, and tasteless. In 1997, the manufacturer, Hoffmann-La Roche Ltd., in response to growing awareness of the misuse of this drug for sexual assault, announced a new formulation. Rohypnol now has a green outer coating that dissolves very slowly and releases as blue when placed in a beverage. Rohypnol can be added covertly to either alcoholic or nonalcoholic drinks; however, the effects are more pronounced when mixed with alcohol. The adverse effects of Rohypnol are dizziness, confusion, impaired judgment, amnesia, and prolonged blackouts, all of which lower the resistance of the victim. Street names for Rohypnol are rophies, roofies, rufies, R2, roofenol, Roche, roachies, la rocha, rope, and rib (52–54).

GHB was once sold over the counter in health food stores as a "steroid alternative" for body building. As a result of toxic side effects including seizures and several deaths linked to the drug, it was removed from the market in 1997 with warnings issued by the Food and Drug Administration. The drug moved underground and gained favor as a recreational drug because of its intoxicating effects. Although it is illegal for any person to produce or sell GHB in the United States, the drug can be obtained through clandestine laboratories or the Internet, where "home brewing" recipes are available as well as the chemical ingredients and supplies needed to make the drug. The "high" obtained from the use of GHB varies: the drug may act as a central nervous system depressant or stimulant. GHB comes in a liquid form and is commonly used with other drugs or alcohol. Its street name is "ecstasy" (MDMA) or the "smart drug." After ingestion of GHB, the victim of sexual assault may be confused, disoriented, or even amnesic about the event (55,56).

## Photography

Photographs are a valuable form of evidence, especially for situations that cannot be documented adequately in diagrams (e.g., bite marks or massive injuries). Ideally, photographs should be taken before medical treatment of the wounds. Any camera may be used, as long as it can be focused for nondistorted close-up shots and provide an accurate color rendition. A 35mm camera is recommended. Adequate lighting is essential, whether the source is natural, flood, or flash. Close-up photographs of wounds and bite marks should be taken. The camera should be held perpendicular to the body surface being photographed. This is essential to avoid photographic distortion of wounds or bite marks, especially those on curved surfaces of the body. Tilting of the camera should be minimized to avoid distortion of the picture. The photograph should be arranged to include an accurate ruler or scale in close proximity to the injury for size reference and a label with the patient's name for identification purposes. The lesion must not be obscured with the ruler or label. At least one or two photographs should be taken without the scale to orient the lesion and to demonstrate that the scale has not obscured important evidence. The scale should be retained for later reference to enable the photographic lab to produce an accurate, life-size (1:1) photograph. The photograph(s) can then be compared with evidence [e.g., suspect dental casts for bite marks or object(s) that may have inflicted the injury]. The name of the photographer should be recorded on the film evidence envelope.

The photographs may be taken in the hospital by the sexual assault examiner or by the crime lab, in accordance with local law enforcement policies. The patient's rights need to be remembered when the photographs are taken. The patient must understand that the photographs taken will be used in court as evidence. The patient's sensitivity about being undressed for photography must be addressed. Patients should always be draped appropriately. Also, the person taking the photographs should be the most likely to minimize the victim's discomfort (e.g., a female law enforcement officer or crime laboratory staff member, or a nurse trained in forensic photography).

### Follow-up

After the evidentiary examination is completed, the patient should be given options for follow-up counseling and be encouraged to obtain it. Address and telephone numbers should be given for rape crisis centers and victims programs. Information should be provided about crime victim compensation. The medical and counseling follow-up plans should be established clearly before the patient leaves the facility. Counseling improves the patient's long-term prognosis. The hope is to help the victim regain a sense of well-being and to limit the effects of posttraumatic stress syndrome, which develops in many victims of sexual assault. Posttraumatic stress syndrome is discussed in Chapter 2.

### ADULT MALE SEXUAL ASSAULT VICTIM

During the past 30 years, concerns about the violent crime of rape have focused on female victims—the "forced vaginal penetration of the woman by a male assailant." That definition ignores the possibility of a male being a rape victim. The term *rape* is now accepted in some states to include forced penile penetration of either male or female victims. In efforts to be gender neutral and encompass a broader range of violent sexual acts (e.g., fellatio and sodomy), the term *sexual assault* is now used.

Although female victims of sexual assault outnumber males 3:1 each year in the United States, the number of sexual assaults against males is alarming. In 1998, the National Institute of Justice reported that approximately 93,000 males are forcibly raped in the United States each year (57). Adult men represent only 5% of reported adult sexual assault cases, but they often sustain more severe physical injury (21). Making this type of assault gender neutral has allowed more treatment options for male victims (e.g., treatment in a sexual assault center). However, a group of sexual assault victims that still cannot obtain the benefit of sexual assault centers and follow-up care is male victims in prisons (58).

The protocols for the evaluation of the male sexual assault victims are similar to those for female victims. The victim should be triaged as a priority to protect the quality of the evidence (Fig. 5-13). He should remain clothed until the

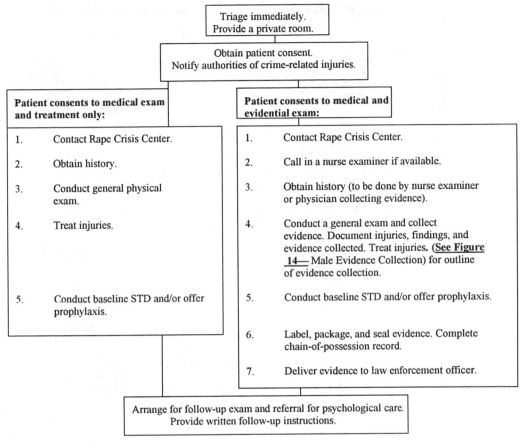

**FIG. 5-13.** Male sexual assault examination.

time of the evidence examination. An advocate for the victim should be involved early on. The victim needs to sign a consent form after being informed of his rights. The police must be notified. A thorough history should be obtained, including the victim's name, age, and race. The date, time, location, and physical surroundings of the assault should be noted. Details about the assailant(s) should be documented, such as name(s), race, and number of assailants involved. The use of physical force or threats should be noted, as well as the use of physical or chemical restraints. The patient's description of the physical or sexual acts committed by the assailant(s) should be documented, including whether penetration or ejaculation occurred.

The victim's symptoms and sites of physical injury should be reported. On the main emer-

gency department chart, pertinent medical history is noted along with other information such as allergies, medications, and use of alcohol or drugs.

The physical and evidence examinations are conducted simultaneously (Fig. 5-14). The clinician should note the patient's general appearance and demeanor. His vital signs, height, weight, and color of eyes and hair should be documented. The condition of the patient's clothing and any signs of rips, tears, stains, and other foreign materials should be noted. The clothing should be scanned with Wood's lamp for fluorescent exudates and the positive areas documented. Clothing is collected in the same manner as for female sexual assault victims, using two sheets of paper. The collection of clothing should be documented. Any evidence of non-

**All swabs and slides must be air dried before packaging. Corresponding swabs and slides are coded, e.g., oral swab #1, oral slide #1.**
**Expansion of #4, Figure 13**

| CLINICAL SPECIMENS FOR LAB (TO GO TO HOSPITAL LAB) | | EVIDENCE FOR CRIME LAB (TO BE GIVEN TO LAW ENFORCEMENT) |
|---|---|---|
| | **4a.** Note condition of clothing on arrival. Collect outer and under clothing worn during or immediately after assault. Collect fingernail scrapings if indicated. | |
| | **4b.** Conduct general physical exam. Scan entire body with Wood's lamp. Collect dried and moist secretions and foreign materials from body including head, hair, and scalp. Document findings. | **4a2.** Put clothing in separate bags. Fingernail scrapings, foreign material on clothing and body. |
| **4c1.** GC | **4c.** Examine oral cavity for injury. Document findings. If indicated by history, swab area around mouth. Collect four oral swabs. Take specimen for GC. | **4c2.** Four swabs from oral cavity |
| **4d1.** GC & *Chlamydia* | **4d.** Examine external genitalia for injury. Scan with Wood's lamp. Collect dried and moist secretions and foreign materials. Document findings. Comb pubic hair to collect foreign materials. Swab shaft of penis and glans penis area. | **4d2.** Any dried secretions, foreign material, pubic hair combings, and the comb: one swab from shaft and one swab of glans penis |
| **4e1.** GC, rectal | **4e.** Examine buttocks, perianal skin, and anal folds for injury. Collect dried and moist secretions and foreign materials. Document findings. If indicated by history or findings; collect two rectal swabs of external area. Conduct an anoscopic or protoscopic exam if rectal injury is suspected, and collect two swabs of internal rectal area. One dry mount slide. | **4e2.** Dried secretions, foreign materials, rectal swabs, wet mount slide, dry mount slide |
| **4f1.** Syphilis tests | **4f.** Clinical tests Syphilis serology (red-topped tube) | |
| **4g1.** Alcohol and toxicology samples | **4g.** Other evidence collected at the discretion of the examiner and law enforcement officer. Blood alcohol (red-topped tube)/toxicology from blood (grey-topped tube) Urine toxicology screen (urine specimen, 50 ml) | **4h2.** Reference samples |
| **SEND CLINICAL SPECIMENS TO LAB.** | **4h.** Collect reference samples (these can be collected at a later date if patient refuses at time of exam): blood typing (yellow-topped tube), saliva specimen, 25 head hairs, 25 pubic hairs | **GIVE EVIDENCE TO LAW ENFORCEMENT OFFICER.** |

**FIG. 5-14.** Male evidence collection.

genital trauma should be reported and evidence collected when indicated. As with female victims, male victims may have findings of severe, moderate, or minimal nongenital trauma. Evidence of abrasions, bruises, lacerations, bite marks, restraint marks, and other signs of trauma should be sought. The findings should be described in the text, including measurements, color, depth, and tenderness. Any visible findings of trauma should be photographed with proper technique. Bite marks, if noted, should be swabbed for saliva using the two-swab technique, and a forensic odontologist should be involved in accordance with local protocol. Any evidence of foreign material should be collected properly using a tweezer, glass slide, or the dull side of a scalpel; the source site must be documented. Each foreign material should be placed in a separate envelope. Foreign materials include fibers, hair, grass, dirt, and thicker stains of semen, saliva, and blood. While checking the patient's hair for evidence of foreign materials, the examiner may find it time efficient to collect the reference scalp hair samples if that procedure is part of the local sexual assault forensic examination protocol (20–30 hairs should be collected from different sites on the scalp).

If the victim gives a history of scratching the assailant or if foreign material is noted under the nails, fingernail scrapings should be collected. The right- and left-hand specimens must be packaged separately. The sexual assault kit contains two fingernail scrapers and the collection envelopes required for the procedure. Evidence specimens of thin secretions and stains from blood, semen, and saliva need to be collected. If the secretion is dried, the two-swab technique is indicated (first swab moistened with distilled water followed by a dry swab in the same area). If the secretion is moist, then only one swab is needed to collect the evidence. The sites of evidence collection are documented in the text. The collection envelopes must be labeled properly. The patient's body should be scanned with a Wood's lamp and the two-swab technique used to collect dried secretions that fluoresce. Sites of fluorescence should be indicated on the male traumagram and labeled "W.L."

If the patient reports fellatio, then the perioral area and the oropharynx need to be examined for evidence of trauma. The lips should be inspected for contusions, lacerations, and moist or dried collections of seminal fluid. In the oral cavity, any sign of ecchymosis, petechiae (most notably in the posterior pharynx or the soft palate), tears of the frenulum under the tongue, other lacerations, and loose teeth should be noted. For evidence collection, the perioral area is swabbed as for dried secretions. If the assault occurred within 6 hours, two swabs should be collected from the oral cavity. With both swabs used simultaneously, the left inside cheek area and the left upper gum line are swabbed with gentle pressure. Two dry mount slides, one from each swab, are prepared and labeled as swab/slide

no. 1 and swab/slide no 2. The swabs are air-dried for at least 1 hour, then the slides are packaged and the envelopes are labeled and sealed. After the oral swabs are collected, cultures for *N. gonorrhoeae* and *Chlamydia* are obtained.

Prior to examining the victim's external genitalia, the clinician should place a sheet of paper beneath the patient's buttocks. The penis and the scrotum are examined for signs of trauma. Injuries to the penis may include abrasions of the glans, tears of the mucocutaneous junction of the meatus, or lacerations. There may also be evidence of bites or linear abrasions caused by nails or teeth. Microscopic or magnified examinations can be performed with a magnifying lens or colposcope to confirm signs of minor injury. Any findings of trauma are photographed using an L-scale and a 35mm camera. The presence of dried and moist secretions, lubricants, feces, and foreign materials must be noted as well as any venereal lesions. In uncircumcised males, foreign materials may be retained on the penis, particularly on the glans or in the sulcus. Any foreign material noted, including matted pubic hair, should be collected and placed in the appropriate envelope, which is then labeled and sealed. Dried secretions are collected with the two-swab technique and moist secretions with the one-swab technique. The area is scanned with a Wood's lamp and the fluorescent areas swabbed. The sites of secretions should be documented on the male traumagram; secretions detected with a Wood's lamp should be marked with "W.L."

The patient's pubic hair should be combed, after which the comb is placed on the paper sheets under the patient's buttocks for later collection. At this time, the reference samples of the pubic hairs (20–30 hairs) should be collected. Penile swabs must also be collected. The number of swabs varies with different protocols; the majority of protocols require one swab from the urethral meatus and one from the glans. A swab taken from the penile shaft may be indicated. The swabs are moistened before evidence is collected. The presence of fecal matter is noted. The swabs are air-dried for at least 1 hour and then labeled as to location. If indicated, a specimen is obtained for *N. gonorrhoeae* and *Chlamydia*

culture from the urethra as a baseline and prophylactic medication offered to the patient. Other
STD cultures are obtained as indicated.

If the patient reports anal penetration, then a
thorough anorectal examination is indicated to
expose evidence of trauma, such as bleeding,
abrasions, ecchymoses, edema, contusions, petechiae, lacerations, and fissures. Again, microscopic or magnified examinations can be
performed with a magnifying lens or colposcope to confirm signs of minor injury. Any
trauma should be photographed. Any dried or
moist secretions noted in the perianal area with
either gross visualization or a Wood's lamp
should be collected using the two-swab technique if dried and one-swab technique if moist.
The swabs are air-dried for at least 1 hour. The
collections are documented in the text and the
sites of the collections marked on the male
traumagram. If the secretion was noted only
with the Wood's lamp, "W.L." is marked next
to it on the traumagram. Any foreign material
is collected in a "debris" envelope, which is
then labeled and sealed. Two anorectal swabs
are collected, and two dry mount slides are prepared from them, labeled swab no. 1/slide no.
1 and swab no. 2/slide no. 2.

An anoscopic examination is performed. An
anoscope lubricated with only water is used to
inspect the rectum for trauma. If a colposcope
is available, trauma can be photographed and
the findings noted in the text. Rectal cultures
should be collected for gonorrhea and possibly
*Chlamydia* infection. When the examination is
completed, the paper beneath the patient's buttocks is folded with the comb inside and placed
in a miscellaneous evidence collection envelope, which is then labeled and sealed.

During the male sexual assault forensic examination, blood should be collected for reference samples for DNA, serum alcohol testing,
rapid plasmin reagin (RPR), hepatitis panel, and
HIV testing. The patient must sign a separate
HIV consent form before HIV testing can be
conducted. A sample of the patient's urine needs
to be obtained for the toxicology screen for illicit drugs.

After the examination is complete, the protected evidence should be given to the police and
the transfer documented. Until the evidence is
given to the police, the primary examiner cannot allow it to be accessed by anyone else. This
secures the chain of custody that is necessary to
have the evidence be valid in court. The patient
should be referred for follow-up for both physical and psychological sequelae of the assault.
The aftermath on the male victim can be devastating, so all patients should be referred for
counseling by professionals trained to address
the psychological trauma related to sexual assault.

## SUSPECT EXAMINATION PROTOCOL

Most sexual assault suspects are male. The
forensic examination of the suspect is similar to
that of the male victim of sexual assault, with a
few modifications (Fig. 5-15). The suspect is
usually brought to a sexual assault evaluation
center by the police. For the safety of the staff,
the police should be present during the entire
evaluation and collection of evidence. Either
consent is obtained from the suspect or the
court-ordered search warrant is reviewed prior
to beginning the examination. The court-ordered
search warrant should specifically order the
medical examination, collection of specimens,
and screens for STDs and HIV. Except in rare
circumstances, it is best to have a search warrant when collecting evidence on a suspect and
to collect only what is specified on the search
warrant. (The sexual assault forensic examiner
should nurture a good working relationship with
the police department so that the clinician can
advise the officers regarding what information
should appear on a search warrant with respect
to different situations that arise with suspects.)
The examiner is allowed to record any utterances
from the suspect during the examination. If a
search warrant is not provided, the suspect can
later state that he did not agree to give the evidence. Then any evidence collected is not admissible in court.

The examination requires the use of a sexual
assault examination kit. The examiner obtains
the history from the police and the patient. Information from the patient should include medications, allergies, major medical history, STD

**All swabs and slides must be air dried before packaging. Code corresponding swabs and slides, e.g., oral swab #1, oral slide #1.**

Obtain history and authorization for exam
from law enforcement officer.
**Establish security.**
**Prevent contact between the victim and the suspect.**

| **CLINICAL SPECIMENS FOR LAB (TO GO TO HOSPITAL LAB)** | | **EVIDENCE FOR CRIME LAB (TO BE GIVEN TO LAW ENFORCEMENT)** |
|---|---|---|
| | **1.** Note condition of clothing on arrival. Collect outer and under clothing worn during or immediately after Assault. Collect fingernail scrapings if indicated. | |
| | **2.** Conduct general physical exam. If within 24 hr scan entire body with Wood's lamp. Collect dried and moist secretions and foreign materials from body including head, hair, and scalp. Document findings. | **1a.** Clothing (in separate bags.) Fingernail scrapings, foreign material on clothing and body. |
| **3b.** GC | **3.** Examine oral cavity for injury. Document findings. If within 24 hr and indicated by history, swab area around mouth. Collect two oral swabs and prepare a dry mount slide. Take specimen for GC. | **3a.** Two swabs from oral cavity, two dry mount slides, one swab from around mouth. |
| **4b** . GC & *Chlamydia* | **4.** Examine external genitalia for injury. If within 24 hr: scan with Wood's lamp, collect dried and moist secretions and foreign materials, document findings, cut matted pubic hair, comb pubic hair to collect foreign materials, swab shaft of penis and glands penis. | **4a.** Any dried secretions, foreign material, matted pubic hair cuttings, pubic hair combings, and comb; one swab from shaft and one swab from glands penis. |
| | **5.** If within 24 hr: Examine buttocks, perianal skin, and anal folds for injury. Collect dried and moist secretions and foreign materials. Document findings. If indicated by history or findings; collect two rectal swabs of external area with two dry mount slides. | **5a.** Dried secretions, foreign materials, and rectal swabs |
| **6b.** Syphilis tests | **6.** Collect: three blood samples, syphilis serology (red-topped tube), blood alcohol/toxicology (grey-topped tube), blood typing (yellow-topped tube), urine specimen, 50ml. Collect reference samples: saliva specimen, 25 head hairs, 25 pubic hairs, 25 body hairs. | **6a.** Blood alcohol/tox, blood typing, urine specimen; reference samples |
| **SEND CLINICAL SPECIMENS TO LAB.** | **7.** Document injuries, findings, and evidence collected. Label, package, and seal evidence. Complete chain-of-possession record. | **GIVE EVIDENCE TO LAW ENFORCEMENT OFFICER.** |

**FIG. 5-15.** Male suspect sexual assault evidential examination.

history, HIV screening history (if the patient is willing), vasectomy history, and recent history of urinary tract infections and anogenital problems. The suspect's clothing should be collected in the same manner as in a sexual assault victim evaluation. When a suspect is brought in within 48 hours after the assault, the physical examination and the evidence examination are conducted like the sexual assault forensic examination of the male victim. For suspects brought in after 48 hours, appropriate modifications of the examination should be implemented. When a suspect is brought in after 72 hours, it may be necessary to collect only reference samples (pubic, head, and body hair and blood).

The examiner must remember to look for physical identifiers of the suspect (e.g., tattoos or scars) and for physical signs of high-risk behavior that would place the victim at greater risk for contracting a disease from the suspect (e.g., needle marks from intravenous drug abuse). Evidence of physical trauma inflicted by the victim's resistance attempts should be sought (e.g., scratches). The rest of the nongenital and genital evidence examination is identical to the sexual assault examination protocol. Photographs should be taken of evidence of trauma. Laboratory specimens are obtained: blood alcohol, urine toxicology, syphilis serology, HIV testing,

hepatitis panel. Cultures for *N. gonorrhoeae* are taken from the throat, the urethra, and, if indicated, the rectum. *Chlamydia* cultures from the urethra and the rectum may be obtained if this procedure is part of the local protocol. The examination should be documented in great detail and a male traumagram should be used to note the sites of the findings. When summarizing the findings, the examiner should not render an opinion as to whether the suspect is indeed the assailant. The evidence should be carefully collected, dried, labeled, and sealed. A copy of the court-ordered search warrant should be enclosed in the evidence envelope. The chain of custody must be maintained during the entire process and the transfer of evidence must be documented.

---

### APPENDIX.  *Female sexual response*[a]

---

Masters and Johnson first described the human sexual response in 1966, and their work was updated in 1988 by Kolodny.[b] These authors describe the physiologic response that occurs in men and women when they engage in consensual sexual intercourse. The entire process can be separated into five phases: desire, excitement, plateau, orgasm, and resolution. The lack of the normal response in the female explains some of the vaginal injuries that occur in rape victims.

The desire phase is referred to as the "springboard for sexual arousal" and is initiated by cognitive cues (such as interpersonal attraction), general mood, situational receptivity, and general health. Approximately 70% of sexual arousal is believed to be psychological. The desire phase induces no physical changes, but serves as the trigger for the excitement phase. During the excitement phase, vaginal lubrication begins: the labia majora flatten and move back from the vaginal orifice; the labia minora thickens; the cervix and the uterus move upward; and the heart rate, blood pressure, and respiratory rate increase. After the excitement phase is the plateau phase, in which there is continual lubrication, the inner two thirds of the vagina lengthens and expands, and the cervix and the uterus are further elevated. The plateau phase is followed by orgasm, when heart rate, blood pressure, and respiratory rate reach a peak. Then follows the resolution phase, when the woman's physiology returns to normal. When these physiologic changes do not occur, a woman is more likely to sustain vaginal trauma during a sexual assault.

---

[a]The female sexual response is often referred to by lawyers during trial, and is frequently used to explain why vaginal injuries occur as a result of sexual assault. The authors of this chapter do not like to use this argument in a court of law. Masters and Johnson used consensual partners for their study, and did not look for any trauma on the women in their study. By using their material, the defense may try to imply that the lack of any trauma means that the act was consensual, which is definitely not the conclusion one should make from the above-discussed study.

[b]Masters WH, Johnson VE, Kolodny RC. Heterosexuality. New York: HarperCollins, 1992.

---

### Sexual Anatomy Terminology

---

**Male**

| | |
|---|---|
| Circumsized male | Male whose foreskin has been removed from the penis. |
| Corona | The upper portion of a body part. |
| Cowper's gland | Two pea-sized structures connected to the urethra below the prostate gland. They produce small amounts of fluid, which may appear at the glans during sexual arousal. This preejaculatory fluid may contain a few live sperm. |
| Dorsal vein | Vein that runs along the dorsal surface of the penile shaft. |
| Epididymis | A highly coiled tubing network folded against the back surface of each testis. Sperm cells spend several weeks in the epididymis while they mature. The epididymis then passes to the vas deferens. |

| | |
|---|---|
| Glans | Head of the penis, covered by a loose skin (foreskin or prepuce), which enables it to expand freely during erection. |
| Midline raphe | Seam-like union extending from the scrotum to the rectum. |
| Penis | External organ consisting of three parallel cylinders of erectile tissue that run the length of the penis; consists of the glands, prepuce, corona, shaft, and frenulum. Two of the masses lie alongside each other and end behind the head of the penis. The third mass lies beneath them and contains the urethra. The average length of a nonerect penis is 8.5–10.5 cm and the length of an erect penis averages 16–19 cm, with a diameter of 3.5 cm. |
| Prepuce or foreskin | Fold of skin that covers the glans of the penis; circumcision removes this skin surgically. |
| Prostate | Normally about the size of a chestnut and consists of a muscular and glandular section. The prostate is located directly below the bladder and surrounds the urethra. The prostate produces about 30% of the seminal fluid. The remaining 70% is produced by the seminal vesicles. |
| Rectum | Terminal part of the intestine from the sigmoid flexure to the anus; not sensitive to pain. |
| Scrotum | Thin loose sac of skin under the penis, which contains the testicles. |
| Seminal fluid | Carries mature sperm from the body. At climax of coitus, the semen is discharged. A single discharge, about 3.5 mL of semen, contains 120 million to 600 million spermatozoa. Seminal fluid is a whitish sticky material. (After a vasectomy, sperm is no longer present in the ejaculate, but the quantity of seminal fluid remains the same.) |
| Shaft | Long cylindric area of the penis below the glans. |
| Spermatozoa | Mature male sperm cells. A sperm is only 1/1,500 in. long and is visible only by microscope. A spermatozoon resembles a tadpole and is made up of three sections: a head, a midpiece, and a tail that propels the sperm with a lashing movement. |
| Testes | The male sex organs. The testes have two functions: production of hormone and production of sperm. The entire process of sperm production takes 70 days. Unlike the female, who creates no new eggs after birth, the male produces billions of sperm annually from puberty until death. |
| Urethral meatus | External orifice for the urethra. |
| Vas deferens | 16-inch tube that connects the epididymis to the urethra; this tube is cut and sutured off during a vasectomy. |
| **Female** | |
| Acts committed | Coitus, penile-labial (aka vulvar coitus or simulated vaginal intercourse); coitus, full penetration; fellatio, oral-penile; cunnilingus, oral-vaginal; sodomy, usually refers to penile-anal, but has many definitions; analingus, oral contact with the anal area. |
| Anus | Terminal orifice of the alimentary canal; opening to the rectum 4 cm in length; pain-sensitive; surrounded by the sphincter muscles. |
|   Anal ampulla | Dilated portion of the rectum just proximal to anal canal. |
|   Anal rugae | Skin folds. |
|   Anal verge | Tissue that overlies external anal sphincter. |
|   Fold | Redundant skin often found at 12 and 6 o'clock. |
|   Pectinate line | Anal papilla and columns interdigitate with the anal verge tissue (where squamous meets columinar cells). |
|   Tag | Extra skin that usually develops after trauma or laceration. |
|   Venous pooling | Dilatation and sometimes bulging of the veins around the anus (aka venous engorgement). |
| Cervical os | Opening of cervix. |
| Cervix | Narrow lower or outer end of the uterus; neck of uterus. |
| Clitoris | Small erectile organ at the anterior or ventral part of the vulva homologous to the penis; sole purpose is for sexual stimulation. |
| Fossa navicularis | Concave area immediately below the hymen, extending outward to the posterior fourchette. |
| Glands (Bartholin's) | Two oval racemose glands lying one to each side of the lower part of the vagina at 4 and 8 o'clock, secreting a lubricating mucus. Skeins toward the urethra area. |
| Hymen | Fine membrane or tissue that separates the external genitalia from the vagina. *All* females have this structure; however, wide anatomical variations exist. |
|   Shapes | |
|     Annular | Ring shape: smooth unfolded 360 degrees. |
|     Crescent | Half moon; anterior rim of tissue extending from 1 to 11 o'clock may be absent. |
|     Cribriform | Multiple small openings. |

| | |
|---|---|
| Elongated | Vertical diameter longer than horizontal. |
| Imperforate | No opening. |
| Microperforate | Small opening. |
| Septated | Bridge of tissue. |
| Sleeve-like | Opening ventrally displaced orifice, "kangaroo pouch." |
| Edges | |
| Bump | Small rounded projections, may indicate where a septate bridge once attached, area of attachment vaginal rugae, or caused by chronic inflammatory change (aka mound). |
| Cleft | V-shaped indentation, not extending to base (junction of the hymen and vestibule) (aka notched). |
| Fimbriated | Uneven edges with small projections. |
| Gaping | Extra large hymenal diameter without stretching. |
| Rolled | Tissue folded over on itself either inward or outward. |
| Scalloped | Rounded series of half-circle tissue (aka ruffled). |
| Smooth | No breaks, bumps, or notches (aka regular). |
| Thickened | Fatter and less elastic. |
| Transection | Tear, cut, or division (usually used to describe healed tear that does not grow back together). |
| Tissue | |
| Attenuated | Decrease in amount of tissue (aka thinning). |
| Estrogenized | Pubertal changes to hymen: light pink/white color, with increased redundancy and elasticity. |
| Flap | Loose movable tissue protrusion. |
| Nonestrogenized | Translucent. |
| Redundant | Containing an excess or superfluous amount. |
| Remnant | Residual tissue left after chronic trauma. |
| Tag | Finger-like projection may occur after break/separation of septated bridge. |
| Thickened | Fatter and less elastic. |
| Velamentous | Veil-like, thin, delicate (aka membranous, translucent, wispy). |
| Intervaginal rugae | Transverse folds of the mucus membrane of the vagina (aka longitudinal folds or ridges). |
| Labia majora | Outer lips to vagina; covered with pubic hair after menarche. |
| Labia minora | Inner lips to vagina. |
| Midline commissure | Midline fusion external from the posterior fourchette; used in anatomical descriptions of children. |
| Midline raphe | Toward the anus; *not* a scar. |
| Midline sparing | White avascular linear area posterior to hymen at 6 o'clock. |
| Mons pubis | Rounded eminence of fatty tissue on the pubic symphysis. |
| Perihymenal tissue | |
| Vestibular papillae | Area lateral to hymen from base of hymen to labia minora; nipple or finger-like projections involving medial aspects of labia, introitus, and lower vagina (aka micropapillamatosis labialis). |
| Perineal body | Mass of muscle and fascia that separates the lower end of the vagina and the rectum in females and the urethra and the rectum in males. |
| Perineum | Region between the thighs, bounded by the scrotum/vulva and anus median raphe palpable line midline extending from the posterior fourchette/scrotum to anus; sometimes raised, rough, pigmented. |
| Periurethral tissue | The immediate 360-degree area around the urethra, not including the urethral meatus. |
| Posterior fourchette | Area below the fossa navicularis, the point of fusion of the posterior labia minora. |
| Tanner stage by pubic hair | |
| 1. No or fine vellus (peach fuzz) hair | |
| 2. Sparse, long pigmented hair | |
| 3. Increased density, dark course curly hair | |
| 4. Abundant hair, sparing medial thighs | |
| 5. Abundant hair, spreading to medial thigh | |
| Urethral meatus | Orifice for the urethra |
| Periurethral/ vestibular bands | Bands lateral to the urethra connected to the vestibule wall; support bands. |
| Vagina | Tubular structure or canal of the female extending from the hymen to the cervix. |
| Ridges | |
| External | Longitudinal ridge of the vestibular hymen from the rim to the fossa navicularis or urethra. |

| | |
|---|---|
| Internal | Longitudinal intravaginal ridge, which extends to or beyond the rim; frequently seen at 10, 2, and 6 o'clock. |
| Vestibule | Space between the labia minora into which the urethra and vagina open (aka vestibulum vaginae). |
| Vulva | Region of the external genital organs of the female (including labia majora and minora and mons pubis). |

Contents of a generic sexual assault kit produced by Tri-Tech Inc. (Tri-Tech produces approximately 90% of all kits used in the United States). Frequently, a given state asks Tri-Tech to customize a kit for that state, which Tri-Tech will do. They produce suspect kits as well.

1. Kit envelope, which is presealed
2. Kit instruction sheet
3. Outer clothing bags
4. Underpants bag
5. Debris collection envelope with two sterile swabs and one plastic fingernail scraper
6. Pubic hair combing envelope containing one towel and one black comb
7. Pulled pubic hair envelope
8. Pulled head hairs envelope
9. Known saliva sample envelope (some places have stopped obtaining these samples because DNA is more reliable)
10. Known blood sample tubes
    7-mL ACD—yellow top
    7-mL EDTA—lavender top
    (These tubes are what expires when a kit has an expiration date. If you have a kit that has expired, simply replace these two tubes with tubes from your department and use the rest of the kit)
11. Anatomical drawings form
    Many places use more detailed drawings that they either produce themselves or have
    Tri-Tech produce for them.

# REFERENCES

1. Bureau of Justice Statistics. *National crime victimization survey.* Washington, DC: U.S. Department of Justice, December 1998.
2. Bureau of Justice Statistics. *Uniform crime report.* Washington, DC: U.S. Department of Justice, 1997.
3. National Institute of Justice and Center for Disease Control Research in Brief. *Findings from the National violence against women survey,* 1998.
4. Ringel C. *Criminal victimization in 1996, changes 1995–96 with trends: 1993–1996.* NJC-165812. Washington, DC: Bureau of Justice Statistics, November 1997:3.
5. Senate Judiciary Report. *Responses to rape,* 1993.
6. National Center for Victims of Crime, 1996.
7. Dansky et al. *National women's study: relationship of victimization PSD to bulimia and nervosa,* 1997.
8. National Center for Victims of Crime, 1991.
9. National Center for Victims of Crime and Crime Victims Research and Treatment. *Rape in America,* 1992.
10. National Institute of Justice. *Victim costs and consequences: a new look,* January 1996.
11. Talbert S. Improving emergency department care of the sexual assault victim. *Ann Emerg Med* 1980;9:293.
12. Holmes RM. *Sex crimes.* New York: Sage Publications, 1991.
13. American College of Obstetricians and Gynecologists. *Sexual assault.* Tech. Bull. No. 101. Washington, DC: 1987.
14. Green WM. *Rape: the evidential examination and management of the adult female victim.* Lexington, MA: DC Health, 1988.
15. Jackson CM, Groleau G, Kimmel C. Comparison of the quality of medical documentation for findings related to sexual assault prior and post the development of a sexual assault forensic examination program (abstract). Presented ACEP Research Forum, Las Vegas, October 11–12, 1999.
16. Satin AJ, Hemsell DL, Stone IC, et al. Sexual assault in pregnancy. *Obstet Gynecol* 1991;77(5):710.
17. Rambow B, Adkinson C, Frost T, Peterson G. Female sexual assault: medical and legal implications. *Ann Emerg Med* 1992;21:727.
18. Rogers D. Physical aspects of alleged sexual assaults. *Med Sci Law* 1996;36(2):117.
19. Deming JE, Mittleman RE, Wetli CV. Forensic science aspects of fatal sexual assaults on women. *J Forensic Sci* 1983;28:572.
20. Marchbanks PA, Lui KJ, Mercy JA. Risk of injury from resisting rape. *Am J Epidemiol* 1990;132(3):540.
21. Geist RF. Sexually related trauma. *Emerg Med Clin North Am* 1998;6(3):439.
22. Tintinalli JE, Hoelzer M. Clinical findings and legal resolution in sexual assault. *Ann Emerg Med* 1985;14(5):447.
23. Cartwright P, Moore R, Anderson J, et al. Genital injury and implied consent to alleged rape. *J Reprod Med* 1986;31:1043.
24. Bowyer L, Dalton ME. Female victims of rape and their genital injuries. *Br J Obstet Gynecol* 1997;104(5): 617.
25. Slaughter L, Brown C, Crowley S, Peck R. Patterns of genital injury in female sexual assault victims. *Am J Obstet Gynecol* 1997;176(3):609.
26. Lenahan LC, Ernst A, Johnson B. Colposcopy in evaluation of the adult sexual assault victim. *Am J Emerg Med* 1998;16(2):183.

27. Ramin S, Satin A, Stone I, Wendel G. Sexual assault in postmenopausal women. *Obstet Gynecol* 1992;80(5): 860.
28. Cartwright P, Moore R. The elderly victim of rape. *South Med J* 1989;82:988.
29. Cartwright PS. Factors that correlate with injury sustained by survivors of sexual assault. *Obstet Gynecol* 1987;70(1):44.
30. Ruback RB, Ivie DL. Prior relationship, resistance, and injury in rapes: an analysis of crisis center records. *Violence Vict* 1988;3(2):99.
31. McLay WDS. Sexual violence. In: Mason JK, ed. *The pathology of trauma,* 2nd ed. Boston: Little, Brown and Company, 1993:138–149.
32. Bowers C, Bell G. *Manual of forensic odontology*, 3rd ed. Montpelier, VT: Printing Specialists, 1995:347.
33. Gresham GA. Violent forms of asphyxial death. In: Mason JK, ed. *The pathology of trauma,* 2nd ed. Boston: Little, Brown and Company, 1993:204–213.
34. Bart PB. A study of women who both were raped and avoided rape. *J Social Issues* 1981;37:123.
35. Ulman SE, Knight RA. Multivariate model for predicting rape and physical injury outcomes during sexual assaults. *J Consult Clin Psychol* 1991;59(5):724.
36. Damm D, White D, Brinker M. Variations of palatal erythema secondary to fellatio. *Oral Surg* 1981;52: 417.
37. Biggs M, Stermac LE, Divinsky M. Genital injuries following sexual assault of women with and without prior sexual intercourse experience. *Can Med Assoc J* 1998; 159(1):33.
38. Kindermann G, Carsten PM, Maassen V. Ano-genital injuries in female victims of sexual assault. *Swiss Surg* 1996;1:10.
39. Lauber A, Souma M. Use of toluidine blue for documentation of traumatic intercourse. *Obstet Gynecol* 1982;60(5):644.
40. McCauley J, Guzinski G, Welch R, et al. Toluidine blue in the corroboration of rape in the adult victim. *Am J Emerg Med* 1987;5(2):105.
41. Slaughter L, Brown CR. Colposcopy to establish physical findings in rape victims. *Am J Obstet Gynecol* 1992;166(1 Pt 1):83.
42. Sweet D, Lorente M, Lorente JA, et al. An improved method to recover saliva from human skin: the double swab technique. *J Forensic Sci* 1997;42(2):320.
43. Ferrell J. Foley catheter balloon technique for visualizing the hymen in female adolescent sexual abuse victims. *J Emerg Nurs* 1995;21:585–586.
44. American Medical Association. *Strategies for the treatment and prevention of sexual assault.* Chicago: October 1995.
45. Hochbaum SR. The evaluation and treatment of the sexually assaulted patient. *Emerg Med Clin North Am* 1987; 5(3):601.
46. Hampton H. Care of the woman who has been raped. *N Engl J Med* 1995;322(4):234.
47. Jenny C. Sexually transmitted diseases in victims of rape. *N Engl J Med* 1990;322(11):15.
48. Evrard JR, Gold EM. Epidemiology and management of sexual assault victims. *Obstet Gynecol* 1979;53:381.
49. Schwarc SK, Whittington WL. Sexual assault and sexually transmitted diseases: detection and management in adults and children. *Rev Infect Dis* 1990;12[Suppl 6]:S682.
50. Everett RB, Jimerson GK. The rape victim: a review of 117 consecutive cases. *Obstet Gynecol* 1977;50(1):88.
51. 1998 CDC Guidelines for treatment of sexually transmitted diseases. *MMWR* 1998;47(1):108–111.
52. The Metro Toronto Research Group on Drug Abuse. *Facts on Rohypnol,* August 30, 1996;1(3).
53. National Institute on Drug Abuse. *Epidemiologic trends in drug abuse: advance report by the Community Epidemiologic Work Group,* June 1995.
54. Fact sheet on Rohypnol. Hoffmann-La Roche Inc., September 1998.
55. U.S. Department of Health and Human Services, Food and Drug Administration. *FDA Talk: FDA warns about GBL-related product,* May 11, 1999.
56. U.S. Department of Health and Human Services, Food and Drug Administration. *FDA Talk: FDA reissues warning on GHB,* February 18, 1997.
57. National Institute of Justice and Center for Disease Control. Research in Brief, *Findings from the National violence against women survey,* November 1998.
58. Schiff AF. Examination and treatment of the male rape victim. *South Med J* 1980;73(11):1498.

## SUGGESTED READINGS

Aiken MM, Speck PM. Sexual assault and multiple trauma: a sexual assault nurse examiner (SANE) challenge. *J Emerg Nurs* 1995;21(5):466.

Beebee DK. Initial assessment of the rape victim. *J Miss State Med Assoc* 1991;32(11):403–406.

Bureau of Justice Statistics. *The crime of rape.* Bull. No. NCJ-96777. Washington, DC: U.S. Department of Justice, 1985.

Bush RA Jr, Owen WF Jr. Trauma and other noninfectious problems in homosexual men. *Med Clin North Am* 1986;70(3):549.

Collins C, Hansen L, Theriot E. A clinical stain for use in selecting biopsy sites in patients with vulvar disease. (reviews false positive toluidine results). *Obstet Gynecol* 1966;28(2):158.

DiNitto DM, Martin PY, Maxwell MS, Norton DB. Rape treatment programs: delivering innovative services to survivors. *Med Law* 1989;8(1):21–30.

Douglas JE, Burgess AW, Burgess AG, Nessler R. *Crime classification manual.* San Francisco: Jossey-Bass, 1992.

Fagan JA, Stewart DK, Hansen KV. Violent men or violent husbands? In: Finkelhor D, Gelles FJ, Hotaling GT, Staus M, eds. *The dark side of families.* Beverly Hills, CA: Sage Publications, 1983:1–25, 49–67.

Golden G. Use of alternative light source illumination in bite mark photography. *J Forensic Sci* 1994;39(3):815.

Hazelwood RR, Burgess AW. *Practical rape investigation.* Boca Raton: CRC Press, 1995.

Ledray L, Netzel L. DNA evidence collection. *J Emerg Nurs* 1997;23(2):156.

Ledray LE. *Recovering from rape.* New York: Henry Holt, 1994.

Lenehan GP. Sexual assault nurse examiners: a SANE way to care for rape victims. *J Emerg Nurs* 1991;17(1):1–2.

Mauser TI. Findings in medical examination of victims of serious sexual offenses. *Police Surgeon* 1991;38(4).

Osborn M, Bryan S. Evidentiary examinations in sexual assault. *J Emerg Nurs* 1989;15(3):284–290.

Perloff W, Steinberger E. In vivo survival of spermatozoa in cervical mucus. *Am J Obstet Gynecol* 1964;88:439.

Pollack O. Semen and seminal stains: review of methods in medicolegal investigation. *Arch Pathol* 1943;35:140.

*SART/SANE orientation guide.* Santa Cruz, CA, 1993.

*SART/SANE preceptorship guide.* Santa Cruz, CA, 1994.

Short J, DeLuca M, DiVasto P, et al. Detection of sperm in victims of rape. *N Engl J Med* 1978;229:424.

West M, Barsley R, Friar J, Stewart W. The detection and documentation of trace wound patterns by use of an alternate light source. *J Forensic Sci* 1992;37(6):1480.

West M, Barsley R, Friar J, Stewart W. Ultraviolet radiation and its role in wound pattern documentation. *J Forensic Sci* 1992;37(6):1466.

Williams RM. Few convictions in rape cases: empirical evidence concerning some alternative explanations. *J Criminal Justice* 1981;9:29.

# 6

# Sexual Abuse and Sexual Assault of Adolescents

V. Jill Kempthorne

## DEFINITIONS AND EPIDEMIOLOGIC CONSIDERATIONS

Determining the true incidence and prevalence of sexual abuse and sexual assault in adolescents is difficult due to definitional issues and underreporting. There are no standardized definitions for such terms as sexual abuse, sexual assault, and rape, and legal definitions may vary from one state to another (1). For instance, the National Center on Child Abuse and Neglect defines child sexual abuse as "involvement of a child in sexual activity to provide sexual gratification or financial benefit to the perpetrator, including contacts for sexual purposes, prostitution, pornography, or other sexually exploitative practices" (2). In the State of Maryland, however, sexual abuse means "any act that involves sexual molestation or exploitation of a child by a parent or other person who has permanent or temporary care or custody or responsibility for supervision of a child, or by any household or family member." Although rape is a legal term referring to sexual victimization of women by male assailants (3), in common usage the term has also been used for male victimization (3a). A commonly used definition of sexual assault is genital, anal, or oral penetration or attempted penetration by a part of the perpetrator's body or by an object, without the consent of the victim. This definition does not include fondling, but in Maryland statutes, fondling is considered a type of sexual assault. Statutory rape is yet another subset of sexual assault in which there is sexual intercourse between a female under a certain age and an assailant who is older. Specific guidelines regarding victim age and age difference vary from one state to another.

In this chapter, *sexual assault* refers to sexual contact that is exploitative, due to either age or power discrepancies, and that may or may not involve penetration or attempted penetration. *Sexual abuse* refers to sexual assault or sexual exploitation by a family member or by an individual with responsibility for the child or adolescent.

Since sexual abuse is a form of child abuse and therefore is reported to child protection, data from child protection can be useful in assessing sexual victimization of children. However, depending on the state reporting laws, sexual assault by nonfamilial perpetrators may or may not be included. The distinction between sexual abuse and sexual assault is especially important for the adolescent patient. For both males and females, the relative proportion of extrafamilial sexual assault increases as the adolescent grows older (Fig. 6-1). In a 1994 crime data brief from the U.S. Department of Justice, almost half of reported sexual assaults involved a family member with girls younger than 12 years, whereas with girls aged 12 to 17 this percentage dropped to 20% and with women 18 and older to 12% (5). In addition, males are more often victimized by non-family perpetrators (4). Hence, if child protection statistics only include perpetration by family members or those responsible for care of the child, then they will underestimate the scope of sexual victimization in children and adolescents, more so for the adolescent than for the younger child, and more so for the male than for the female victim.

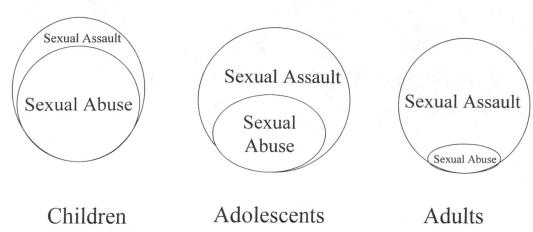

**FIG. 6-1.** Relative prevalence of sexual abuse in different age groups.

Nondisclosure or delayed disclosure also result in underestimation. In the 1997 Commonwealth Fund Survey of the Health of Adolescent Girls, 30% of girls surveyed and 50% of boys surveyed with a history of physical or sexual abuse had told no one (6). Data from the National Crime Victimization Survey indicate that only 30% of rapes are reported to the police and that only 50% are disclosed at all (7). For adolescents, only 20% of sexual assaults are reported to the police (8). Finkelhor found in a national telephone survey of children aged 10 to 16 years that the rate of sexual assault was three times higher for 12- to 15-year-olds than the rate reported in the comparable National Crime Survey (9). In one study of sexual aggression on college campuses, 27% of college women reported experiencing and 7.7% of college men reported perpetrating sexual assault, but almost none of these events had been reported to the police (10).

Nondisclosure is more common if the victim knows the perpetrator (11). This underreporting bias needs to be considered in evaluating sexual abuse reports to child protection and in evaluating rape statistics, since most rape victims know their attacker. Nondisclosure is more common for males than for females for both rape (12) and sexual abuse (6). Delayed disclosure is also common. In one study of adolescent girls, there was a mean time of 2.3 years from onset of unwanted sexual experience to disclosure (13).

There are multiple reasons for nondisclosure and delayed disclosure. First is the adolescent's failure to recognize victimization (14). This may apply both to intrafamilial abuse, where the adolescent assumes that it is her fault, and to peer-sexual relationships in which the adolescent may assume that coercion is a normal part of the sexual experience (15,16). In one study, nearly one third of adolescents interpreted violent behavior as love, and fewer than 5% related it to hate (3,17). In cases of statutory rape involving adolescents, the adolescent may experience intimacy and receive material comforts from the perpetrator. She may ignore or not understand any coercive qualities in the relationship and may not view herself as a victim. In such cases, even parents may acknowledge and accept these relationships, particularly if they themselves have difficulty meeting the needs of the adolescent. Hence, in many cases statutory rape is not disclosed or reported to either child protection or the police.

Nondisclosure happens if the adolescent does not remember being assaulted. This typically happens when he or she is under the influence of drugs or alcohol. Recently, there has been increasing use of the "date rape drug" flunitrazepam (Rohypnol), a benzodiazepine with significant sedative and amnesiac effects (18).

For those adolescents who recognize that they have been victimized, there may be a reluctance to disclose due to shame, guilt, or fear.

Disclosure following date rape is not common, primarily due to self-blame (19). Some of this reflects the high rate of coincident drug and alcohol use in date rape and the victim's sense of responsibility for both the drug use and the consequent assault (11,20).

Anticipated parental reaction may be important. In one study of adolescents who did not tell their parents, only half thought the parents would believe them (13). Fear of parental anger and parental blame are also significant factors, and may be magnified if the adolescent has used drugs or alcohol. The higher nondisclosure for male victims may be related to fears of homosexuality, since more than 90% of perpetrators are male, for both female and male victims (4).

Despite the epidemiologic challenges, it is recognized that adolescent sexual victimization is a significant problem. It is estimated that by age 18 years, 10% to 30% of females and 5% to 10% of males will have been sexually victimized (8). Although many sexual abuse victims are under the age of 5, the risk of sexual abuse increases markedly between the ages of 6 and 10 (21). The average age of onset of sexual abuse of girls ranges from 7 years to 12 in many studies. Moreover, the duration of the abuse can extend for several years. In one study, the average age of onset was 7.5 years and the average age at the end of molestation was 13 (22). The early signs of pubertal maturation coupled with a continued strong dependence on parental figures may offer some explanation for this age-dependent finding.

Although the incidence of sexual abuse begins to taper in the early to mid-adolescent years, the incidence of sexual assault increases. In the July 1999 Bureau of Justice Statistics report on the National Crime Victimization Survey, the number of violent crimes per 100 persons aged 12 or older was highest for the ages 12 to 15 and 16 to 19. The same survey shows that the rate of sexual assault increases through the teen years and peaks around age 20 (23).

Although there are limited statistics on statutory rape due to underreporting, data regarding the age of fathers of babies born to teen mothers indicate the significance of this problem. In a 1988 National Maternal and Infant Health Survey, fathers of newborn babies were at least 5 years older for 24% of births to 17-year-olds, 27% of births to 16-year-olds, and 40% of births to 14-year-olds (3,24).

## UNIQUE VULNERABILITIES OF THE ADOLESCENT

The adolescent patient is vulnerable to sexual victimization in ways that differ from both the child and the adult. These differences are outlined in the following discussion.

### Puberty

The process of puberty, with its physical and hormonal maturation, heightens the adolescent's interest in sex and in forming his or her sexual identity. Sexual curiosity and some sexual experimentation are natural consequences. They also place the adolescent at increased risk of sexual victimization.

### Risk Taking Behavior

Risk taking is a necessary part of the identity formation that occurs during adolescence and allows the adolescent to learn from consequences (24a). However, risk taking can also result in serious consequences, including sexual victimization. Curiosity, impulsivity, and peer pressure may all cloud judgment. Sexual encounters that seem consensual initially may rapidly evolve into coercive experiences.

### Heightened Needs for Privacy and Confidentiality

A necessary part of the individuation process in adolescence is the heightened awareness of privacy issues and the need for confidentiality. The need for confidentiality may override any other concerns in deciding to disclose or seek care following sexual abuse or sexual assault. Numerous studies have documented that adolescents would not seek medical care, particularly for reproductive health issues, if parental consent were required (25,26). In recognition of this, position statements from the American Academy of Pediatrics, the American

## PERMISSIVE

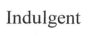

Indulgent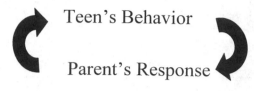

Teen's Behavior

Parent's Response

Risk-taking behavior

## AUTHORITARIAN

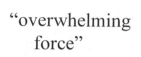

"overwhelming force"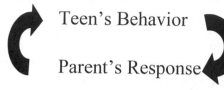

Teen's Behavior

Parent's Response

Risk-taking behavior

**FIG. 6-2.** Parenting styles.

Academy of Family Physicians, and the American Academy of Obstetricians and Gynecologists have all endorsed the importance of confidentiality in adolescent health care (27,27a). In addition, state-specific minor consent statutes allow the provision of reproductive health care services to adolescents without parental consent (27b). These statutes not withstanding, many teens and parents do not understand minor consent, and some providers may not be comfortable providing confidential care to adolescents.

### The Teen–Parent Relationship

The early and middle adolescent years are marked by increasing identification with peers and separation from parents. Parents appropriately view their teen as more responsible for his or her behavior and the consequences thereof. Some degree of parent–teen conflict is a necessary part of this individuation and separation process (28). However, in authoritarian families, this conflict can be extreme and lead to increased risk taking by the adolescent. In permissive families, parents may offer very little guidance and monitoring during the adolescent years. This parenting style also can lead to increased risk taking. In either family type, if the adolescent is victimized consequent to perceived risk taking behavior, the parent's

response may be anger or blame toward the adolescent. In such situations, the parent is often less likely to seek help for the adolescent, and the adolescent is more likely to engage in further high-risk behavior in response to the parent's anger. Hence, a cycle of behaviors and parental response may actually increase the adolescent's risk for subsequent victimization (Fig. 6-2).

### The Myth of Adolescent Turmoil

Early adolescent behaviorists assumed that adolescent turmoil is a necessary part of adolescent individuation. However, recent studies have shown that adolescence is typically not a tumultuous experience (29), and that the rate of behavioral disturbance in adolescence is similar to the rate at other life stages (30). Although the term *adolescent rebellion* is commonly applied to the adolescent experience, most adolescents do not rebel to the point of engaging in disruptive and dangerous patterns of behavior. Although some conflict and risk taking are normal, intense conflict and extreme risk taking behaviors are not. To the extent that adults assume that extreme risk taking behavior is a part of the normal adolescent experience, they may fail to provide guidance or protection or search for underlying causes of the behavior. In particular, there may be a history of sexual abuse.

## Access to Health Care

There are many access to care issues unique to the adolescent patient. Principle among these is the adolescent's concern with confidentiality and privacy, as discussed earlier.

Financial issues are also important in access to care. Adolescents and young adults are more likely to be uninsured than individuals from any other age group (31–33). Although there are programs that subsidize medical care for victims of crime, these programs are often limited to acute care and are accessible only at certain sites of care, and adolescents and their parents may not be aware that such programs are available. Even insured adolescents face barriers. Parents have no obligation to pay for confidential services rendered to their adolescent without parental consent, unless emergency care is provided (27,34). Many providers or clinics may require insurance or payment before seeing a patient. Since adolescents have limited financial resources, they may be refused care, particularly in a nonurgent clinical setting. Billing considerations also can be important. If the adolescent is covered under his or her parent's insurance but wants confidential care, he or she may need to cover the cost of the visit to avoid itemized bills being sent to the parent. This typically applies if the insurance is fee for service.

In addition, some clinics may require parental consent to register, even if the adolescent is seeking care for reproductive health issues. Parental access to medical records, phone follow-up, and appointment reminders also may compromise confidentiality.

## Service Delivery Systems

Even though the rates for adolescent maltreatment are equal to or higher than the rates for younger children, adolescent maltreatment is less likely to be reported to child protection and the adolescent is more often viewed as responsible for the maltreatment (2) (Fig. 6-3). The perceived normalcy of parent–teen conflict and adolescent rebellion may obscure underlying issues of maltreatment. The perception that adolescents may provoke their parents and that parents may be justified in their response may interfere with investigative efforts.

These issues underline the importance of adolescent-focused programs within child protection. Such programs are hard to find. A survey of the 24 county-based child protection offices in the state of Maryland in 1996 did not

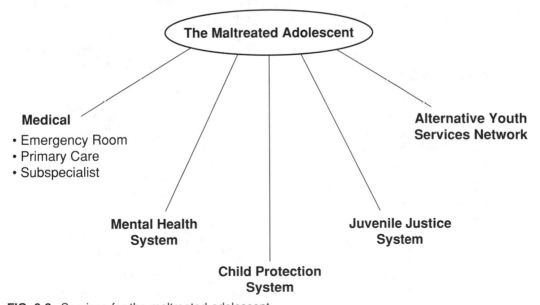

**FIG. 6-3.** Services for the maltreated adolescent.

reveal any evaluation and treatment programs specifically designed to serve maltreated adolescents (Elaine Kelly, personal communication, 1996).

In cases accepted by child protection, options for effective intervention are often limited. Foster home placements often do not work for these youth. Their issues of separation from their own family are so overwhelming that they may not tolerate a strange family and the new family may not tolerate them. Comprehensive services may be hard to find, and the adolescent and his or her family may not be willing to participate.

For the adolescent victim of abuse, it is often the case that mental health, juvenile justice, or youth runaway systems, not child protection agencies, are involved (35). For instance, up to 80% of runaway youth come from abusive families. Such youth typically come to attention through the juvenile court as status offenders. Although the court mandates services, the underlying issues of abuse may never be addressed.

## ESPECIALLY VULNERABLE ADOLESCENTS

In discussing adolescent vulnerability to sexual victimization, it is important to highlight specific adolescent subpopulations. In addition to facing the issues discussed earlier, these adolescents are at heightened risk for victimization and for inadequate treatment.

### Adolescents Living in Poverty

Adolescents living in poverty, particularly in the inner city, are more exposed to violence and more likely to be victims of crime, including sexual assault. Sexual abuse also is more common in poor families (36).

### Adolescents with a History of Childhood Sexual Abuse

Adolescents who have been sexually abused when they were younger are at increased risk for sexual victimization. Moreover, these adolescents are less likely to seek help with subsequent victimization.

### The Male Adolescent

Male adolescents are less likely to disclose or seek help following sexual victimization, for the reasons outlined earlier. With less disclosure, the male adolescent is at risk for continued sexual victimization. Eventually, runaway or delinquent behavior may result. In addition, health care providers are less likely to ask male patients about possible victimization (4), reflecting a larger societal underrecognition of male victimization.

### Gay Youth

It is estimated that 10% of the adolescent population is bisexual or gay. Many of these adolescents are confused about their sexual identity and are afraid to discuss their concerns with anyone. Disclosure by gay youth following sexual abuse or sexual assault may be compromised by concerns about disclosing sexual orientation. Nondisclosure leads to increased risk of repeat victimization and, in many cases, runaway or delinquent behavior.

### Adolescents Who Use Drugs or Alcohol

Sexual activity is more common in adolescents who use drugs and alcohol (33). In addition, drug or alcohol use increases the risk of sexual assault and is associated with at least half of date rapes. Disinhibition, impaired judgment, and, in the case of alcohol, increased aggression all contribute to this association. The Centers for Disease Control (CDC) 1999 Youth Risk Behavior Survey found that more than 80% of high-school students had consumed alcohol in the past, and 42% of high-school seniors had engaged in binge drinking (33,37). The survey also reveals that up to 40% of high-school seniors admit to past use of marijuana, and cocaine use is reported by 3% of seniors.

### Adolescent Children of Parents with Mental Health or Substance Abuse Issues

Parents who are mentally ill or who abuse drugs and alcohol provide less supervision and guidance to their children, and this leads to increased risk taking by the adolescent (36). In addition, teens whose parents abuse drugs and alcohol are themselves more likely to do the same and thereby further increase their risk of sexual victimization.

## Adolescents with Developmental Disabilities or Mental Retardation

Adolescents with developmental disabilities or mental retardation are at increased risk for sexual victimization (38,39). Such adolescents may be easily engaged in voluntary sexual activity by peers or adults. Although there may not be coercion, there is exploitation because the adolescent may not fully understand the implications of the sexual experience.

## ADOLESCENCE AND PUBERTY: AN OVERVIEW

Adolescents are not young adults or large children. In particular, adolescent decision making, attitudes, and behavior are all shaped by significant developmental considerations (40). Adolescence is a period of life marked by cognitive, psychosocial, and pubertal maturation as the child transforms into the adult. There are no standardized age limits for adolescence partly because the timing and tempo of these maturational changes vary widely. Puberty tends to occur in early to mid-adolescence for girls and in mid-adolescence for boys. Cognitive maturation occurs in early to mid-adolescence, whereas psychosocial maturation can extend into late adolescence and young adulthood.

The developmental hallmark of adolescence is puberty. Puberty constitutes the physical changes of secondary sexual development occurring during adolescence. The first signs of normal puberty can come as early as age 8 or 9 and as late as age 14 or 15. Most pubertal development is completed by age 16 to 17 in both boys and girls. In general, puberty begins earlier in girls than in boys.

In the late 1960s, Tanner and Marshall studied several thousand schoolchildren in England and devised the Tanner stage classification scheme to describe pubertal changes. Use of the Tanner stages when examining pubertal children is helpful in assigning degrees of pubertal maturation. For both boys and girls, pubic hair quality and distribution are characterized in the following ways:

Tanner 1: prepubertal; no coarse or dark pubic hair
Tanner 2: sparse, dark, slightly coarse pubic hair, not extending onto the mons pubis
Tanner 3: darker, coarser hair extending onto the mons pubis
Tanner 4: more dense hair pattern, covering most of the external genitalia but not extending to the inner thighs
Tanner 5: dense hair extending to the inner thighs

For girls, breast development is also assigned a Tanner stage:

Tanner 1: prepubertal
Tanner 2: breast bud with minimal breast development beyond the areola
Tanner 3: breast development extending beyond the areola
Tanner 4: more breast development with elevation of the areola above the breast contour (the "double mound")
Tanner 5: more breast development with loss of the double mound

For boys, genital development, as measured by penile and testicular size, is also assigned Tanner staging. Although there are not absolute measurements to guide this staging, a testicular length of 2.5 cm is considered pubertal.

There is marked variation in the timing and duration of the pubertal event (Figs. 6-4 and 6-5) (42,43). For girls, the interval from the first sign of puberty to completion of puberty ranges from 1.5 years to 8 years, with a mean duration of 4 years (41). The first sign of puberty in three of four pubertal girls is the onset of breast development, and in one of four the appearance of pubic hair. The onset of menses in girls is a late pubertal event, typically occurring on average 2.5 years following the onset of breast development and during Tanner stage 3 or 4 breast or pubic hair development. The average age is 12.7 years.

For boys the duration of puberty is from 2 to 5 years, with a mean of 3 years (41). The first

| | Onset | Completion | Duration |
|---|---|---|---|
| Females | 8-13 Years | 13-18 years | 2.5-4 years |
| Males | 9.5-13.5 Years | 13.5-17.5 years | 3-5 years |

**FIG. 6-4.** Pubertal timing.

sign of pubertal maturation is typically testicular enlargement. It is very unusual for pubic hair to appear before genital development in boys. Spermarche, or the onset of sperm production, starts at an average age of 13.4 years. Cognitive maturation is marked by improved abstract reasoning, improved understanding of consequences, and more mature judgment and decision making capabilities. The maturation of the frontal lobe in early adolescence is linked to cognitive maturation (41,41a). One study demonstrated that when 14-year-olds were asked about theoretical medical dilemmas, they were capable of adult-level abstract reasoning in forming their responses (41b).

Psychosocial maturation is marked by identity formation, separation from parents and family, an increased alliance with friends and peer group, the need to experiment, and heightened concerns about privacy and confidentiality. For most adolescents, psychosocial maturation probably shapes the adolescent experience more than cognitive or

---

**FEMALES   Breast Budding** (11.15 ± 1.10)

**Appearance of pubic hair** (11.69 ± 1.21)

**Growth Spurt** (12.5 ± 1.21)

**Menarche** (13.3 ± 1.3)

---

**MALES  Onset of enlargement of scrutum & testes** (11.64 ± 1.07)

**Onset if enlargement in penis** (12.85 ± 1.04)

**Appearance of pubic hair** (13.44 ± 1.09)

**Voice break** (13.5 ± 1.0)

**Growth Spurt** (13.8 ± 1.1)

---

**FIG. 6-5.** Pubertal progression (average age in years, standard deviation).

pubertal maturation. Although by mid-adolescence the teen is capable of mature reasoning and, in essence, has the ability to think before acting, he or she may fail to do so. Exercising mature judgment may be impaired by psychosocial maturational issues, emotional distress, or drug and alcohol use.

The evolving sexuality of the adolescent must be viewed within the context of pubertal, cognitive, and psychosocial maturation. Pubertal timing may influence behavior. Several studies have shown higher deviance and school behavior problems in early maturing girls and in late maturing boys (44,45). Major compounding factors include the life experiences of the adolescent and the emotional framework of any past sexual experiences. Adolescents who have a history of sexual abuse, either as a child only, as a child and adolescent, or as an adolescent only, will have different views of sexuality than the adolescent who has not experienced sexual abuse. It is crucial that the health care provider appreciate these differences when approaching the adolescent patient. The key is, first, to elicit any history of prior sexual victimization and, second, to use any such information in a nonjudgmental manner to guide evaluation and intervention.

## APPROACHING THE ADOLESCENT PATIENT

### Consent and Confidentiality

Adolescents who seek care following sexual abuse or sexual assault may consent for their own care; parental consent is not needed. Confidentiality is usually implicit when consent is given. However, there are limits to confidentiality, and those limits are more extensive and complex for the adolescent patient than for the adult patient. Since confidentiality is extremely important to the adolescent patient, it is important that the physician discuss confidentiality and the limits therein during the visit. If sexual abuse or sexual assault has occurred because of parental neglect, then child protection must be notified. In such cases, it may be appropriate to discuss this with the adolescent. In addition, if screening tests for sexually transmitted diseases (STDs) are performed, it may be appropriate to review reporting guidelines to public health departments. If the patient is covered under the parent's health insurance, the possibility of itemized bills being sent to the parent should be discussed, and alternative billing arrangements should be made if the adolescent does not want the parent to receive a bill.

A final consideration in confidentiality is that of parental notification. Parental notification is contingent on the physician's assessment of the specific situation, what is in the best interests of the adolescent, and the relevant statutory guidelines. For adolescents younger than 18 who request that their parents not be notified, the physician must first ascertain whether sexual abuse occurred or whether sexual assault occurred due to parental neglect. If either is the case, then a report to child protection must be made, and parental notification by the physician may be appropriate, depending on the situation. If neither is the case, then in some states the health care provider has the right, but not the obligation, to notify parents if he or she feels that it is in the best interests of the teen to do so. This may be appropriate in a number of situations as follows:

- The parent expresses concern about possible sexual abuse or sexual assault.
- Significant medical or mental health issues are identified and the physician is concerned about the safety and appropriate follow-up of the adolescent.
- The adolescent needs to be hospitalized.
- The situation warrants a pelvic examination or conscious sedation and the adolescent is unable or refuses to give consent.
- The competence of the adolescent is questioned due to mental state, drug or alcohol intoxication, or developmental delay.

In cases where notification of the legal guardian is deemed important despite the expressed objections of the adolescent, it is very important to address why the teen is resistant to telling his or her parent. The physician should tell the adolescent if the parent is going to be contacted and to assess whether it is best to first talk with the parent alone or to talk with the teen and parent together. In many cases, the parent may need to express feelings of anger, shame, or guilt without the teen being present.

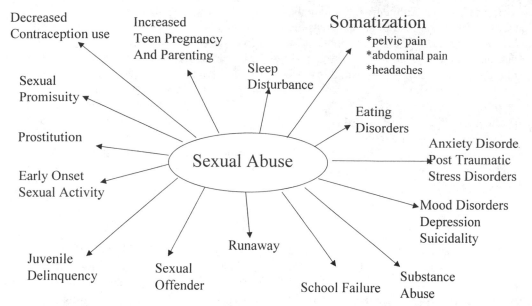

**FIG. 6-6.** Psychosocial consequences of sexual abuse in the adolescent patient.

In some cases, the legal guardian for the adolescent is not the parent. If the adolescent is living with a nonparental legal guardian, or is in foster care or the juvenile justice system, then the designated legal guardian should be involved. If the adolescent does not have a legal guardian or is in an alternative youth service (e.g., home for runaway youth), then the mature minor doctrine may be applied, depending on the clinical situation. If the physician feels that such an adolescent is in need of assistance, social service agencies can be contacted.

In summary, consent and confidentiality are very important considerations in caring for the adolescent victim of sexual abuse or sexual assault. It is important that providers be familiar with the statutes that apply in their particular state. The state attorney's office may be consulted in cases that need clarification.

### The History

Most adolescent victimization is identified through the history. Specific circumstances vary widely. Spontaneous disclosure whereby the adolescent volunteers a history of victimization without being asked is not typical. Although disclosure may occur in most cases presenting to an emergency department following acute sexual trauma, in other settings it is uncommon. During the routine history and physical, adolescents should be asked about any history of sexual victimization. They should be asked this on a yearly basis, even if prior responses were negative. In the 1997 Commonwealth Fund Survey of the Health of American Girls, almost 50% of the girls surveyed felt that their physician should ask about an abuse history, yet only 13% reported that their physician had done so (6). In addition, a history of sexual victimization should be considered for patients presenting with specific medical and/or psychological issues. Figure 6-6 details some of the medical and psychological consequences of victimization. Patients presenting with any of these complaints should be asked specifically about a history of sexual victimization. In addition, youth who are cared for within mental health facilities, the juvenile justice system, the foster care system, or runaway shelters are more likely to have a history of sexual victimization. Health care providers caring for these young people should inquire about victimization, even if past histories were negative.

In taking the history from the adolescent patient, the clinician should follow these guidelines:

- The history should be obtained with the adolescent fully clothed and comfortable.
- Good eye contact should be maintained, and the seating for the examiner and the adolescent should place them at the same eye level.
- Note taking should be limited so as to avoid distracting the adolescent.
- Limits of confidentiality should be discussed, and no promise of unconditional confidentiality should be given.
- The teen should be interviewed without the parent present for matters regarding sexuality, history of abuse, and high-risk behaviors.
- In approaching the psychosocial interview, least intimate questions, such as those pertaining to the home, education, and activities, should be asked initially. These can be followed by questions regarding sexual activity and abuse.

The sexual history should include the following:

- *Any consensual sexual activity;* if so, age at first sexual experience; type of sexual contact (e.g., exchange of bodily fluids; penetration or attempted penetration, including oral-penile, vaginal-penile, or anal-penile); number of partners in lifetime; sexual orientation; use of barrier methods; age of partners; use of drugs or alcohol by partners or patient prior to sexual experience; any coercive element in the sexual experience.
- *Any history of STDs.* Most adolescents with STDs have acquired them through consensual, peer-based sexual experiences. In the patient who has an STD and who denies any history of sexual activity, the possibility of sexual abuse should be seriously considered. The risk of STD is higher with coercive sexual experiences. In one study, there was an association between the adolescent's fear of partner aggression and failure to negotiate condom use (45a).
- *Any history of clinical signs suggesting STD,* including a history of genital ulcers, warts, or other lesions; any history of painful urination or rectal complaints; and any abdominal pain.

Girls should be asked about any history of vaginal discharge or pelvic pain, and boys should be asked about any history of penile discharge or scrotal pain.

- *For girls, a good menstrual history,* including age at first menses, menstrual pattern (frequency, duration, regularity), any heavy or painful menses, and dates of last menstrual period. In addition, a thorough contraceptive history should be obtained, including use of condoms and hormonal contraception.
- *Any history of sexual abuse or sexual assault.* If so, what were the frequency, the duration, and the degree of sexual contact? Were force or threats used? Has there been prior disclosure and, if so, what was the response of the parents? Did the patient receive counseling? Was a report made to child protection or the police? What happened to the perpetrator? Is there continued contact with the perpetrator?

Specific points in the abuse or assault history will help determine specific testing for STDs and the need for prophylactic treatment. The history will also be important in pressing charges. The use of force or weapons may lead to higher criminal charges. Also, if there was actual penetration of an orifice, charges may be higher. Some adolescents may be able to state clearly whether penetration did or did not happen. However, especially for the sexually inexperienced adolescent, the history may be vague. Sometimes vulvar coitus occurs, whereby the penis is forced between the labia majora and the labia minora but not past the hymen into the vaginal vault. Similarly, intercrural coitus may occur whereby the penis is forced between the buttocks but not into the rectum. The patient's perception of whether there was ejaculation also may not be reliable. In one study, in 7 of 16 patients who denied vaginal penetration or ejaculation, seminal fluid was detected (46).

### The Physical Examination

With pubertal maturation during adolescence comes a heightened sense of privacy and increased embarrassment with the physical examination. The following guidelines should be used when examining the adolescent patient:

- A chaperone should be present whenever possible.
- If the patient expresses a gender preference for the examiner, then this should be accommodated if possible.
- If the patient prefers that a parent be present, then this should be accommodated.
- A focused examination is appropriate for patients with specific complaints. However, for those who may have been sexually assaulted or abused, a complete physical examination should be performed.
- The adolescent should be asked whether he or she has ever had a genital exam. If not, the physician should outline the examination before proceeding.
- If the adolescent refuses any or all of the genital or perianal examination, gentle counseling may be appropriate to relieve any anxiety. However, if the patient still refuses, then the examination should be performed at a later time. In cases where serious injuries may need evaluation and treatment, then conscious sedation or general anesthesia may be considered.

### The General Physical Examination

A general physical examination should be focused on finding any signs of trauma or extragenital manifestations of STDs. Specific attention should be focused on the skin, looking for any rash, bruising, or old scars; the oropharynx, looking for intraoral signs of infection; and the abdomen, checking for any abdominal tenderness.

### The Breast Examination

The breast examination is an important part of Tanner staging in adolescent girls. This examination should also be included for adolescent boys. The breast examination in the male adolescent is important primarily because gynecomastia is so common in this population, occurring in more than 60% of individuals (41). It is important to ask about marijuana use and to check for testicular masses, since marijuana and testicular tumors are both associated with gynecomastia. However, the vast majority of persons with gynecomastia have no underlying pathology, and reassurance regarding normalcy of this finding may be important, particularly in the sexually abused male. Gynecomastia resolves within 1 year in 70% of patients and within 2 years in more than 90%.

### The Female Genital Examination

The pelvic examination includes the external examination, a speculum examination, and a bimanual examination. The patient should be draped appropriately and examined in the dorsal lithotomy position. The frog-leg position, used for younger patients, is less ideal once the patient is 11 or 12 years old. If a patient has never had a pelvic examination, it is important to provide an overview of the exam and to show her the speculum before proceeding.

In performing the pelvic examination, the examiner should note the Tanner stage and any signs of injury or infection. The external examination should begin with touching the thigh, then proceeding to the inguinal area and, finally, the vulva. The mons pubis and labia majora should be inspected systematically, followed by the labia minora and the vestibule. The pattern and distribution of pubic hair should be noted and a Tanner stage assigned. In addition, the physician should note any findings that suggest an endocrinologic problem (e.g., clitoromegaly) or a congenital malformation (e.g., transvaginal septum). Although such findings are rare, appropriate evaluation and follow-up should be arranged.

The hymen should be inspected carefully. In response to the increasing estrogen levels in early puberty, the hymen becomes thick and pink (Fig. 6-7). In addition, it becomes more distensible, though there is significant individual variability in the degree of elasticity. The normal pubertal hymen may have a smooth curvilinear edge or extensive folds and notches. The terms used to describe the prepubertal hymen, that is, annular and crescentic, are not typically appropriate for the thickened, often redundant pubertal hymen. Distinguishing notches from healed tears may be difficult. Those notches, which extend through the base of the hymenal rim (so-called complete transections), are highly

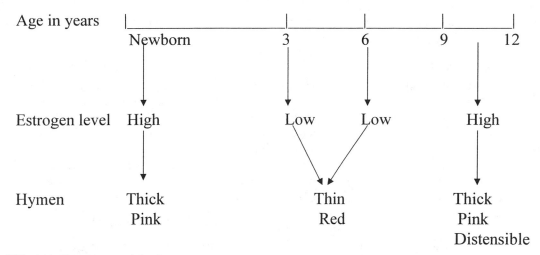

**FIG. 6-7.** Estrogen and the hymen.

suggestive of blunt trauma and penetration. Detecting complete transections may require "running the hymen" with a Q-tip or using a Foley catheter to expose the hymenal border (47). Either technique may be uncomfortable for the sexually inexperienced teen.

The presence of any discharge at the hymenal orifice should be noted. Normal vaginal discharge is typically mucoid or white and without odor. Patients may note a marked increase in normal vaginal discharge in the year or two before menarche. This is called *physiologic leukorrhea.*

The possibility of an STD should be considered with any discharge that is yellow or green, is frothy, or has an odor.

Although the speculum examination is a standard part of the examination in the adult female, there may be extenuating circumstances for the adolescent girl. The speculum examination need not be performed on all adolescent girls who have been sexually victimized. This is especially true for the adolescent who is less than a Tanner 3. Adequate sampling of the vaginal pool and cervix can be performed without a speculum. In the acute setting, if there are signs or symptoms suggesting possible intravaginal injury, such as vaginal bleeding or pelvic pain, then the speculum exam should be attempted, even in the absence of any history of attempted penetration. If the patient refuses the exam or if attempts at speculum insertion are unsuccessful, then conscious sedation may be needed so that adequate inspection of the vaginal vault and cervix can be insured. If there was attempted or completed penile vaginal intercourse, the speculum exam affords access to the vaginal fornices and the endocervix, which are the preferred sampling sites for laboratory tests. This is particularly important for patients who may wish to press charges. In such situations, the importance of the speculum exam should be explained to the patient. However, it should not be performed without the adolescent's consent.

In the patient who is willing to have a speculum examination, it is helpful to first perform a digital examination with a gloved finger, explaining to the patient that you are feeling for her cervix. In addition, this part of the examination allows the examiner to assess the laxity of the vaginal opening, the length of the vagina, and the position of the cervix. If the introitus barely admits one finger, then a speculum exam may be difficult. In such cases, if there is pain or bleeding and an examination of the vagina and cervix is needed, a vaginoscope should be used. Assessing laxity of the introitus and the length of the vagina also helps determine the size speculum to use. When a digital examination is performed, the examiner should obtain a swab sample from the vaginal pool before doing the digital examination, and a set after the speculum is inserted. When a forensic examination is being performed for the police, the digital examination is usually deferred or done after the speculum examination.

Before inserting the speculum, it is often helpful to exert downward pressure with the examining finger, thereby helping to create a space for the speculum. As the speculum is inserted, the examining finger is removed. The position of the speculum is adjusted based on the position of the cervix determined by the digital exam. During the digital and the speculum exam, any lubrication should be achieved with water. K-Y Jelly can interfere with the growth of gonorrhea and should be avoided.

During the speculum exam, the vaginal walls and the cervix should be examined for any signs of injury or infection. The following laboratory tests should be performed:

Wet prep, obtaining vaginal discharge from the vaginal walls
Pap smear in the nonurgent setting
Endocervical gonorrheal and chlamydial infection testing
Additional forensic tests, if appropriate

Following the speculum examination, a bimanual examination should be performed to assess the size and shape of the adnexa and the uterus. In addition, the examiner should determine whether there is any cervical motion tenderness or any adnexal or uterine mass or tenderness. A brief explanation of this examination should be given before undertaking this part of the exam. Although two intravaginal fingers will allow a better examination than one, the relative tightness of the introitus, particularly in the younger adolescent, may necessitate the use of one finger. If there are any concerns regarding a pelvic mass or intrapelvic injury, a pelvic sonogram and/or consultation by a gynecologist should be obtained.

### The Male Genital Examination

As with the female, examination of the male patient should include Tanner staging and a systematic examination for any signs of injury or infection. Signs of injury include ecchymosis,

swelling, and lacerations. The glans and shaft of the penis, the scrotal sac, the perineum, and the perianal region must be examined for any signs of ulceration or wart-like lesions. The urethral meatus also must be checked for lesions and/or discharge. The testes must be palpated for size and tenderness. The physician should also check for any testicular mass or congenital anomaly (e.g., hypospadias; undescended testicle). Although rare, these findings should be noted and evaluation or follow-up should be arranged.

### The Perianal Examination

The perianal exam is particularly important in the male victim of sexual abuse or assault given the high rate of sodomy in such cases. The skin and anal verge should be examined for signs of injury or infection. Any tears, erythema, or ecchymosis should be noted. Reflex anal dilatation should be assessed with lateral traction. If there is bleeding or rectal pain, a proctoscopic exam should be performed.

### Interpretation of Physical Examination Findings

The significance of the physical examination rests on the history of abuse. Was there vaginal penetration? How many times and over what time period? Did the abuse start in childhood and end before adolescence? Did it start in childhood and continue into adolescence, or did it start in adolescence? Although there have been some longitudinal studies following childhood sexual abuse (48), additional studies are needed, following such patients through adolescence.

### Tanner Staging

Tanner staging is very important in sexual abuse and assault evaluation. The sexual activity of the adolescent is very loosely correlated with his or her Tanner stage. Adolescents who mature earlier tend to be sexually active at an earlier age. Hence, if a young adolescent has immature Tanner staging but is sexually active, a history of sexual victimization may be more likely. Tanner staging is also helpful in cases that pursue litigation. It lets the jury know the developmental stage of the adolescent at the time of the assault. Finally, of note is the descriptive study of several female children with premature thelarche or adrenarche who had a history of sexual abuse (49). Although most cases of premature thelarche or adrenarche are idiopathic, this reported association is of interest.

### Signs of Injury in the Female Patient

With adolescent girls, genital injuries are seen with both consensual and forced intercourse. One study examined the presence of genital lacerations of the posterior fourchette in sexually abused adolescents using toluidine blue application, and found that there were no significant differences between these adolescents and the sexually active control group of adolescents (50). In another study of adolescent girls without a history of sexual abuse, attenuation of the hymen, defined as narrowing of the hymen to less than 1%, was found in 37% of sexually active adolescents and hymenal remnants (myrtiform caruncles) in 21%. Complete hymenal clefts, defined as notches extending through the entire rim to the vestibule, were found in 84% of the sexually active adolescents (51). The prevalence of attenuation was higher in girls who were sexually active for more than 3 years, and neither attenuation nor myrtiform caruncles were found in girls who had no history of sexual activity (51). Hence, it seems a reasonable conjecture that attenuation of the hymenal rim occurs only after repetitive trauma.

It is likely that very serious genital injuries, such as intravaginal tears, are more likely to result from a coercive experience. Any signs of anogenital trauma in the adolescent who denies any sexual experience should raise suspicions of possible sexual abuse or sexual assault.

There are very few studies that examine genital findings in adolescents who have been abused and attempt to correlate those findings with the frequency, duration, and timing of abuse. In one study that correlated the sexual act with genital findings in sexually abused girls aged 1 to 17 years, the most common finding following penile penetration in prepubertal and adolescent girls was a hymenal tear (52). In another study of 204 sexually abused girls aged 9 to 17 years, with a mean age of 13, who gave a clear history of penile-vaginal penetration, the most common findings were complete hymenal transections, seen in 8%, and hymenal notches (defined as sudden narrowings of the hymen to less than 1 mm in width), seen in 25%. These were most often found in the lower half of the hymen. Genital injury was seen in 69% of adolescents seen within 3 days after the assault and in only 15% seen more than 6 months after the assault (53).

### Significance of a Normal Examination in the Female Patient

As with prepubertal children, adolescents who have been sexually victimized often have normal examinations. In the Adams and Knudson study of adolescent girls with a clear history of penile-vaginal penetration (but no outside corroboration), 31% of the patients examined within 3 days of the assault had normal examinations, and 85% examined more than 6 months after the assault had normal examinations.

There are multiple reasons for normal findings in the sexually assaulted adolescent female. Like prepubertal girls, adolescents may think they have experienced vaginal penetration but instead may have been fondled or experienced vulvar coitus without attempted intravaginal penetration. If there was penetration, the estrogenized adolescent hymen, due to its relative elasticity, may not tear with vaginal penetration. If there were tears, it is often difficult to distinguish normal convolutions from healed tears. Although tears that extend through the hymenal rim result in a permanent discontinuity in the hymenal edge, evidence of this requires careful examination which may be difficult to perform.

### Signs of Injury in the Male Patient

The prevalence of anal and rectal injury following consensual or forced sodomy is not well documented. Erythema is a nonspecific finding. Fissures can be seen following sodomy but are also a normal finding. Reflex anal dilatation is more likely to occur with repeated acts of sodomy, although this finding is also seen with chronic constipation. Rectal tears and rectal bleeding are more associated with forced anal intercourse.

### Significance of a Normal Examination in the Male Patient

In studies of boys who have been sexually assaulted, most examinations either have nonspecific findings or are normal. The same is likely the case for adolescent males.

## DIAGNOSIS AND TREATMENT OF STDS

Adolescents are uniquely vulnerable to STDs. Sexually active adolescents have higher rates of STD than any other age group. A greater percentage of adolescents are sexually active now than several decades ago. In the 1995 Youth Behavior Risk Survey conducted by the CDC, more than two thirds of high-school seniors reported having had intercourse by their senior year of high school, and more than 15% had at least four partners up to that point (37). These percentages are even higher for adolescents who are not in school. Up to one third of the STDs reported annually occurs in adolescents, and it is estimated that at least 25% of adolescents will develop an STD before graduating from high school (33). In the past 10 years, these observations have resulted in STD screening guidelines for adolescents issued by the American Medical Association and the American Academy of Pediatrics (54,55). These guidelines include yearly PAP smears and syphilis, chlamydial infection, gonorrhea, and human immunodeficiency virus (HIV) testing. Recently, twice-yearly screening for chlamydial infection has been recommended for inner-city youth (56).

Despite heightened awareness and recommended screening guidelines, adolescents remain uniquely vulnerable to STDs. The younger the adolescent, the higher is the risk of acquiring an STD (57,58). Cognitive, behavioral, and biologic factors are all important. Adolescents' understanding of STDs is limited. They often do not understand the high prevalence of asymptomatic disease or the relative risk of transmission, and may not seek care unless they are sympto-

matic. Even if they understand STDs, they may underestimate their own personal risk and engage in high-risk behavior, assuming that they are somehow invincible.

In addition, there is a biologic vulnerability. In prepubertal girls, *Chlamydia* and *Neisseria gonorrhoeae* typically infect the vaginal mucosa, and vaginitis results. In pubertal or postpubertal girls, the more acidic vaginal environment prevents vaginal colonization by these organisms. However, the adolescent cervix is uniquely susceptible to chlamydial infection and gonorrhea. With pubertal maturation, the columnar cells lining the endometrium and the cervical canal extend onto the face of the cervix, forming a ring of "ectopy" surrounding the cervical os. This ectopy is prominent during adolescence and becomes less so during later adult years. Since the *N. gonorrhoeae* and *Chlamydia* organisms preferentially attach to this columnar epithelium and not the squamous epithelium, there is a higher chance of infection following exposure in the adolescent patient (59,60). In addition, cervical ectopy may pose an increased risk of HIV acquisition due to the increased vascularity and consequent vulnerability to trauma following intercourse (60).

In addition to having more prominent cervical ectopy, the adolescent cervix has a prominent squamocolumnar junction. This junction, also called the transitional zone, is the boundary between the squamous and columnar cells on the cervix. It is characterized by a high rate of cellular turnover and transformation from squamous to columnar epithelium. This so-called transformation zone is more susceptible to infection with human papillomavirus (58).

Testing and treatment for STDs are a critical part of the care of the adolescent sexual assault victim. The following points must be considered (see also Table 6-1):

1. Any prior sexual experience, consensual or coercive, can lead to infection.
2. The adolescent who has engaged in prior consensual sexual activity may be reluctant to disclose this.
3. Adolescents have a relatively high incidence and prevalence of STDs. Many are

**TABLE 6-1.** *Characteristics of sexually transmitted diseases*

| Disease | Transmission/risk after sexual assault[a] | Incubation | Percentage asymptomatic |
|---|---|---|---|
| Trichomoniasis | 85%–30% (m to f > f to m) | 5–28 d | Women 25%–50% Men >50% |
| Chlamydia | 30%–70% (m to f > f to m) | 7–21 d | Women 2/3 Men 1/3 |
| Gonorrhea | 20%–90% (m to f > f to m) | 1–14 d | Women 20%–80% Men <20% |
| Syphilis | 30%–60% | 10–90 d (chancre) 1–6 mo (rash) | >90% |
| HPV | 60%–70% | 1.5–20 mo | >90% |
| HSV-2 | Probably <5% | 3–14 d | >90% |
| Hepatitis B | Probably <5% | 45–160 d (average 120 d) | >90% |
| HIV | Probably <5% | 3–6 mo | >90% |

HIV, human immunodeficiency virus; HPV, human papillomavirus; HSV, herpes simplex virus.
[a]Risk depends on type of sexuality activity, number of sexual acts, concurrent sexually transmitted diseases (65).

undiagnosed due to the relatively high rate of asymptomatic infection and inadequate screening of patients at risk.

4. Specific testing and prophylactic treatment may be tailored to the patient's history to the extent that the history is reliable. For instance, if there is no mucosa-to-mucosa contact or exchange of bodily fluids, as in fondling, then testing for STDs may not be needed if the patient is asymptomatic.

5. Knowledge of the incubation periods of the various STDs will help the physician tailor the specific STD tests based on the time elapsed since the assault.

6. In most patients, testing for chlamydia, gonorrhea, and trichomoniasis is performed.

7. For asymptomatic patients seen several months after an assault, testing should also include serologies for HIV and syphilis, and a Pap smear.

8. Some have recommended that in an acute evidentiary examination, the routine testing of asymptomatic patients is not needed. Positive findings are frequently interpreted as an indication that there was prior sexual activity (which is not necessarily true), and this could be used against the patient in court (61). This point notwithstanding, many centers perform these tests in asymptomatic patients receiving an evidentiary examination. It is important to remember that a positive

gonorrheal or chlamydial culture in an asymptomatic patient is just as likely to be from a recently deposited vaginal specimen (i.e., from the assault) that has not had a chance to become symptomatic.

9. Recent research has suggested that self-collection of introital specimens may be as sensitive as cervical specimens for detection of trichomoniasis and bacterial vaginosis, and that urine-based testing for chlamydial and gonorrheal infection is more sensitive than endocervical sampling. Hence, for those patients without signs or symptoms of intravaginal injury or upper tract genital infection, the speculum exam may not be needed for STD testing in the acute setting (64).

10. For patients seen in the acute setting, the need for additional follow-up testing either in that setting or in the primary care office should be discussed. This is particularly important for patients with infections with relatively long incubation periods, e.g., syphilis, human papillomavirus infection, and HIV.

11. In the acute situation following attempted or actual penile penetration of the mouth, the vagina, or the rectum, the CDC guidelines for treatment following sexual assault should be followed: ceftriaxone, 125 mg IM, plus metronidazole, 2 g PO, plus azithromycin, 1 g PO, or doxycycline, 100 mg PO b.i.d. for 7 days (64a).

12. In nonacute situations, there are no firm guidelines on whether to test and treat or to test and wait for results in the asymptomatic patient. The physician should base the decision on patient compliance and willingness regarding follow-up.

13. In nonacute situations, if patients have signs or symptoms suggestive of specific STDs, treatment should be initiated before test results are back, and the examiner should screen for additional STDs, specifically, chlamydial infection, gonorrhea, syphilis, HIV, and, possibly, hepatitis B or hepatitis C.

There are now more than 30 distinct sexually transmitted or transmissible pathogens (65). The most common infections are discussed below.

## Chlamydia and Gonorrhea

### Epidemiology and Clinical Presentation

Chlamydial infection is the most common bacterial STD in adolescents. The prevalence among males has been estimated at 5% to 20%; in females, 10% to 25%. The higher numbers apply in inner-city schools and STD clinics. Gonorrhea is not as common as chlamydial infection, but is still prevalent in sexually active adolescents. Overall rates of gonorrheal infection have been declining in the United States, though not as quickly for adolescents as for older populations.

There is considerable overlap in the signs and symptoms of chlamydial and gonorrheal infection. For both there is a high rate of asymptomatic infection. For both, the most common clinical presentations are vaginal discharge, mucopurulent cervicitis, and pelvic inflammatory disease in the female and urethritis in the male. Both can cause epididymitis, the male equivalent of pelvic inflammatory disease. Both gonorrheal and chlamydial organisms may cause a perihepatitis infection, known as Fitz-Hugh—Curtis syndrome. Typically these patients are ill appearing and have sharp, pleuritic, right upper quadrant pain. However, lesser degrees of symptomatology may also be present. Both gonorrheal and chlamydial infections can cause proctitis in homosexual men and in heterosexual women who practice anorectal intercourse. Such individuals may present with symptoms of tenesmus, rectal pain, and bloody or purulent rectal discharge. The rate of asymptomatic infection is high (66).

Pharyngeal infections with *Chlamydia* and *N. gonorrhoeae* occur, but are usually asymptomatic. The prevalence depends on the population studied. Pharyngeal infection with *Chlamydia* was found in 1% of adolescents attending an adolescent clinic (65). The prevalence of pharyngeal gonococcal infection ranges from 3% to 25%, the latter figure applying to active homosexuals. Gonococcal infection of the pharynx is a primary cause of disseminated gonococcal infection; hence, it should be treated, even in asymptomatic individuals. Chlamydial infection in the pharynx appears to be self-limited, and in several studies has not been linked to pharyngitis.

Gonococcal infection tends to present with a shorter incubation time and more impressive signs and symptoms, whereas chlamydial infection may present in a more indolent manner. Chlamydial infection specifically can cause chronic inflammation of the upper genital tract in women with minimal signs and symptoms. These include inter-menstrual spotting and menorrhagia without signs of pelvic inflammatory disease.

### Testing

In the sexual assault victim, testing for gonorrheal and chlamydial infection should be guided by the history and the physical examination.

In general, attempted or actual penetration of a body orifice requires testing of that site for gonorrheal and chlamydial infection. The one exception is oropharygeal testing for chlamydial infection. Typically, this is not performed because of the low incidence of infection and the failure to link pharyngitis to chlamydial infection. In addition, even if there is no history of sexual contact, any signs or symptoms of vaginal, urethral, or rectal infection in a sexually assaulted adolescent should lead to testing for chlamydial and gonorrheal infection at those sites.

Several different testing methodologies have been developed for both gonorrheal and chlamydial infection. These include culture, enzyme immunoassay (EIA), direct fluorescent antibody (DFA), nucleic acid hybridization (GenProbe), and amplification of *Chlamydia* DNA or RNA by ligase chain reaction (LCX) or polymerase chain reaction (PCR). The EIA and DFA tests have unacceptably low sensitivities and specificities, especially in children, and therefore the courts have recognized culture results only for child sexual abuse cases. The performance characteristics of GenProbe are comparable to those of EIA and DFA. The LCX and PCR tests have not been tested adequately for rectal or pharyngeal screening but are excellent for cervical, urethral, and urinary sites and have specificities exceeding 99%. Recent studies have shown the urine LCX test to be superior to endocervical tests for detecting chlamydial infection, and some centers have adopted this test as the routine screen for chlamydial and gonorrheal infection in sexually active adolescents (67). In addition, one study demonstrated superior sensitivity and specificity of a self-collected introital specimen using the PCR test for chlamydial infection (68). Rectal swabs for gonorrheal and chlamydial infection ideally should be taken from the columnar epithelium in the anal columns just proximal to the pectinate–dentate line. In some adolescents, this test is very uncomfortable, and the physician may have difficulty inserting the swab far enough to reach the columnar epithelium. Hence, negative test results do not necessarily rule out the presence of anorectal chlamydial or gonorrheal infection.

### Treatment

In the absence of penile-vaginal, penile-anal, or oral-genital contact, the risk of exposure to chlamydial or gonorrheal organisms is small. Hence, if there is a history of fondling only, prophylactic treatment for these infections may not be needed. For any patient who had oral-genital, anal-genital, or genital-genital mucosal or body fluid contact, prophylactic treatment for gonorrheal and chlamydial infection should be given. This should be offered regardless of the time elapsed since the contact. The avail-

ability of one-dose oral regimens have simplified prophylaxis and ensured compliance. Specifically, administration of 400 mg of cefixime and 1 g of azithromycin ensures adequate treatment for asymptomatic or lower genital tract infections caused by *N. gonorrhoeae* and *Chlamydia,* respectively. If there is any sign of upper genital tract infection, including pelvic pain, intermenstrual spotting, or menorrhagia in the female patient, or scrotal pain in the male patient, then the longer treatment course recommended for pelvic inflammatory disease or epididymitis should be followed. In particular, outpatient treatment should include ceftriaxone (250 mg IM) or, for patients 18 or older, ciprofloxacin, for gonorrhea, and 2 weeks of doxycycline (100 mg PO b.i.d.) for chlamydial infection. More specific treatment guidelines have been summarized by the CDC.

### Follow-Up Testing

Test of cure is not recommended by the CDC. However, rescreening for both chlamydial and gonorrheal infection 1 or 2 months following an initial positive result may be indicated in teens who engage in high-risk sexual activity or who may have been re-exposed.

## Syphilis

### Epidemiology and Clinical Presentation

Syphilis is often asymptomatic. A chancre, typically painless, appears at the site of inoculation within 3 weeks of infection. This ulcer is typically 1 to 2 cm in diameter and has an indurated margin. It lasts for 3 to 6 weeks, but because it is painless and often intravaginal in women, it frequently goes unnoticed by the patient. Without treatment, the diffuse rash of secondary syphilis, typically maculopapular and involving the palms and soles, will appear, on average, 6 weeks later. Secondary syphilis is a systemic disease, and patients may have symptoms such as malaise, fever, sore throat, and lymphadenopathy. Without treatment, this rash resolves in 3 to 12 weeks. Signs and symptoms of tertiary syphilis are unusual in the adolescent patient. However, in persons infected with HIV, up to 30% may have neurosyphilis by cerebrospinal fluid analysis without any clinical signs (69). Hence, testing for HIV is important for any patient with syphilis.

### Testing

Syphilis testing should be performed on any victim of sexual abuse or assault in which there has been mucosal contact or exchange of bodily fluids. The usual screening test is the rapid plasma reagin (RPR) test. This is not as sensitive as the tests that measure antibody to surface proteins of *Treponema. pallidum* [fluorescent treponemal antibody (FTA) or *Treponema pallidum* hemoagglutination (TPHA)], so most laboratories will do this test to confirm the diagnosis of syphilis in patients with a positive RPR. Both tests should be ordered if the patient has a chancre and primary syphilis is a possibility. In such cases, the RPR is negative 20% of the time, and the FTA is negative 10% of the time and turns positive before the RPR. The preferred method for diagnosing syphilis in the patient with a chancre is examination of fluid obtained from the surface of the chancre with a darkfield microscope. The appearance of treponemes establishes the diagnosis. However, most emergency departments and clinics do not have ready access to such a microscope, and only serologic tests are performed. In cases of secondary syphilis, serologic tests are positive. HIV testing is particularly important in patients who may have syphilis because the diagnostic testing and treatment differ for the HIV-positive patient.

### Treatment

Ceftriaxone is the preferred prophylactic treatment for syphilis following sexual assault. The dosage recommended by the CDC is 125 mg. If the patient has a positive serology or has primary or secondary syphilis, then one dose of benzathine penicillin, 2.4 million units, is adequate treatment in the HIV-negative patient. If the patient has a chancre and the clinical suspicion for syphilis is high, then the patient should be given penicillin without waiting for the serology results. If the patient has positive serologies

and no history or prior negative tests or prior syndromes suggestive of syphilis, then it must be assumed that the infection is potentially of more than 1 year's duration, and treatment with three separate weekly shots of benzathine penicillin is recommended. In addition, patients who have HIV are at risk for treatment failure and for asymptomatic neurosyphilis. Consultation with an infectious disease expert should be obtained in such cases.

### Follow-up Testing

Since the incubation period for syphilis can be as long as 3 months, repeat testing should be considered if the initial screen was negative and the sexual assault happened within the previous 3 months. For patients who do have positive serologies, serial testing every 3 months following treatment should be performed for at least a year to assess treatment response.

## Human Immunodeficiency Virus

### Epidemiology and Clinical Presentation

Adolescents are at substantial risk for HIV infection. From 1993 to 1995, the increase in acquired immunodeficiency syndrome (AIDS) cases among 15- to 19-year-olds was 177% greater than the rate of diagnosis for the previous 5 years. During the same period, the rate of diagnosis for older individuals increased by 122% (58). AIDS statistics do not adequately capture the importance of HIV infection in adolescents because most adolescents with HIV infection are asymptomatic, and the average time from HIV acquisition to the diagnosis of AIDS is at least 10 years (60).

Although most victims of child sexual abuse do not acquire HIV either as children or as adults, adolescent patients who are infected with HIV have a very high incidence of childhood sexual abuse. In addition, adolescents who engage in anal intercourse are at increased risk for HIV. Since male adolescents who are sexually abused are most likely to be victims of sodomy, this subgroup is at particularly high risk of HIV infection. HIV infection following receptive oral exposure to ejaculate has also been reported but appears to be rare (70,71).

### *Testing*

HIV testing should be considered in any adolescent sexual abuse or sexual assault victim. The testing requires written informed consent in most states and should be performed with appropriate pretest counseling. If the patient is unable to provide informed consent, then HIV testing should not be performed unless the patient is developmentally challenged and the guardian requests the testing. If the patient is unable to return for posttest counseling, then HIV testing should not be performed. Also, if the patient states that he or she would commit suicide if infected, the test should be postponed. In most states, parental consent is not required for HIV testing. In Connecticut when parental consent requirements were dropped, the requests for HIV testing doubled, reflecting the concerns teens may have in letting their parents know they are being tested (71a). HIV test results should be delivered in person with appropriate posttest counseling.

HIV testing using the enzyme-linked immunosorbent assay (ELISA) screening test performed shortly after an assault will not reflect infection acquired from the assault because antibody response to the infection takes several weeks to develop. Moreover, it can take up to 6 months for seroconversion to occur after initial infection. Hence, patients seen immediately following sexual assault need to be advised that repeat testing at 3 and 6 months may be appropriate. HIV testing may be offered in the acute setting with the understanding that positive results may not be related to a recent sexual encounter.

If the patient is seen in the nonacute setting, HIV testing should be offered with the same stipulations: informed consent, ability to follow up, appropriate counseling, and no expressions of suicidal thoughts.

### *Treatment*

Risk of seroconversion following percutaneous exposure to blood for an infected individual is about 0.3%, and less following mucous membrane exposure (including contact with bodily fluids) (72). Hence, uniform postexposure prophylaxis following sexual assault is controversial. However, since postexposure prophylaxis is very effective, it should be considered in circumstances where the perpetrator is known to be HIV positive or at presumed high risk for HIV (71). The risk of HIV transmission increases with receptive anal intercourse, with mucosal tears or bleeding, and with ulcerative STD syndromes. These should also be factored into the decision making. Finally, the patient may request HIV prophylaxis following sexual assault, and this should be honored. The fear of contracting HIV following sexual assault is considerable; one study of adult women survivors of rape found that 40% feared contracting HIV from the rape (71,73).

The value of prophylaxis declines rapidly following the initial several hours following exposure and is negligible after 72 hours. The CDC has formulated guidelines for postexposure prophylaxis for health care workers, and these can be used for victims of sexual assault if appropriate (74). For adolescents specifically, compliance issues may be significant, and prophylaxis should not be offered unless there is a reasonable guarantee of good compliance.

### *Follow-up Testing*

It can take up to 6 months following exposure and initial infection for a serologic response to yield a positive ELISA and Western blot test. Hence, any negative tests in this interval should be followed with additional testing at 6, 12, and 24 weeks after the assault.

### Trichomoniasis and Bacterial Vaginosis

#### *Epidemiology and Clinical Presentation*

In one review of adult female victims, trichomoniasis and bacterial vaginosis were the most commonly acquired infections following sexual assault (62). The most common symptoms associated with trichomoniasis are dysuria and urethral or vaginal discharge, although in sexually active males and females up to 60% of trichomoniasis infections may be asymptomatic.

The incubation period for trichomoniasis is 5 to 28 days, so tests done shortly after the assault will likely reflect previous sexual activity. The most commonly used test for trichomoniasis is the wet mount microscopic examination of vaginal discharge, although this test has a sensitivity of only 60%. *Trichomonas* can also be detected in urinalysis. The spun urine sample increases the yield, and its sensitivity is almost as good as the vaginal swab. In addition, the spun urine may show *Trichomonas* when the wet prep is negative (75). *Trichomonas* culture kits are available, but are not used routinely at most centers.

Bacterial vaginosis is limited to female patients; there is no pathogen yet identified in male partners. This infection is more common in sexually active adolescents but can also be found in patients who have never had sexual intercourse (76). Hence, its significance in a legal sense is limited. Most commonly, the patient with bacterial vaginosis complains of a fishy odor, particularly around the menses or following sexual intercourse. The diagnosis rests on a combination of physical exam and laboratory findings. A thin gray vaginal discharge, a fishy odor (particularly with KOH applied to the discharge), and the presence of clue cells on the wet mount all support the diagnosis. Recent studies suggest that patient-applied vaginal swabs yield detection rates for trichomoniasis and bacterial vaginosis at rates comparable to those of physician-obtained vaginal swabs during a speculum exam (77).

### Treatment

Treatment with metronidazole can be offered to the acute sexual assault victim. A single dose of 2 g is adequate treatment for trichomoniasis and for most cases of bacterial vaginosis. A 7-day course of metronidazole is as effective for trichomoniasis and more effective for bacterial vaginosis. Some patients experience nausea after taking the single dose of metronidazole. In addition, significant emesis may result in patients who take this medication within 24 hours of alcohol ingestion. For both reasons, it may be appropriate to delay treatment until the follow-up visit. Metronidazole vaginal cream or clindamycin cream may be used for bacterial vaginosis, but neither has demonstrated efficacy for trichomoniasis.

### Follow-up Testing

Follow-up testing and treatment should be performed only if there are clinical signs or symptoms of infection.

### Human Papillomavirus

### Epidemiology and Clinical Presentation

Human papillomavirus (HPV) is the most common STD in the United States (58). In a review of the medical literature from 1988 to 1998 on STDs in sexually abused children and adolescents, one of the most striking observations was the increased diagnosis of condyloma acuminatum and HPV infection over that time span (78). Additional studies have shown a high prevalence of abnormal Pap smears in both inner-city and suburban youth (79). Genital HPV infection is also common in men.

Most HPV transmission occurs via receptive vaginal or anal intercourse. Both complete and attempted penetration pose a significant risk for transmission. Although oral infection may occur following oral-genital sex, this is typically asymptomatic. Digital transmission may occur but is not common in pubertal or postpubertal individuals. It is not known whether condoms prevent transmission of HPV, though infection is correlated with number of sexual partners and earlier age of sexual activity.

The two primary clinical manifestations of HPV infection are squamous intraepithelial lesions of the cervix and genital warts. Cervical dysplasia is relatively common in adolescents, reflecting not only increased possible exposure (higher number of sexual partners) but also the vulnerability of the cervix due to cellular turnover in the transformation zone. Cervical lesions almost never yield symptoms, but 20% will progress to invasive cervical cancer over a several-year period. Genital warts may be found on the vulva, vagina, penis, or perianal area.

They are much less common than cervical lesions and may or may not be apparent to the patient. Hence, the adolescent with cervical dysplasia or genital warts may be totally unaware that he or she is infected.

### Testing

The Pap smear is the primary screening tool for cervical HPV infection; comparable screening tools for penile or anal HPV infection have not been developed. Although the Pap smear is recommended annually for sexually active adolescents, it is underutilized in the adolescent population. Most adolescents do not appreciate the need or rationale for routine Pap smears. Moreover, many health care providers do not appreciate the importance of annual Pap smear screening in sexually active adolescents (80). Although the risk of HPV infection following sexual assault and sexual abuse is significant, many sexual assault protocols fail to mention the need for follow-up Pap smears.

Unlike tests for chlamydial infection, gonorrhea, trichomoniasis, and bacterial vaginosis, the Pap smear requires a speculum examination. In patients who refuse the speculum exam, there are no other ways to assess cervical infection. Since the incubation for HPV infection is up to 3 months, a Pap smear is not important in the acute setting. Moreover, due to follow-up issues, the Pap smear is not typically performed in emergency departments. However, due to the high prevalence of HPV and the relatively high incidence of abnormal Pap smears in adolescents, the Pap smear should be performed on victims of attempted or completed vaginal or anal penetration within 3 to 6 months of the initial assault. Patients should be alerted to this at the time of the initial evaluation.

### Treatment and Follow-up

There is no prophylaxis for HPV infection. Patients who present with condyloma acuminatum can be treated with patient-applied imiquimod cream (Aldara) or podofilox. The provider also can apply trichloroacetic acid (TCA) or topical podophyllin. Since podophyllin should not be used during pregnancy, Aldara and TCA are preferred treatments for adolescent patients. Follow-up and retreatment may be needed on a weekly or biweekly basis, and referral to a gynecologist is important if the condyloma does not respond to treatment within 6 weeks. Patients with large condyloma may need referral to gynecology for cryosurgery or laser treatment.

Patients with mildly abnormal Pap smears require repeat smears in 3 to 6 months and referral for colposcopy if the abnormalities persist. Patients with more significant abnormalities should be referred for colposcopy.

## Herpes Simplex Virus

### Epidemiology and Clinical Presentation

There are two antigenic types of herpes simplex virus (HSV). Type 1 is more often associated with oral infection, but it can also cause genital infection; type 2 is more often associated with genital infection, but it can also cause oral infection. Genital HSV-1 infections have been reported with increasing frequency, perhaps a reflection of increasing oral-genital sexual practices. In both the population as a whole and in adolescents, the prevalence of genital herpes has increased markedly in the past 30 years (60).

The most common clinical presentation is the genital ulcer. In first episodes of infection, these ulcers are typically extensive and very painful; in addition, these episodes are typically associated with fever and malaise. Subsequent clinical relapses are usually less painful. Although the risk of transmission is highest with exposure to ulcerative lesions, shedding of the virus can occur in asymptomatic individuals, particularly in the few days preceding and the few days following active ulceration.

The differential diagnosis for herpes simplex genital ulcers includes syphilis, chancroid, lymphogranuloma venereum, and granuloma inguinale. Unlike the ulcers associated with syphilis, the herpetic ulcer is typically shallow, painful, and without indurated edges. With chancroid, the ulcer is painful and lasts longer than the 7 to 10 days seen with HSV. With lymphogranuloma venereum, the ulcer is transient, lasting only a few days, and not very painful, but followed by severe pain and enlargement of inguinal lymph nodes. With granuloma inguinale, the ulcer becomes larger and deeper over many months. Chancroid and lymphogranuloma venereum are seen in adolescents in the United States but are not common.

### Testing

HSV testing should be considered with any genital ulcerative lesion. A viral culture from the base of a new lesion is the only definitive way to diagnose HSV infection. Neither the Tzanck preparation nor serologic tests are helpful in acute disease (58).

### Treatment

The primary treatment modality for ulcerative genital herpes is acyclovir. Various treatment regimens are recommended for acute and recurrent disease. These are summarized in the CDC's most recent STD treatment guidelines. Since the treatment of genital ulcers associated with herpes simplex is not curative and the treatment of the ulcerative syphilitic chancre is curative, it is important for the physician to check for syphilis, even if he or she suspects herpes, and treat for syphilis if there is a reasonable degree of uncertainty.

### Follow-up

No specific testing is needed in follow-up once HSV infection has been diagnosed and syphilis ruled out. If the patient has recurrent herpetic outbreaks, suppressive therapy with daily acyclovir should be offered as outlined by the CDC.

## Hepatitis B

### Epidemiology and Clinical Presentation

Hepatitis A, B, C, and D can all be transmitted sexually, some more so than others. The most significant pathogen in sexual abuse and sexual assault is hepatitis B. Although it is most often transmitted by inapparent percutaneous or mucosal exposure, it is associated with vaginal and anal intercourse. Most cases are asymptomatic, and up to one third are associated with self-limited acute hepatitis that appears 40 to 100 days following exposure. One percent of patients will develop acute hepatitic failure and of these 75% will die. Chronic hepatitis B occurs in approximately 5% of cases. This, in turn, is associated with subsequent primary carcinoma of the liver. The risk of transmission following exposure is significantly higher for hepatitis B than for HIV.

### Testing

Serologic testing usually allows the physician to distinguish between acute, subacute, resolved, and chronic infection. In approximately 5% of cases, hepatitis B can lead to chronic infection, characterized by a positive hepatitis B surface antigen and no antibody to hepatitis B surface antibody. In the remainder, hepatitis B infection is cleared and there is no hepatitis B surface antigen but there are hepatitis B surface and core antibodies. The process of resolution or progression to a chronic infection can take up to 6 months. In patients who have been immunized, there is antibody only to hepatitis B surface antigen and not to the core antigen.

### Treatment and Follow-up

With the introduction of hepatitis B vaccine more than 10 years ago and the recent adoption of universal vaccination guidelines, most adolescents who have received preventative health care have been vaccinated against hepatitis B. This offers considerable protection against acquiring hepatitis B following sexual abuse or sexual assault, and persons who have completed the vaccination series do not need any preventative treatment following possible exposure. Recommendations vary regarding the appropriate management of the patient with no clear history of receiving or completing the vaccination series. The American Academy of Pediatrics recommends giving the hepatitis B vaccine as soon as possible. In addition, if the alleged offender is known or suspected to have hepatitis B, then hepatitis B immune globulin should also be given, since it is 75%

effective in preventing infection. There are no firm guidelines regarding maximum time interval following exposure, but the hepatitis B immunoglobulin should be given preferably within 14 days after exposure (81). The CDC guidelines for treatment following sexual assault do not mention hepatitis B prophylaxis. Sexual assault centers vary in their approach. As more and more adolescents become immunized in childhood, postexposure prophylaxis will become less important over time.

## EVIDENTIARY LABORATORY TESTS

If the examination is performed within 72 hours of the sexual assault, various tests may be administered as a part of the rape kit. Meticulous attention to detail and documentation are needed, and a standardized form and protocol are used. Care must be exercised to maintain the "chain of evidence." These tests are discussed further in other chapters.

## PREGNANCY TESTS

Any female adolescent who has been sexually victimized may be at risk for pregnancy. The following points should be considered:

1. Adolescents who have not yet had menses may still be at risk for pregnancy, although this is unusual.
2. Adolescents who report regular menses should have a pregnancy test because menses occasionally will occur in a regular fashion in early pregnancy.
3. Adolescents who have had vulvar coitus without vaginal penetration may still be at risk for pregnancy.
4. For adolescents who have a history of consensual and coercive sexual experiences, it may be difficult to ascribe a positive pregnancy test to a specific event, unless there is a significant time interval between them.
5. Any female adolescent being evaluated following sexual assault should undergo a pregnancy test.
6. A pregnancy test should be performed on any female adolescent with delayed menses, vaginal bleeding, pelvic pain, or vaginal discharge.

Pregnancy may be diagnosed by a urine test or a serum test. The urine test detects a pregnancy as early as 12 days after conception, whereas a serum test detects a pregnancy as early as 8 days after conception.

If patients are seen within 72 hours of a sexual assault, emergency contraception should be offered. This method involves two large doses of oral contraceptives given 12 hours apart. It decreases the risk of pregnancy by up to 75%. Nausea occurs in up to 80% of patients and emesis in up to 25% of patients, so an antiemetic should be offered if this treatment is prescribed. In addition, a urine pregnancy test should be performed prior to administration, and a follow-up visit should be scheduled for 2 to 3 weeks.

## REPORTING SEXUAL ABUSE AND ASSAULT

All states require the physician to report sexual abuse to a child protection agency. Beyond this, generalizations are difficult because state laws vary considerably. In some states, there is a statute of limitations whereby child abuse that occurred beyond a certain time frame does not need to be reported. In other states there is no statute of limitations. For some states, there is mandatory reporting to child protection if a teen younger than a certain age, typically 12 or 13, is diagnosed with an STD (34). In other states, there is no lower limit, and the health care provider must exercise judgment in deciding whether given circumstances warrant a report to child protection. In some states, suspicion of domestic violence requires the physician to report to the police. In some states, suspicion of domestic violence requires the physician to refer the patient for mental health and/or social services.

The reporting guidelines for statutory rape also vary widely. In some states, statutory rape need not be reported unless it is due to parental neglect. In other states, this may require reporting to child protection or the police.

## MENTAL AND SOCIAL CONSEQUENCES OF SEXUAL ASSAULT AND SEXUAL ABUSE

### Acute Mental Health Needs

Crisis counseling should be offered to all adolescent victims seen acutely following sexual assault. Crisis counseling also should be offered to the parents of the adolescent. Studies have shown that adolescents' most immediate concerns following rape are fears of bodily harm, shame, and fears of pregnancy and STDs (58,82). In providing counseling, issues of safety should be addressed. If the adolescent is suicidal, he or she should be admitted. If the adolescent seeks care alone, without the company of a parent, the adolescent should be discharged only if there is a responsible adult who can be with him or her and provide comfort and monitoring. After discharge, a follow-up phone call should be made within 24 hours and a follow-up visit should be scheduled within 1 week. Supportive counseling should be arranged if needed.

In addition to acute mental health needs, more than 80% of adolescent victims may experience reactions similar to posttraumatic stress syndrome, with long-term hypervigilance, avoidance, and flashbacks. In a study of adolescent rape victims, Felice et al. described a sequence of behaviors whereby rape was followed by phobias, denial, and psychosomatic complaints (83).

### Long-Term Mental Health Consequences

The adolescent who experienced sexual abuse as a child may not suffer apparent mental health consequences until adolescence, with its attendant sexual identity formation (84,85). After a "denial-numbing latency period," often extending for many years, the adolescent may suffer symptoms consistent with posttraumatic stress syndrome. In a study comparing depressed adolescents with and without a history of sexual abuse, Brand et al. found that posttraumatic stress syndrome was much more common in those with a history of sexual abuse and that chronicity and severity of abuse were strongly correlated with the risk of developing posttraumatic stress syndrome symptoms (86).

Depression and suicidal ideation are also linked to a history of sexual abuse. In a study of attempted suicide in gay and bisexual youth, Remafedi et al. found that suicide attempters were more likely to have a history of sexual abuse (87). In the 1997 Commonwealth Fund Survey of Adolescent Girls, it was found that adolescent girls with a history of physical or sexual abuse were twice as likely to have depressive symptoms or low self-esteem as adolescent girls without this history (6). The same survey found that a history of sexual abuse was an especially strong risk factor for depression in adolescent boys. In another study of 5,780 students in the 7th through 12th grades, self-reported physical or sexual abuse was associated with an increased relative risk of considering or attempting suicide (88). A study by Riggs et al. found by anonymous survey that high-school students with a history of sexual abuse were more than three times as likely to attempt suicide (89). Eating disorders are also more common in adolescents with a history of sexual abuse (6,88).

The long-term mental health consequences of childhood sexual abuse underscore the importance of longitudinal and comprehensive primary care. If the child is seen in the urgent care setting, it is appropriate to ask the parent to sign a release of information so that the primary care physician can be notified. The primary care physician can then provide more frequent monitoring of mental health and psychosocial needs, particularly as the child enters puberty.

In addition, the co-occurrence of childhood sexual abuse and subsequent somatization, anxiety disorders, and depressive symptomatology argues for the provision of integrated medical and mental health services for the adolescent patient.

### Behavioral and Psychosocial Consequences

The behavioral and psychosocial consequences of child and adolescent sexual victimization are far reaching (Fig. 6-6). Some of the more significant consequences are outlined below.

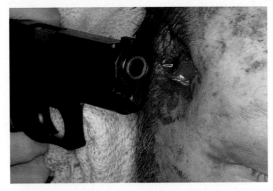

**FIG. 4-9B.** Forceful expansion of the skin overlying the right temple resulted in a muzzle contusion from the barrel of a 9-mm semi-automatic handgun.

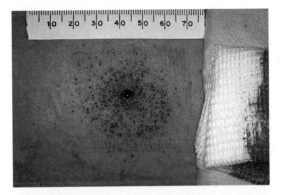

**FIG. 4-12A.** "Tattooing" is the result of partially burned or unburned gunpowder impacting skin. The "tattoos" are punctate abrasions and are associated with an intermediate-range gunshot wound. Tattooing has been seen with wounds as close as 1 cm and as far away as 1 m.

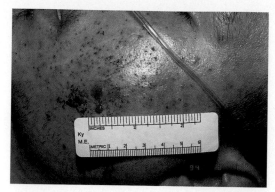

**FIG. 4-12B.** This patient stated that he was shot with a .22 caliber handgun at a distance of 12 in. His cheek exhibited punctate abrasions or "tattooing" associated with intermediate-range gunshot wounds.

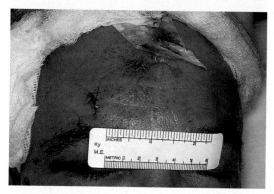

**FIG. 4-12C.** Forehead "tattooing" from an intermediate-range gunshot wound. The patient reported he was shot with a .38 caliber revolver from a distance of 18 in.

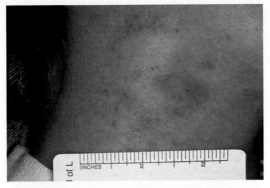

**FIG. 4-29C.** Horseshoe-shaped petechial hemorrhage with central clearing is associated with pressure applied by the pad of the finger. This victim of sexual assault displayed two horseshoe-shaped contusions with petechial hemorrhage with central clearing on the lateral aspect of her neck.

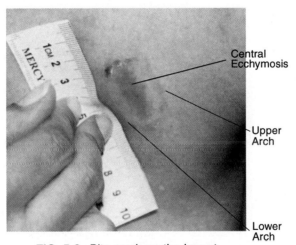

**FIG. 5-3.** Bite mark on the breast.

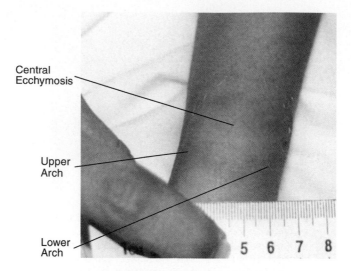

Central Ecchymosis

Upper Arch

Lower Arch

5 6 7 8

**FIG. 5-4.** Bite mark on the wrist.

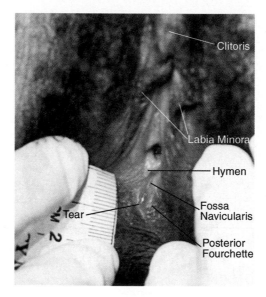

Clitoris

Labia Minora

Hymen

Tear

Fossa Navicularis

Posterior Fourchette

**FIG. 5-5.** Tear to posterior fourchette. Female Tanner 4 sexual assault patient.

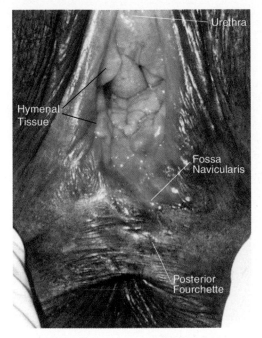

FIG. 5-6. Female sexual assault victim Tanner 5 before toluidine blue dye testing.

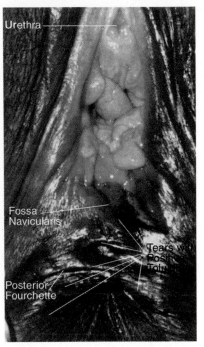

FIG. 5-7. Female sexual assault victim Tanner 5 after toluidine blue dye testing.

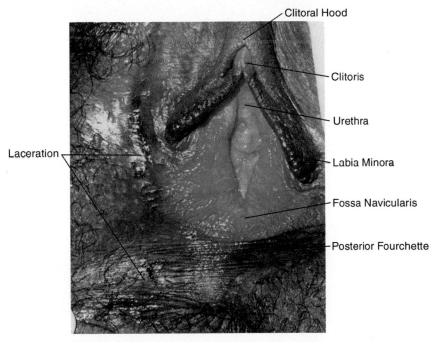

FIG. 5-8. Female sexual assault victim Tanner 5 after toluidine blue dye testing.

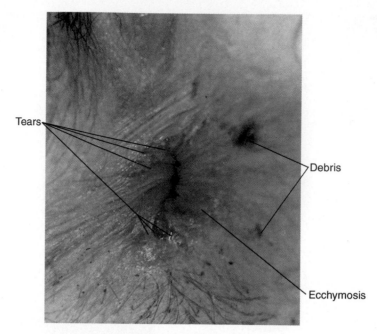

**FIG. 5-9.** Anal trauma in a female with a history of anal penetration.

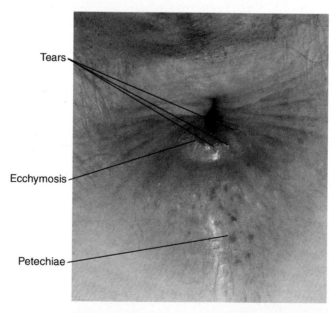

**FIG. 5-10.** Anal trauma in a female with history of anal penetration.

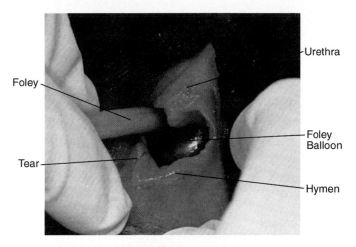

**FIG. 5-12.** Use of a Foley balloon to show hymen tear on a 14-year-old sexual assault patient.

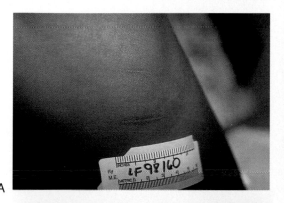

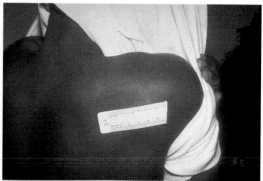

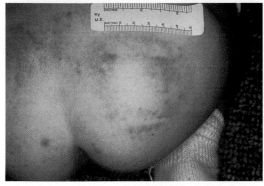

**FIG. 7-1.** Pattern injuries. **A:** A looped-belt injury. **B:** Another looped-belt injury. **C:** A fly-swatter injury. Note the square pattern produced from two overlapping blows through a diaper. (Courtesy of Chief Medical Examiner's Office, Louisville, Kentucky.)

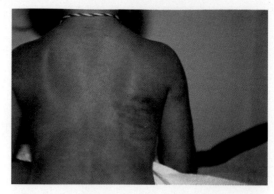

**FIG. 7-2.** Hand-slap mark. Note parallel linear contusions with central sparing that highlight the imprint of fingers. (Courtesy of Dr. William Smock, University of Louisville School of Medicine.)

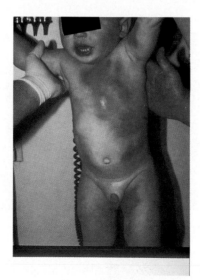

**FIG. 7-3.** A V-shaped scald burn caused by hot liquid cooling as it poured down this child's body. This scald caused both first- and second-degree burns. (Courtesy of Chief Medical Examiner's Office, Louisville, Kentucky.)

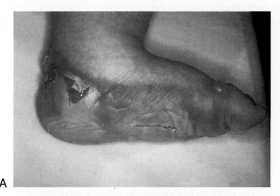

A

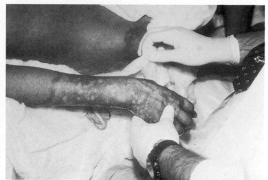

B

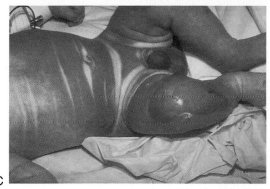

C

**FIG. 7-4.** Immersion burns. **A:** Immersion or "dunk" burn caused by dipping foot in hot liquid. Note the clear delineation of burned and normal skin along with the uniform degree of burn (here a second-degree burn) throughout the burn distribution. **B:** Immersion burn caused by dipping infant in hot liquid. **C:** Note where skin folds protected underlying tissue from serious burn. (Courtesy of Dr. William Smock, University of Louisville School of Medicine.)

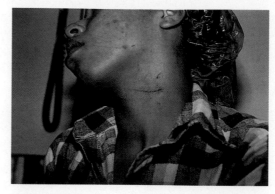

**FIG. 9-6.** Patterned, fingernail-like scratch abrasions to right lateral neck from strangulation mechanism of injury.

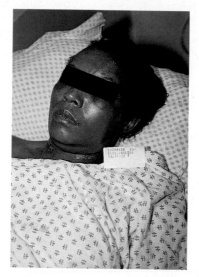

**FIG. 9-7.** Patterned, punch-like abrasion from a ring with stone to the mid-forehead; sutured partial avulsion injury to the nose; punch-like contusion to the left eye involving the sclera; and strangulation-related abrasions to the neck.

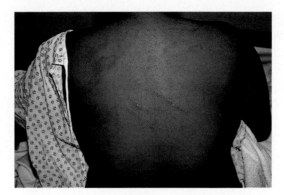

**FIG. 9-8.** Newer, patterned, looped, cord-like contusions to the right upper posterior shoulder and left lower posterior shoulder; patterned, looped, cord-like scar to the right mid-lateral back; patterned, scabbed, cord-like abrasions to the mid-back; patterned, kick/stomp heel-like contusion to the left mid-back; and patterned foot kick/stomp-like, with heel imprint and sole imprint to upper left posterior, superior shoulder.

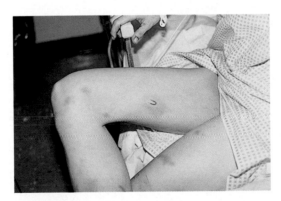

**FIG. 9-9.** Patterned, punch-like contusion to right medial thigh with a patterned imprint abrasion from ring with a stone; patterned, fingertip-like contusions to right medial knee and left anterior medial thigh from a reported marital rape.

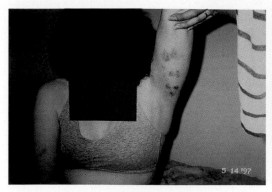

**FIG. 9-10.** Multiple, patterned, fingertip-like contusions to the left upper arm.

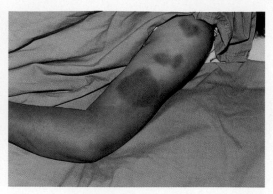

**FIG. 9-11.** Multiple, patterned, punch-like contusions to the left upper arm.

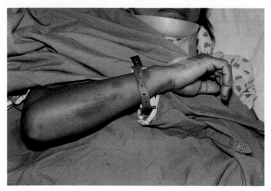

**FIG. 9-12.** Patterned, defensive posture-like contusions to ulnar surface of the left arm.

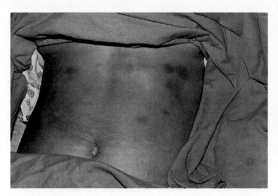

**FIG. 9-14.** Patterned, hidden, punch-like contusions to the upper abdomen, lower anterior chest.

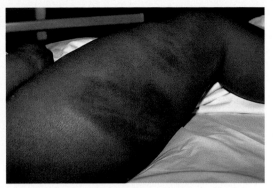

**FIG. 9-16.** Patterned, foot kick/stomp-like contusion to the right, superior lateral thigh pushing blood outward from the point of impact and patterned, foot kick/stomp-like contusion to the right inferior lateral thigh.

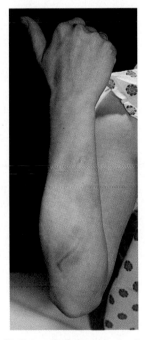

**FIG. 9-13.** Patterned, defensive posture-like contusions to the right lower arm.

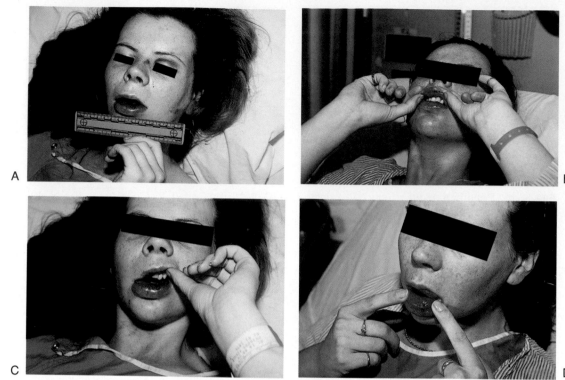

**FIG. 9-17.** Series of four photographs to illustrate how photographs can be used to demonstrate mechanisms of injuries. **A:** Victim has obvious facial trauma to her left eyelid, left lateral nose, and mouth. The left lateral nose contusion was caused by the nosepiece of her glasses being forcefully pushed into the nose from a punch injury to left eye. The patient's glasses absorbed much of the punch force and were broken (not pictured). Hence, the actual trauma to her left eye was limited to left upper eyelid. A second punch produced the mouth trauma. **B:** The force of the punch caused the upper teeth to leave patterned contusion, abrasion, and minor laceration trauma to oral mucosa. **C:** A few of the victim's upper teeth are shown to demonstrate the source of the trauma in the fourth photo. **D:** The victim has a patterned puncture wound to the lower oral mucosa that corresponds to the teeth shown in part C.

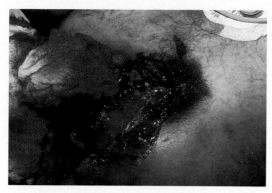

**FIG. 13-2.** The soot present on this close-range shotgun wound is short-lived. When the wound is scrubbed, debrided, and closed, the soot, which indicates a close range of fire, will have been destroyed.

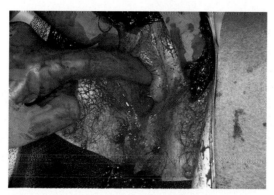

**FIG. 13-7.** A large vaginal laceration that occurred as a result of sexual assault. The presence of blood and the graphic nature of the injury resulted in the judge ruling the photograph inflammatory and not admissible.

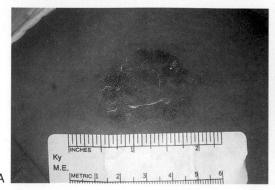
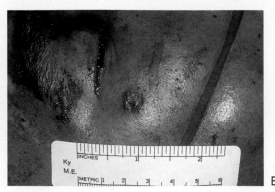

**FIG. 13-13. A:** Healing bite mark to breast. **B:** Gunshot entrance wound with the associated abrasion collar. The injuries are well lighted by the ring flash.

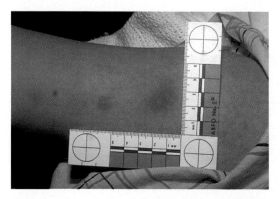

**FIG. 13-22.** A photograph with a scale and without perspective distortion permits accurate measurement of a wound. These fingertip contusions on the upper left arm are from a domestic assault.

### High-Risk Sexual Activity

Many studies have linked high-risk sexual behavior with a history of childhood sexual victimization (88a,90,92). High-risk sexual behavior, in turn, can lead to sexual revictimization:

Sexual abuse → high-risk sexual behavior → sexual revictimization

Sexual activity is more common in adolescents with a history of abuse. A 1990 anonymous survey of high-school students found that students with a history of sexual abuse were $3\frac{1}{2}$ times as likely to be sexually active (89). A 1990 study of adolescents with open cases at child protection showed that those who had been sexually abused were more likely to voluntarily engage in sexual activity (90).

Adolescents who have been sexually abused are also more likely to be accepting of coercive sexual relationships. Their communication skills may be limited and their ability to negotiate condom use may be compromised (91). Adolescent drug and alcohol use are associated with a history of abuse (6). Moreover, drug and alcohol use are associated with high-risk sexual activity and increased risk of sexual victimization.

Finally, sexual abuse increases behavioral risk factors for HIV (92). More than 50% of HIV-infected youth have sexual abuse histories.

### Teen Pregnancy

Many studies have shown an increased risk of pregnancy in adolescents with a history of sexual abuse (93,93a). One study found that adolescents with a history of abuse were more likely trying to conceive, to have boyfriends pressuring them to conceive, or to have concerns about fertility (94).

### Juvenile Delinquency

Adolescent boys who have a history of sexual abuse are at risk for delinquency. Adolescent boys, more so than girls, will exhibit externalizing behaviors, particularly if they are depressed. These behaviors often lead to problems with the law and subsequent involvement with the juvenile justice system (95). In addition, sexual abuse also is a risk factor for drug and alcohol use which, in turn, can lead to delinquent and criminal behaviors (96).

### Runaway Behavior

For both adolescent girls and boys, there is a very strong association between runaway behavior and sexual abuse histories (97,95).

### Prostitution

Prostitution is linked to childhood sexual abuse (98–100). The peak age for entering prostitution is 14 or younger, and in most cases runaway behavior precedes the prostitution. In turn, runaway behavior is often due to sexual abuse. So prostitution reflects the cycle of sexual victimization. Male prostitutes are less likely to be arrested than female prostitutes and hence are less likely to come to medical attention through the juvenile justice system (100).

### Coercive Sexual Behavior

In a study of 9th through 12th graders in a midwestern state who completed an anonymous risk taking survey, Lodico et al. found a striking correlation between a history of abuse and likelihood of engaging in sexual aggression or being sexually victimized. Self-reported sexual aggression was twice as common in adolescents who had been sexually abused, and self-reported sexual victimization was six times as common (101). Sexual coercion may take many forms. It may present as the adolescent female who is hesitant to talk about condom use for fear of physical or sexual aggression in response. It may present as the adolescent female pressuring an acquaintance to have intercourse so that she can become pregnant.

### Sex Offenders

Adolescents are perpetrators in at least 20% of child sexual abuse cases (102). In addition, up to 80% of adult sex offenders began their sexually aggressive behavior in adolescence (99). More than half of adolescent child molesters were themselves sexually abused as children (103), and a substantial number of imprisoned child molesters have a history of child sexual abuse (104). Hence, there is a sexual victimization cycle wherein the victim is at risk to become the victimizer.

## SUMMARY

Adolescence offers unique and difficult challenges in successful identification and treatment of sexual victimization. More often than not, sexual victimization is linked to antecedent and subsequent high-risk behaviors. Effective intervention requires an understanding of how the adolescent processes information; how this is affected by emotion, stress, and life experience; and how sexual behavior shapes identity and risk taking. Effective anticipatory guidance regarding important decision making skills requires that the provider address the knowledge, attitude, and behaviors of the adolescent. This takes time, patience, and skill. These challenges are all magnified in the acute care setting, where the specific provider's window of opportunity may be limited to a 1-hour visit. On the other hand, during a single visit, the adolescent may hear new ideas or the same old idea expressed in a new way. In subsequent weeks, he or she may remember the compassion and care provided, and this memory may help sustain her through the emotional upheaval that can follow a sexual assault. In addition, the adolescent sexual assault victim needs comprehensive longitudinal care. If she or he is seen in the emergency department, the examining physician should attempt to get a release to talk with the primary doctor so that optimal care can be provided and the intergenerational cycle of violence can be interrupted.

## REFERENCES

 1. Finkelhor D, Hotaling GT. Sexual abuse in the national incidence study of child abuse and neglect: an appraisal. *Child Abuse Neglect* 1984;8:23–33.
 2. AMA Council on Scientific Affairs. Adolescents as victims of family violence. *JAMA* 1993;270:1850–1856.
 3. ACOG. Educational bulletin: adolescent victims of sexual assault. *Int J Gynecol Obstet* 1999;64:195–199.
 3a. Scarce M. Same-sex rape of male college students. *J Am Coll Health* 1997;45:171–173.
 4. Black DA, DeBlassie RR. Sexual abuse in male children and adolescents: indicators, effects, and treatments. *Adolescence* 1993;109:123–132.
 5. Langan PA, Harlow CW. Crime data brief: child rape victims, 1992. U.S. Department of Justice, Bureau of Justice Statistics. NCJ-147001, 1994.
 6. The Commonwealth Fund. *Survey on the health of adolescent girls.* New York: 1997.
 7. ACOG. Educational bulletin: sexual assault. *Int J Gynecol Obstet* 1998;60:297–304.
 8. Stewart D. Adolescent sexual abuse, sexual assault, and rape. In: Hofman AD, Greydanus DE, eds. *Adolescent medicine.* Stamford, CT: Appleton & Lange, 1997.
 9. Finkelhor D, Dziuba-Leatherman J. Children as victims of violence: a national survey. *Pediatrics* 1994;94:413–420.
10. Koss MP, Gidycz CA, Wisniewski N. The scope of rape: incidence and prevalence of sexual aggression and victimization in a national sample of higher education students. *J Consult Clin Psychol* 1987;55:162–170.
11. ACOG. Committee opinion: adolescent acquaintance rape. *Int J Gynecol Obstet* 1993;42:209–211.
12. Scarce M. Same-sex rape of male college students. *J Am Coll Health* 1997;45(4):171–173.
13. Kellogg ND, Huston RL. Unwanted sexual experiences in adolescents: patterns of disclosure. *Clin Pediatrics* 1995;34:306–312.
14. Berliner L, Conte JR. The process of victimization: the victims' perspective. *Child Abuse Neglect* 1990;14:29–40.
15. Kershner R. Adolescent attitudes about rape. *Adolescence* 1996;31(121):29–33.
16. Blumberg ML, Lester D. High school and college students' attitudes towards rape. *Adolescence* 1991;26(103):727–729.
17. Koval JE. Violence in dating relationships. *J Pediatr Health Care* 1989;3:298–304.
18. Wiemann CM. Rohypnol—the "date-rape" drug. *NASPAG News* 1998;12:1–5.
19. Finkelson L, Oswalt R. College date rape: incidence and reporting. *Psychol Rep* 1995;77(2):526.
20. Davis TC, Peck GQ, Storment JM. Acquaintance rape and the high school student. *J Adol Health Care* 1993;14:220–224.
21. Finkelhor D. The victimization of children: a developmental perspective. *Am J Orthopsychiatry* 1995;65(2):177–193.
22. Kendall-Tackett KA, Simon AF. Molestation and the onset of puberty: data from 365 adults molested as children. *Child Abuse Neglect* 1988;12:73–81.
23. Rennison CM. *Criminal victimization 1998.* U.S. Department of Justice, Bureau of Justice Statistics. NCJ 176353, 1999.
24. Small SA, Kerns D. Unwanted sexual activity among peers during early and middle adolescence: incidence and risk factors. *J Marriage Family* 1993;55:941–952.
24a. Ponton LE. *The romance of risk: why teenagers do the things they do.* New York: Basic Books, 1997.
25. Cheng TL, Savageau JA, Sattler AL, DeWitt TG. Confidentiality in health care: a survey of knowledge, perceptions, and attitudes among high school students. *JAMA* 1993;269:1404–1407.
26. Marks A, Malizio J, Hoch J, et al. Assessment of health needs and willingness to utilize health care resources

of adolescents in a suburban population. *J Pediatrics* 1983; 102:456–460.

27. AMA Council on Scientific Affairs. Confidential health services for adolescents. *JAMA* 1993;269: 1420–1424.

27a. AAP. Confidentiality in adolescent health care. Policy statement. *AAP News,* 1989.

27b. Morrissey JD, Hofmann AD, Thrope JC. *Consent and confidentiality in the health care of children and adolescents: a legal guide.* New York: Free Press, 1986.

28. Montemayor R. Parents and adolescents in conflict. *J Early Adol* 1983;3:83–101.

29. Rutter M, Graham P, Chadwick OF, Yule W. Adolescent turmoil: fact or fiction? *J Child Psychol Psychiatry* 1976;7:35–56.

30. Offer D, Ostrov E, Howard KI. Adolescence: what is normal? *Am J Dis Childh* 1989;143:731–736.

31. Newacheck PW, McManus MA, Brindis C. Financing health care for adolescents: problems, prospects, and proposals. *J Adol Health Care* 1990;11:398–403.

32. Klein JD. Adolescence, the health care delivery system, and health care reform. In: Brindis C, Irwin C, Langlykke K, Holt K. Health care reform: opportunities for improving adolescent health. Washington, DC: Bureau of Maternal and Child Health, 1994; cited in Ozer et al., 1997.

33. Ozer EM, Brindis CD, Millstein SG, et al. America's adolescents: are they healthy? San Francisco: University of California, San Francisco, National Adolescent Health Information Center, 1997.

34. English A. Treating adolescents: legal and ethical considerations. *Med Clin North Am* 1990;74:1092–1112.

35. Fisher B, Berdie J. Adolescent abuse and neglect: issues of incidence, intervention, and service delivery. *Child Abuse Neglect* 1978;2:173–192.

36. Moore KA, Nord CW, Peterson JL. Nonvoluntary sexual activity among adolescents. *Family Planning Perspect* 1989;21:110–113.

37. Centers for Disease Control and Prevention. CDC Surveillance Summaries. Youth Risk Behavior Surveillance—United States, 1999. June 9, 2000. *MMWR* 2000;49(No. SS-5).

38. Tharinger D, Horton CB, Millea S. Sexual abuse and exploitation of children and adults with mental retardation and other handicaps. *Child Abuse Neglect* 1990; 134:301–312.

39. Chamberlain A, Rauh J, Passer A. Issues in fertility control for the mentally retarded female adolescents: sexual activity, sexual abuse, and contraception. *Pediatrics* 1984;73:445–450.

40. Frieberg KL. *Human development: a life-span approach.* Boston: Jones and Barlett, 1987.

41. Slap G. Normal physiologic and psychosocial growth in the adolescent. *J Adol Health Care* 1986;7:13S–23S.

41a. Eeg-Olofsson O. Longitudinal developmental course of electrical activity of brain. *Brain Dev* 1980;2(1):33–44.

41b. Weithorn LA, Campbell SB. The competency of children and adolescents to make informed treatment decisions. *Child Dev* 1982;53:1589–1598.

42. Marshall WA, Tanner JM. Variation in the pattern of pubertal changes in girls. *Arch Dis Child* 1969;44: 291–303.

43. Marshall WA, Tanner JM. Variations in the pattern of pubertal changes in boys. *Arch Dis Child* 1970;45: 13–23.

44. Duke PM, Carlsmith JM, Jennings D, et al. Educational correlates at early and late sexual maturation during adolescence. *J Pediatrics* 1982;100(4): 633–637.

45. Duncan PD, Ritter PL, Dornbusch SM, et al. The effects of pubertal timing on body image, school behavior, and deviance. *J Youth Adol* 1985;14:227–235.

45a. Rosenthal SL, Cohen SS. Primary prevention of sexually transmitted disease: self-efficacy in the context of sexual coercion. *Adolesc Pediatr Gynecol* 1994;7: 63–68.

46. Hook SM, Elliot, DA, Harbison SA. Penetration and ejaculation: forensic aspects of rape. *N Z Med J* 1992; 105:87–89.

47. Starling SP, Jenny C. Forensic examination of adolescent female genitalia: the Foley catheter technique. *Arch Pediatr Adol Med* 1997;151:102–103.

48. McCann J, Voris J, Simon M. Genital injuries resulting from sexual abuse: a longitudinal study. *Pediatrics* 1992;89:307–318.

49. Herman-Giddens ME, Sandler AD, Friedman NE. Sexual precocity in girls: an association with sexual abuse? *Am J Dis Child* 1988;142:431–433.

50. McCauley J, Gorman RL, Guzinski G. Toluidine blue in the detection of perineal lacerations in pediatric and adolescent sexual abuse victims. *Pediatrics* 1986;78: 1039–1043.

51. Emans SJ, Woods ER, Allred EN, Grace E. Hymenal findings in adolescent women: impact of tampon use and consensual sexual activity. *J Pediatrics* 1994;125: 153–160.

52. Muram D. Child sexual abuse: relationship between sexual acts and genital findings. *Child Abuse Neglect* 1989;13:211–216.

53. Adams JA, Knudson S. Genital findings in adolescent girls referred for suspected sexual abuse. *Arch Pediatr Adol Med* 1996;150:850–857.

54. Elster AB, Kuznets NJ, eds. *AMA Guidelines for preventive services (GAPS).* Baltimore: Williams & Wilkins, 1994.

55. Green M, ed. *Bright futures: guidelines for health supervision of infants, children, and adolescents.* Arlington, VA: National Center for Education in Maternal and Child Health, 1994.

56. Burstein GR, Gaydos CA, Diener-West M. Incident *Chlamydia trachomatis* infections among inner-city adolescent females. *JAMA* 1998;280:521–526.

57. Cates W. The epidemiology and control of sexually transmitted diseases in adolescents. *Adol Med: State of the Art Rev* 1990;1:409–427.

58. AAP Committee on Adolescence. Sexually transmitted diseases. *Pediatrics* 1994;568–572.

59. Stamm WE. *Chlamydia trachomatis* infections of the adult. In: Holmes KK, Sparling PF, March P, et al., eds. *Sexually transmitted diseases,* 3rd ed. New York: McGraw-Hill, 1999, chapter 29.

60. Berman SM, Hein K. Adolescents and STDs. In: Holmes KK, Sparling PF, March P, et al., eds. *Sexually transmitted diseases,* 3rd ed. New York: McGraw-Hill, 1999, chapter 9.

61. Ledray L. Sexual assault evidentiary exam and treatment protocol. *J Emerg Nurs* 1995;21:355–359.

62. Jenny C, Hooton TM, Bowers A, et al. Sexually transmitted diseases in victims of rape. *N Engl J Med* 1990; 322(11):713–716.

63. Glaser JB, Schachter J, Benes S, et al. Sexually transmitted diseases in postpubertal female rape victims. *J Infect Dis* 1991;164:726–730.

64. Joffe A. Amplified DNA testing for sexually transmitted diseases: new opportunities and new questions. *Arch Pediatr Adol Med* 1999;153:111–113.

64a. Centers for Disease Control and Prevention. Guidelines for treatment of sexually transmitted diseases. *MMWR* 1998;47(RR-1):1–111.

65. Holmes KK, Sparling PF, March P, et al., eds. *Sexually transmitted diseases,* 3rd edition. New York: McGraw–Hill, 1999.

66. Rompolo AM, et al. Diagnosis and treatment of sexually acquired proctitis and proctocolitis: an update. *Clin Infect Dis* 1999;28[Suppl 1]:S84–S90.

67. Shafer MA, Pantell RH, Schachter J. Is the routine pelvic examination needed with the advent of urine-based screening for sexually transmitted diseases? *Arch Pediatr Adol Med* 1999;153:119–125.

68. Wiesenfeld HC, Heine RP, Rideout A. The vaginal introitus: a novel site for *Chlamydia trachomatis* testing in women. *Am J Obstet Gynecol* 1996;174(5):1542–1546.

69. Malone JL, Wallace MR, Hendrick BB, et al. Syphilis and neurosyphilis in a human immunodeficiency virus type-1 seropositive population: evidence for frequent serologic relapse after therapy. *Am J Med* 1995;99:55–63.

70. Lifson AR, O'Malley PM, Hessol NA, et al. HIV seroconversion in two homosexual men after receptive oral intercourse with ejaculation: implications for counseling concerning safe sexual practices. *Am J Public Health* 1990;80:1509–1511.

71. Gostin LO, Lazzarini Z, Alexander D, et al. HIV testing, counseling, and prophylaxis after sexual assault. *JAMA* 1994;271:1436–1444.

71a. Meehan TM, Hansen H, Klein WC. The impact of parental consent on the HIV testing of minors. *Am J Pub Health* 1997;87:1338–1341.

72. Eron JJ, Hirsch MS. Antiviral therapy of human immunodeficiency virus infection. In: Holmes KK, Sparling PF, March P, et al., eds. *Sexually transmitted diseases,* 3rd ed. New York: McGraw-Hill, 1999, chapter 74.

73. National Victim Center, Crime Victims Research and Treatment Center. National Women's Study, reported in *Rape in America: a report to the nation,* 1992.

74. Centers for Disease Control and Prevention. Public health service guidelines for the management of health-care worker exposures to HIV and recommendations for postexposure prophylaxis. *MMWR* 1998;47(N, RR-7).

75. Blake DR, Duggan A, Joffe A. Use of spun urine to enhance detection of Trichomonas vaginalis in adolescent women. *Arch Pediatr Adolesc Med* 1999;12:1222–1225.

76. Bump RC, Buesching WJ. Bacterial vaginosis in virginal and sexually active adolescent females: evidence against exclusive sexual transmission. *Obstet Gynecol* 1988;158:935–939.

77. Blake D, Duggan A, Quinn T. Evaluation of vaginal infections in adolescent women: can it be done without a speculum? *Pediatrics* 1998;102:939–944.

78. Beck-Sague CM, Solomon, F. Sexually transmitted diseases in abused children and adolescent and adult victims of rape: review of selected literature. *Clin Infect Dis* 1999;28 [Suppl 1]:S74–S83.

79. Fisher M, Rosenfield WD, Burk RD. Cervicovaginal human papillomavirus infection in suburban adolescents and young adults. *J Pediatrics* 1991;119:821–825.

80. Igra V, Millstein SG. Current status and approaches to improving preventive services for adolescents. *JAMA* 1993;269:1408–1412.

81. AAP Committee on Infectious Diseases. *Red Book 2000.* Elk Grove, Illinois.

82. Mann EM. Self-reported stresses of adolescent rape victims. *J Adol Health Care* 1981;2:29–33.

83. Felice M, Grant J, Reynolds B, et al. Follow-up observations of adolescent rape victims. *Clin Pediatrics* 1978;17:311–315.

84. Gerlinas D. The persisting negative effect of incest. *Psychiatry* 1983;46:312–332.

85. Massie ME, Johnson SM. The importance of recognizing a history of sexual abuse in female adolescents. *J Adol Health Care* 1989;10:184–191.

86. Brand EF, King CA, Olson E, et al. Depressed adolescents with a history of sexual abuse: diagnostic comorbidity and suicidality. *J Am Acad Child Adolesc Psychiatry* 1996;35(1):34–41.

87. Remafedi G, Farrow JA, Deisher RW. Risk factors for attempted suicide in gay and bisexual youth. *Pediatrics* 1991;87:869–875.

88. Hibbard RA, Ingersoll GM, Orr DP. Behavioral risk, emotional risk, and child abuse among adolescents in a nonclinical setting. *Pediatrics* 1990;86:896–901.

88a. Nagy S, Adcock AG, Nagy MC. A comparison of risky health behaviors of sexually active, sexually abused, and abstaining adolescents. *Pediatrics* 1994;93:570–575.

89. Riggs S, Alario AJ, McHorney C. Health risk behaviors and attempted suicide in adolescents who report prior maltreatment. *J Pediatrics* 1990;116:815–821.

90. Polit DF, White CM, Morton TD. Child sexual abuse and premarital intercourse among high-risk adolescents. *J Adol Health Care* 1990;11:231–234.

91. Beckman LJ, Harvey SM. Factors affecting the consistent use of barrier methods of contraception. *Obstet Gynecol* 1996;88[3 Suppl]:65S–71S.

92. Zierler S. Adult survivors of childhood sexual abuse and subsequent risk of HIV infection. *Am J Public Health* 1991;81:572–575.

93. Kenney JW, Reinholtz C, Angelini PJ. Ethnic differences in childhood and adolescent sexual abuse and teenage pregnancy. *J Adol Health* 1997;21:3–10.

93a. Fiscella K, Kitzman HJ, Cole RE, et al. Does child abuse predict adolescent pregnancy? *Pediatrics* 1998;101(4 pt 1):620–624.

94. Rainey DY, Stevens-Simm C, Kaplan DW. Are adolescents who report prior sexual abuse at higher risk for pregnancy? *Child Abuse Neglect* 1995;19:1283–1288.

95. Famularo R, Kinscherff R, Fenton T, Bolduc SM. Child maltreatment histories among runaway and delinquent children. *Clin Pediatrics* 1990;29:713–718.

96. Burgess AW, Hartman CR, McCormack A. Abused to abuser: antecedents of socially deviant behaviors. *Am J Psychiatry* 1987:1431–1436.

97. Hibbard RA, Brack CJ, Rauch S, Orr DP. Abuse, feelings, and health behaviors in a student population. *Am J Dis Child* 1988;142:326–330.

98. Brannigan A, Brunschot EG. Youthful prostitution and child sexual trauma. *Int J Law Psychiatry* 1997; 20:337–354.

99. Myers JEB. *Legal issues in child abuse and neglect practice.* Thousand Oaks, CA: Sage Publications, 1999.

100. Schetky DH, Green AH. *Child sexual abuse: a handbook for health care and legal professionals.* New York: Brunner/Mazel, 1988.

101. Lodico MA, Gruber E, DiClemente RJ. Childhood sexual abuse and coercive sex among school-based adolescents in a midwestern state. *J Adol Health* 1996; 18:211–217.

102. AMA. *Diagnostic and treatment guidelines on child sexual abuse.* Chicago: 1992.

103. Deisher RW, Wenet GA, Paperny DM, et al. Adolescent sexual offense behavior: the role of the physician. *J Adol Health Care* 1982;2:279–286.

104. Greenfield LA. *Child victimizers: violent offenders and their victims.* Office of Juvenile Justice and Delinquency Prevention. U.S. Department of Justice, NCJ-153258, 1996.

# 7

# Child Abuse/Assault—General

Adrienne Suggs, Richard Lichenstein, Clare McCarthy, and M. Christine Jackson

Child maltreatment is an unfortunate aspect of clinical forensic medicine. Caffey first described child abuse in 1946 when he recognized that some patients with long-bone fractures also had subdural hematomas (1). Kempe et al. elaborated and coined the term "battered child syndrome" in 1962 (2). Since then, health care professionals have become increasingly aware of child abuse and its manifestations, and laws have been enacted that mandate reporting of suspected child abuse by health care professionals, educators, and human service workers.

Although definitions vary by state, child physical abuse is usually defined as the physical injury of a child by a parent, household or family member, or other person who has permanent or temporary custody or responsibility for supervision of that child. Other forms of child maltreatment include neglect, sexual abuse, and emotional abuse.

The National Institute of Child Abuse and Neglect statistics for 1998 document almost 3 million referrals to child protective services for investigation of child maltreatment (3). Of these, about one third were substantiated, translating to a victimization rate of 12.9 per 1,000 children. Of substantiated cases, more than half (53.5%) suffered neglect, whereas almost one fourth (22.7%) suffered physical abuse. Eleven-and-a-half percent were victims of sexual abuse, and 6% or fewer suffered psychological abuse or medical neglect. Twenty-five percent were victims of more than one type of abuse. An estimated 1,100 children died of abuse and neglect, translating to a fatality rate of 1.6 per 100,000 children in the general population.

Victimization rates are highest for the 0 to 3 years age group and decline with increasing age. Rates of victimization are highest for African Americans, followed by American Indians/Alaska Natives, Hispanics, Caucasians, and, finally, Asian/Pacific Islanders (3).

Although overall perpetrators of child maltreatment tend to be female, perpetrators of physical and sexual abuse tend to be male. The majority of perpetrators of child maltreatment are parents (87%) or other relatives. Fewer than 2% are day-care providers or facility staff (3).

Pediatricians and emergency physicians must maintain a high level of suspicion when children present with injuries highly specific for abuse or when children have injuries not explained by the history presented. The physician must be aware of the many risk factors for abuse and must be able to identify clues in the history that raise the suspicion for abuse.

Risk factors for physical abuse and neglect include prematurity, chronic illness, mental retardation, and difficult temperament. Caretaker and environmental risk factors include young parents, abuse of the caretaker as a child, previous removal of a child by protective services, substance abuse, mental illness, lack of family support, and low socioeconomic status (4,5).

Clues in the history that may suggest abuse include a history not consistent with the injury or the developmental age of the child, changing or inconsistent histories, previous history of abuse, delay in seeking treatment, projection of blame onto a third party, and aggressiveness of the caretaker (5).

One must be careful to maintain a high degree of suspicion if the history lends clues and not be fooled by caretakers who do not seem to fit the profile. For example, Jenny et al. reported that young age of the child, white race, less severe symptoms, and an "intact" family were key features that led to missed diagnoses of abusive head trauma (6).

## HEAD TRAUMA/CENTRAL NERVOUS SYSTEM INJURY

Inflicted head trauma constitutes the leading cause of nonaccidental death in child abuse (7). When caregivers provide a history that is inadequate to explain the extent of head injury, child abuse must be considered.

Shaken baby syndrome (SBS) is classically described as occurring in infants younger than 6 months, with minimal or no external signs of trauma, subdural hematomas, and retinal hemorrhages (5). It usually presents as a spectrum of findings, including intracranial, cervical cord, intraocular, skeletal, and cutaneous injuries. Caretakers may be unaware of the specific injuries that can be caused by shaking, but it is reported that the act of shaking or slamming can be so violent that competent individuals observing the shaking would recognize it as dangerous (8). SBS has also been called shaken impact syndrome, based on an autopsy study of infants who were fatally abused in conjunction with biomechanical studies not performed on humans. That study concluded that severe head injuries require impact, not shaking alone (9). However, the majority of the literature supports the lack of need for an impact. Most agree that a constellation of findings exist, as a result of inflicted head trauma, with or without impact (5), thus referring to the general terms of nonaccidental head trauma, inflicted head trauma, or abusive head trauma.

It is important to distinguish between accidental and inflicted head injuries. Short vertical falls in infants, usually less than 4 feet (the majority of childhood falls), usually result in minor injury or no injury at all. Although falls from low heights may cause linear, unilateral skull fractures without intracranial injury, significant force is required to sustain depressed, stellate, complex, bilateral, or basilar skull fractures. Other than the rare reported cases of epidural hemorrhage, falls from low heights do not cause significant intracranial pathology, including subdural or subarachnoid hemorrhage, or retinal hemorrhage (9–14). Outside of a history of motor vehicle trauma, falls from heights greater than 4 feet, or head impact from a moving object, child abuse must be considered in children with intracranial injuries.

In SBS there may be an absence of external findings to implicate nonaccidental trauma (15). The degree of injury depends on the force or severity of the shake or impact and the time elapsed from the event. Symptoms may be vague and occur intermittently, which may be misleading to evaluating physicians (16). The range of manifestations includes poor feeding, vomiting, lethargy, irritability, colic, apnea, seizures, and death (5).

Intracranial pathology encountered in abusive head trauma includes, most commonly, subdural hemorrhages along with parenchymal injuries, including diffuse axonal injury (DAI). During shaking, because the infant's head is heavy and the neck muscles are weak, intracranial bleeding results from a tearing of cortical bridging veins that stretch and shear as the shaken head is subjected to rotational forces. These same forces also permit tearing of axons in the child's incompletely myelinated brain, resulting in DAI and cerebral edema. Other intracranial pathology includes subarachnoid hemorrhage and cerebral contusions. The incidence of epidural hematoma is low (5,7).

Shaken infants are also at risk for cervical cord injury because of the infant's large head-to-torso ratio and weak neck musculature. Spinal cord contusions and subdural and epidural hematomas at the cervicomedullary junction may lead to morbidity and mortality (5).

Retinal hemorrhages are associated with extraordinary force and are rare occurrences in minor accidental trauma (17–19). Unilateral or bilateral retinal hemorrhages are present in 75% to 95% of cases of abusive head trauma (16). Although retinal hemorrhages do occur with accidental trauma, diffuse and severe retinal hemorrhages are considered specific for SBS. In SBS, retinal hemorrhages usually involve the posterior pole in the nerve fiber and ganglion cell layers of the retina, and often are diffuse, extending to the periphery of the retina (20). Retinal folds or detachment may also develop (4). Retinal hemorrhages may occur as a result of birth trauma (approximately 30% of newborns), but they are quickly resolved by age 4 weeks (5). Retinal hemorrhage after cardiopulmonary resuscitation (CPR) has rarely been reported, but not in the absence of previous head trauma or abnormal coagulation and platelet studies. When such hemorrhage is found, it tends to be morphologically different from that associated with SBS (20,21).

Some controversy exists when evaluating the interval between head injury and symptom onset, which may help to identify a perpetrator. Determining whether or not a lucid interval has occurred can be difficult because perpetrators may not be telling the truth (22). Gilliland et al. found that neurologic changes and severe symptoms, such as difficulty breathing, unresponsiveness, and respiratory collapse, occurred less than 24 hours after head injury in the majority of incidents. Of note, whenever information was supplied by someone other than the perpetrator, the child was not described as normal during the period (23). Starling, studying perpetrators, found that 97% of convicted perpetrators who admitted to inflicting head trauma were with the child at the time of onset of symptoms, suggesting that symptoms occur soon after the abuse, as opposed to occurring over hours to days (24). In a retrospective review of 95 accidental fatalities involving head injury, only one patient had a lucid interval; that patient had an epidural hematoma (25).

Another recent controversy is the theory of rebleeding, after minor or no trauma, into chronic or subacute subdural hemorrhages. This theory has implications in identifying a perpetrator. Although this is a very recent topic, Block, after reviewing the literature, contends that "there is no evidence to support the current concept that rebleeding of an organizing subdural hemorrhage can occur from a subsequent trivial injury and cause severe neurologic impairment or death" (20). This appears to be the general consensus of the many experts in nonaccidental head trauma at a recent SBS conference (26).

Physicians should be aware that nonaccidental head trauma is often associated with extracranial signs of abuse. Posterior rib fractures can occur as a result of squeezing the infant's chest while shaking the infant. Other long-bone and cutaneous findings may also be present as a result of repetitive abuse. The physician should perform a careful search for other physical signs of abuse or neglect.

## ABDOMINAL AND THORACIC INJURY

Abdominal trauma is the second most common cause of child abuse deaths (27,28). Unfortunately, children who sustain severe abdominal trauma from child abuse present late to medical attention. Generally, their presentation is in response to the pathology that results from abdominal injury rather than to the injury itself (27). Blunt abdominal trauma can result in no external evidence of injury, even if there is severe organ and tissue damage (29). Initial manifestations may be nonspecific and include abdominal pain, distention, nausea, vomiting, and fever. Peritonitis and associated sepsis may become evident within hours to days after abdominal injury, whereas hematoma and subsequent intestinal obstruction usually take longer, possibly days, to diagnose. Sometimes older children can describe the causative event. In the case of younger children, diagnosis of abdominal trauma may rest on the history provided by the caretaker or on the suspicion of the physician. As with head trauma, the absence of any history, or the report of a minor injury despite evidence of serious trauma, implies that the injury was inflicted.

Multiple injuries are seen in 18% to 37% of children with inflicted abdominal trauma (27). Both solid and hollow organs are at risk for injury in thoracoabdominal trauma. The mortality of blunt abdominal trauma from child abuse is greater than that of abdominal trauma suffered in falls or in automobile or bicycle accidents (28).

Nonaccidental blunt thoracic trauma can result in rib fractures and injury to underlying structures. Lower rib fractures may lacerate the spleen or liver. Rib fractures can cause pneumothorax or pneumomediastinum. Direct blunt anterior trauma can lead to esophageal perforation, pneumomediastinum, or mediastinitis.

The spleen and the liver can sustain damage when there are fractures of the lower ribs. Blunt abdominal trauma may yield contusions of these organs as well. Liver injury can range from small, asymptomatic contusions to fractures that lead to significant blood loss and death. Delay in evaluation of severe liver injury increases pediatric mortality. Diagnosis of liver injury may be determined by a history of blunt abdominal trauma, abdominal pain and tenderness, elevated aspartate aminotransferase/alanine aminotransferase, and computed tomography findings. Elevated liver enzymes can be helpful in evaluating occult liver injuries, even when there is no report of abdominal trauma or clinical evidence of abdominal injury in suspected child abuse (29). The spleen can be injured in both accidental and nonaccidental trauma settings, but inflicted injury should be suspected when the patient is an infant who is not yet able to walk.

In general, pancreatic injury is not common in childhood (28), but when present it may be the result of inflicted trauma. On rare occasions, seat belts or bicycle handlebar accidents may cause damage to this potentially volatile organ. However, injury to the pancreas requires deep abdominal wall indentation (27).

Injury to either or both kidneys can result from blunt thoracoabdominal trauma. The kidneys are generally well protected by the lower ribs but are not completely protected from blunt or penetrating trauma.

Abdominal viscera is also at risk of injury from blunt trauma associated with child abuse. The duodenum, located in the anterior epigastrium, is fixed relative to the more mobile jejunum and ileum. The most common form of duodenal injury from blunt trauma is intramural hematoma, resulting in partial obstruction, nausea, and vomiting. In some cases, there is rupture and/or transection of the duodenum. Since delay in seeking treatment is common after abdominal trauma in child abuse, peritonitis may be significant when the child is brought to the emergency department. The ileum and jejunum are less prone to injury from blunt trauma, prob-

ably because they are not tethered in the same manner as the duodenum. Although they sustain fewer injuries, jejunal and ileal injuries (27) manifest as hematoma or perforation.

Injury to the colon and rectum can occur in blunt trauma, usually resulting in bruising or perforation. In addition, pelvic trauma may lead to rectal injury, as can anal penetration. Substantial blunt force is required to injure these organs. Absence of plausible history and delay in seeking treatment are indicators of abuse.

## CHILD SEXUAL ASSAULT/ABUSE

Dealing with the pediatric sexually assaulted or abused child is extremely difficult because we don't like to admit that it occurs. Any discussion or referral we make to protective services regarding abuse or sexual assault of a child certainly can have major ramifications for the child and his or her family. If we look at medical textbooks from the 1950s, the subject is frequently not mentioned. Today we know that sexual abuse and assault can occur anytime from birth to death. It is difficult for us to imagine a baby or a child being sexually abused or assaulted, so it is frequently not sought or is overlooked. As health care providers we must first get into the habit of looking and putting it into our differential when evaluating the pediatric patient. Remember that every child should have an external genital examination at every routine pediatric visit.

### Perpetrators

We teach "stranger danger," but most of the time the perpetrator is known to the victim and is usually a family member or friend of the family. We need to tell our children to also be cautious of their relatives and teachers. The sexual assault or abuse by strangers along with the kidnapping and/or death of a child is usually what we read about, but it is not the norm.

The use of children for pornography can be a family practice, a particular individual's practice, or part of an organized child sexual abuse ring. Among pedophiles or people with a sexual preference for children, the preferences of child sexual abusers can be broken down into the following categories: individuals or groups preferring children from birth to age 3 years; those who like children from 3 years to around 8 years; those who like children from 8 to 12 years; and, finally, those who like adolescents. The preferences also can be male only, female only, or both.

### Evaluating the Pediatric Patient

As with any evaluation of a pediatric patient, the health-care provider needs to obtain a good history. In the child with equivocal or no injuries noted, this is the most important part of the examination. Interviewing techniques should be age specific. When possible, interview the child without anyone else present. For the preverbal and mentally challenged child, we must rely on others to give us the history. It is important to remember that you may be getting the history from the perpetrator. How to conduct an appropriate interview is covered elsewhere. Knowing what is normal behavior and normal genitalia for a child helps the examiner to pick up what is not normal.

### Physical Examination

Children should never be forced to have an examination. They should be offered choices and prepared prior to coming in for the examination. When an examination is a necessity it may be necessary to sedate the patient, particularly in acute cases. Remember that parents also need to have their concerns addressed.

The physical examination should include a complete physical with particular attention paid to the mouth and nasal area, the genital region, and the anal region. Remember that most pedophiles have no desire to harm their victims. Most wish to continue the abuse. Thus, the presence of a normal examination does not in any way mean that abuse has not occurred. The purpose of the physical examination is to identify any form of abuse or trauma, to identify any medical conditions that are suggestive of sexual assault or abuse, to properly collect medical legal evidence of abuse or assault, and to address the concerns of the patient and family.

Physical indicators of concern are irritation, pain or redness to the genital or anal regions, bed-wetting, bruises, tears, difficulty with uri-

nation, soiling of pants, vaginal or penile discharge, vaginal disease, and pregnancy.

The presence of physical findings depends on the degree of force used if any, the use of lubricants, the type and frequency of abuse, the size and age difference between perpetrator and patient, the use of foreign objects, the degree of resistance, the presence of preexisting injury or disease, and the time between the incident, reporting, and examination of the patient. The genital and anal areas are noted for their quick healing capabilities, frequently leaving little or no indication of trauma. It is important to remember that, in most cases, the examination is normal.

When evaluating the head and neck in babies, remember that babies have a natural inclination to suck. Therefore, in an infant look for sperm or discharge in the mouth, nose, and eyes and swab these areas. In a suspected acute case, the fat folds of the neck and the external ear should be swabbed. Also make note of any tears to the frenula or any mucosal petechiae. There should be a careful evaluation of the entire body for any suck marks or bite marks The extremities should be examined for bruises caused by grasping, pinching, or tying.

The male genitalia should be examined with the child supine and standing. The rectal area is best evaluated in the knee-chest position, but can also be examined in the lateral decubitus position. The female genitalia and anal areas should be examined in the knee-chest position and in the supine frog-leg position with the use of labial separation and traction. Changing examination position and degree of traction allows the examiner to differentiate true abnormalities from hymenal tissue folds that change with position. Remember that all females have a hymen, and that many normal variants exist. It is important to document the exam by photography or videography for later review by an expert if needed.

In 1996, Kini et al. described clinical indicators and level of concern when looking at the physical examination in child sexual abuse cases (30) (Table 7-1). There are numerous skin conditions that can mimic sexually transmitted diseases or child sexual assault or abuse (Tables 7-2 and 7-3). Distinguishing these from sexual assault or abuse requires cultures and, in some cases, consultation with a pediatrician or a dermatologist.

**TABLE 7-1.**  *Clinical indicators and level of concern*

**No Concern**
Normal physical examination or the following features:
  Anatomical
    Anterior, midline anal skin tags
    Perianal erythema
    Labial adhesions or imperforate hymen
    Smooth, anterior hymenal concavities
    Periurethral bands or ridges
    Perineal erythema or erythema of the vestibule
    Normal hymen variants
  Nonanatomical
    Diaper region erythema
    Diaper dermatitis (irritant or candidal)
**Some Concern**
Anal dilatation > 2 cm (without stool in ampulla)
Anal fissures outside the infant age group
Perianal bruising
Friable posterior fourchette
Presence of labial friability or adhesions in girls outside the diaper age group
**Serious Concern**
Anal scars outside the midline
Hymenal border disruptions, such as thinning or absence of hymenal tissue posteriorly in knee-chest position
Anal tags outside the midline
Posterior concavities, scars, or transections
Anal dilatation > 2 cm (without stool in the ampulla)
Obvious genital injury, such as avulsion, laceration, or contusions
**Grave Concern**
Pregnancy
Any sexually transmitted disease that is not perinatally acquired
Presence of semen, sperm, or acid phosphatase
Obvious extensive anogenital injury (30)

**TABLE 7-2.**  *Sexual and nonsexual transmission of infectious organisms*

**Organisms transmitted sexually**
*Neisseria gonorrhoeae* needs to be reported (transmission at birth through an infected birth canal has been reported).
*Chlamydia trachomatis* needs to be reported (neonatal transmission can result in carriage up to 29 months).
*Trichomonas vaginalis* needs to be reported (transmission at birth through an infected birth canal has been reported).
Syphilis.
HIV.
**Organisms transmitted both sexually and nonsexually**
*Gardnerella vaginalis.*
Human papillomavirus/condyloma acuminata, report and work-up (transmission at birth through an infected birth canal has been reported).
Herpes simplex types 1 and 2 report and work-up (transmission at birth through an infected birth canal has been reported).
**Organisms transmitted via the placenta and amniotic fluid**
Syphilis.
HIV.

touch. (This same type of effect also occurs with menopause with changes in estrogen.) Glycogen is no longer present and there are no lactobacilli, so there is no food for organisms to grow. The

**TABLE 7-3.**  *Skin conditions that mimic sexually transmitted disease*

Behcet's syndrome
Bowenoid papulosis
Bullous pemphigoid
*Candida albicans* infection
Contact dermatitis
Crohn's disease
Epidermal nevus
Hemangioma of infancy
Kawasaki's syndrome
Langerhans cell histiocytosis
Labial adhesions
Lichen sclerosus
Molluscum contagiosum
Pemphigus vulgaris
Perianal pseudoverrucous papules and nodules
Perianal streptococcal dermatitis
Pinworms
Posttraumatic injuries
Psoriasis
Seborrheic dermatitis
Vulvovaginitis

From Siegfried EC, Frasier LD. Anogenital skin diseases of childhood. *Pediatr Ann* 1997;26:321–331, with permission.

## Evaluation of the Hymen

When evaluating the hymen and genital area of the female, it is important to remember how these organs change. From birth to approximately 2 years of age, the hymen and vagina are influenced by the presence of estrogen. This means that the hymen is thick and fluffy, with some elasticity both to it and to the vagina. Glycogen is present, which means that there is food for organisms to grow. Lactobacilli are present, and there is a vaginal discharge that is usually white. Occasionally, at birth there can be a bloody discharge. Around age 2 years, the effects of estrogen are no longer present; the vaginal epithelium becomes thin, and the hymen becomes thin, delicate, and very painful to urethra is the food site, and culture swabs of this area frequently are more productive than vaginal swabs. The urethra becomes erythematous and tender, and can cause dysuria when infection is present. Nonspecific indicators of sexually transmitted disease are dysuria, discharge, pruritus, genital sores or lesions, and vulvar or rectal pain. *Neisseria gonorrhoeae* and *Chlamydia trachomatis* rarely produce pelvic inflammatory disease or infectious arthritis in infected children. When puberty begins, estrogen again causes thickening and elasticity of the hymen and the vagina.

Due to the elasticity of the hymen and the vagina resulting from the effect of estrogen, it is possible for the female to accommodate a penis without injury to the genital area. It is also the effect of estrogen that allows the vagina to expand to accommodate the child at birth. Glycogen and lactobacilli are again present. This means that food is available for invading organisms. Prior to menses, leukorrhea is present and can be misdiagnosed as a discharge. This is why it is important to do cultures. The American College of Emergency Physicians recently established guidelines for sexual assault victims (31). With the adult female patient, it is suggested that cultures are not always necessary. However, with the pediatric patient cultures are very important and should always be done. Cultures are the gold standard; the direct fluorescent antibody and the enzyme immunoassay should not be used. If herpes simplex is suspected, be sure to use a cotton or Dacron swab, and do not allow the swab to dry. The time from exposure to disease is usually 2 to 7 days, but can reach 20 days. If human papillomavirus (HPV) is present, viral typing should be done and the result compared with that from viral typing of the perpetrator. The most common types of HPV found in the genital area are types 6 and 11. However, proving sexual transmission is still very difficult. In children there may be more modes of transmission than in adults. When warts are seen, the possibility of sexual abuse should be considered and a sexual abuse workup undertaken (32).

Treatment of acquired sexually transmitted diseases should follow the guidelines of the U.S. Centers for Disease Control and Prevention (CDC) (52).

## Documentation

Conclusions should state whether and what trauma is present or absent. Statements such as "consistent with sexual assault or abuse" or "not consistent with sexual assault or abuse" should be avoided.

## CUTANEOUS MANIFESTATIONS OF CHILD ABUSE

### Skin Lesions

The cutaneous markings of child abuse are many, with some more subtle than others. Injuries involving the dermis and epidermis are the most prevalent injuries seen in child abuse. The skin is a remarkable recorder, and many weapons leave behind specific patterns of injury. These patterns are reproducible (33) and are generally the result of blunt trauma, sharp forced trauma, or thermal injury.

Contusions are the result of blunt trauma and, in many cases, take on the shape of the instrument used to inflict them (i.e., hand slap, belt, loop cord, and so forth) (Fig. 7-1, see Colorplate following page 144). A hand-slap mark may consist of parallel, linear contusions with central clearing; these areas of clearing may result when the skin is impacted with extended fingers, mirroring the appearance of skin struck with a linear, cylindrical object (Fig. 7-2, see Colorplate following page 144). If a specific history of blunt trauma is elicited, it is important for the clinician to understand the nature of the contusion that can result in order to determine if the physical findings are consistent with the history.

Some parts of the body are prone to routine superficial traumas. The extensor surfaces of the arms and legs may have many incidental bruises from minor, accidental trauma in active children. And the protruding bony surfaces of the face, such as the chin, cheekbones, and forehead, are often the recipients of minor blunt trauma from falls or other accidental injuries. On the other hand, certain parts of the body are routinely "protected" during minor falls or injuries; examples of these are the inner arms, submental or throat area, abdomen, lower back, and inner thighs. When children are seen with cutaneous injuries

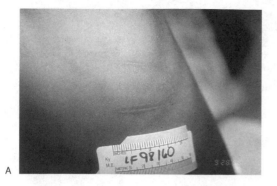

A

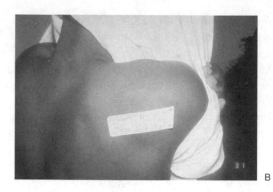

B

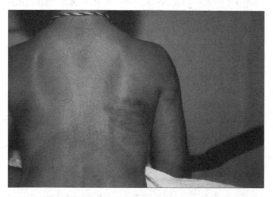

C

FIG. 7-1. Pattern injuries. **A:** A looped-belt injury. **B:** Another looped-belt injury. **C:** A fly-swatter injury. Note the square pattern produced from two overlapping blows through a diaper. (Courtesy of Chief Medical Examiner's Office, Louisville, Kentucky.)

in these protected areas, a careful history must be taken to delineate the nature of the incident.

One frequently asked question is whether bruises can be dated by examination to determine when they were inflicted. Accurate dating of bruises may indeed direct investigators to possible perpetrators. However, formal dating of

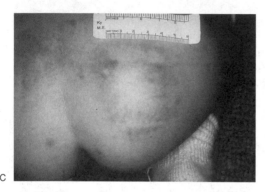

FIG. 7-2. Hand-slap mark. Note parallel linear contusions with central sparing that highlight the imprint of fingers. (Courtesy of Dr. William Smock, University of Louisville School of Medicine.)

bruises is difficult because there are many variables from patient to patient and within each patient. Many factors can determine a bruise's appearance, including depth, location, amount of bleeding into the tissues, and the circulatory status of the bruised area (34). Depth of injury may determine how soon a bruise will appear. Superficial injuries may show skin discoloration sooner than deep injuries, which may not appear for more than 24 hours. Bruise location can affect the timing of the bruise appearance as well. Areas of the body with loose tissue (e.g., periorbital) may show bruising sooner than denser regions (e.g., bony prominences). In addition, the patient's skin color may mask or enhance the appearance of bruises. Children with fair skin will display contusions from small impacts, whereas in dark-skinned children extensive contusions may be obscured. There are histologic evaluations that can help to determine how old a bruise may be. These require skin biopsy to determine whether hemosiderin can be found in macrophages (35), but this is an impractical approach.

Bruises show multiple color changes as they age. Fresh bruises are red or purple, then progress to blue, then to brown or yellow or green. Although these color changes can help to distinguish "early" or recent bruises from "late" or older bruises, the color of a bruise should not be the only determinant of its age and implication in abuse (36). In addition, photographic representation depends on lighting and technique and may portray bruises inaccurately.

Ongoing studies by Wallen et al. incorporate spectrophotometric procedures to determine hemoglobin breakdown in contusions. When viewed at various wavelengths of light, hemoglobin degradation products may help to determine the posttraumatic interval (37). In addition, the use of infrared light may reveal pattern contusions in the skin that are not visual to the naked eye, especially on darkly pigmented skin (33). These techniques are not routinely performed in the emergency department.

Bruises lend themselves to documentation. They can be measured and recorded in the text of a medical report, they can be sketched and diagramed in drawings on the report, and they can be photographed to provide prints or slides as a depiction of the injury. In addition, when the bruise represents a pattern injury that may provide a clue to the object used to inflict it, careful documentation creates a lasting record for future reference long after the wound has healed.

## Burns

Burning is a significant form of child abuse. Inflicted burns may come from hot liquids, flames, contact with hot objects, or caustic agents. Children's skin is thinner than adult skin and less resistant to thermal trauma. Therefore, children are burned more deeply and by less heat, and the burns often involve more body surface area with more scarring (38). Burning can account for 10% to 25% of child abuse injuries (39–41). Abusive burns tend to be more severe, deeper, and larger than accidental burns (40). Distinguishing inflicted burns from accidental burns is a critical duty of the pediatrician or emergency physician evaluating infants and children after thermal injury.

Patterns of burns from hot liquid can help to determine whether the burn was accidental or inflicted. A common scenario that results in accidental burn is when a toddler reaches up to pull a cup or a pan of hot liquid from a table edge or stove. As the hot liquid spills down over the child, it can soak through clothes to leave a characteristic burn pattern. This scald burn pattern typically has irregular, sometimes indistinct, margins. There may be areas of both superficial and partial-thickness involvement. Satellite splash lesions may also be noted. In some cases, the burn may have a V-shaped pattern in which the burn diminishes lower on the child's body, representing cooling of the liquid as it descends during the spill (42) (Fig. 7-3, see Colorplate following page 144).

An inflicted burn from hot liquid may be the result of intentional scalding or immersion. With immersion burns, children's buttocks or limbs are dipped into hot water. When burns have a stocking- or glove-like (circumferential) pattern or bilateral/mirror image distribution, abuse must be considered. Features of immersion burns include distinctly clear margins between burned tissue and intact skin (42), a uniform degree of burn (e.g., second degree) throughout the wound, and sometimes a circumferential distribution of the burn. Satellite splash marks are generally absent, and

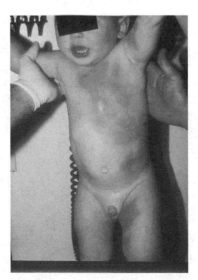

**FIG. 7-3.** A V-shaped scald burn caused by hot liquid cooling as it poured down this child's body. This scald caused both first- and second-degree burns. (Courtesy of Chief Medical Examiner's Office, Louisville, Kentucky.)

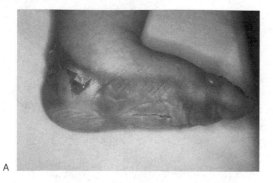

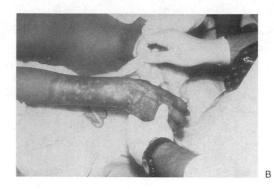

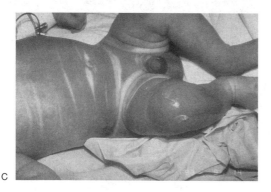

**FIG. 7-4.** Immersion burns. **A:** Immersion or "dunk" burn caused by dipping foot in hot liquid. Note the clear delineation of burned and normal skin along with the uniform degree of burn (here a second-degree burn) throughout the burn distribution. **B:** Immersion burn caused by dipping infant in hot liquid. **C:** Note where skin folds protected underlying tissue from serious burn. (Courtesy of Dr. William Smock, University of Louisville School of Medicine.)

areas of skin pressed against the tub or the container of liquid, as well as skin folds, are spared (42) (Fig. 7-4, see Colorplate following page 144). Hot tap water can cause severe scald burns, especially if hot-water heaters are set excessively high (43). For example, water at 111°F requires 6 hours to produce thermal skin injury, whereas water at 130°F requires only 10 seconds to result in second-degree and third-degree scald burns. At 140°F, the burn can occur after 1 second (40,44).

Contact with hot objects (e.g., curling irons, cigarettes, or chemicals) can also result in thermal injury. Specific hot objects making contact with skin produce pattern burns. Differentiation between accidental and inflicted burns may depend on reconstruction of the event based on the child's story, the caretaker's story, and the pattern itself. Generally, inflicted burns result when rigid objects hot enough to produce a second-degree burn are pressed against the skin (42). The burn degree is uniform throughout the wound. Accidental burns may have variability in their appearance secondary to pulling away from the hot object.

Single burns from steam irons or curling irons must be evaluated carefully in relation to burn location (e.g., buttocks or perineum), age of the burn, age of the child, and the history given (43–45). Cigarette burns (typically measuring 8 mm) especially should spark the investigator's curiosity because lit cigarettes are not common childhood hazards (45,46). Multiple burns are rarely accidental (45,47). Suspicion should also be raised when burns coexist with other injuries or with neglect (45–48). A grasp of burn injuries and their identification and evaluation is a powerful tool for assessing the truth presented in a caretaker's history (42,45).

### Bite Wounds

Bite wounds in child abuse can be located on any body surface. The investigator must first determine if the wound is indeed a bite mark, then whether the bite is human or animal (35). Animals generally possess canine teeth that protrude and can create puncture marks separate from the other smaller teeth in their jaws. This can help distinguish animal bites from human bites, in which generally no one tooth punctures significantly more deeply than the others.

The upper and lower arches help to define a human bite wound. They create an oval wound (if both arches are involved) or an arc-shaped wound if only one arch was used in biting. Bite injuries result from the force of the teeth leaving their imprint in the skin, producing contusions or abrasions. Included in bite wounds is the "suck mark," where suction also causes petechial hemorrhages ("hickey").

Both adults and children can inflict bite wounds. To determine if a bite wound was created by adult jaws the distance between the canine teeth marks can be measured. A distance of greater than 3 cm indicates that the perpetrator was likely an adult.

It is critical that bite wounds be diagrammed, with measurements recorded, as well as photographed, if possible. A measuring indicator, such as a ruler, must be included in the photograph to aid in further evaluations. In some cases, when a bite wound also imparts significant swelling, the measurements and photographs can be repeated 24 hours later for clarity. A forensic dentist can be helpful in the evaluation of bite marks and their unique individual characteristics that help to identify the perpetrator.

Another component of bite wounds that can be overlooked is that recent wounds are contaminated with human saliva. Since 80% of humans secrete their ABO blood group antigens in saliva, swabbing these wounds may secure evidence to help confirm or deny a known suspect as the perpetrator (35).

### Intraoral Soft-Tissue Injuries

Intraoral soft tissue injuries in child abuse can occur when significant external force is applied to the child's mouth. A common example is a contusion or laceration of the mucosal surface of the lip, produced when the child's own teeth imprint on the soft tissue. If the external force produces severe distortion of the upper or lower lips, the delicate frenula of the lip may tear partially or completely. The frenulum of the tongue is less likely to be torn by external force but may be injured by objects thrust into the mouth, such as a bottle, when forced (49). Note that objects forced into the mouth can lead to direct trauma of the buccal mucosa and the hard and soft palates. A careful oral examination should be included in the assessment of child abuse.

## SKELETAL MANIFESTATIONS OF CHILD ABUSE

The incidence of fractures in child abuse ranges from 11% to 55% (50). Associated injuries include head trauma (70% of abused patients with intracranial injuries also have fractures), visceral injuries, and soft-tissue injuries. Caffey's early work identified the connection between long-bone fractures and intracranial bleeding and paved the way for child abuse investigations (1,50,51). Fifty-five to seventy percent of fractures attributed to child abuse are in victims younger than 1 year; 80% are in victims younger than 18 months, and only 2% of fractures in this age group are the result of accidents (50). It is helpful to understand the types of fractures seen in abuse and their mechanisms of injury. Transverse and greenstick fractures result from bending or direct impact: spiral fractures, oblique fractures, and periosteal stripping result from twisting/torsion of an extremity. Metaphyseal fractures are highly suspicious for abuse, resulting from disruption of a relatively fragile, growing portion of the bone. These injuries typically result from twisting or pulling forces, are multiple, and appear on x-ray in a corner or bucket-handle configuration. The physician must compare fracture types, location, number, and mechanism with the history when considering the possibility of abuse.

The clavicle is the most commonly fractured bone in childhood, occurring in 2% to 10% of children, and such a fracture may be accidental or inflicted. The middle third is the most frequently fractured portion. Fractures in the lateral third may be more suggestive of abuse, although not diagnostic (53).

After extremity fractures, the second most commonly fractured bone in child abuse is the skull. Often, but not always, a scalp hematoma is present at the site of impact (53). The most common skull fracture, whether due to abuse or accident, is a linear fracture of the parietal bone (54). A simple, single, linear, nondisplaced fracture of one bone of the skull can result from accidental trauma, especially if there are no findings of intracranial injury. Multiple fractures that are comminuted or involve more than one bone are often a result of child abuse or significant forceful trauma, such as a high-speed motor vehicle collision. The probability of child abuse is increased when there is associated intracranial bleeding. As mentioned earlier, vertical falls from heights of less than 4 feet are not likely to produce substantial injury.

Rib fractures are highly specific for child abuse, accounting for 5% to 27% of child abuse injuries (50,53). They can result from thoracic compression or blunt injury to the chest (55). These fractures are generally found in patients younger than 2 years. They are often multiple and most frequently located posteriorly, at the costovertebral angles. However, they can occur laterally and at the costochondral junction in abused infants. Rib fractures rarely result from accidental trauma. Typically, they are the result of shaking an infant or young child while holding him or her about the torso. Acute rib fractures can be difficult to detect initially and may not be evident on x-ray. It may not be until callous formation develops at around 2 weeks that the fracture is radiologically evident.

Femur fractures account for about 20% of the fractures seen in abused children. Femur fractures in infants are more likely a result of abuse than in older children. In abuse, fractures usually occur as a result of violent twisting or swinging of the leg. Femur fractures can be accidental when a major force is present. However, trivial injury is unlikely to cause a femur fracture in a healthy infant. Therefore, a careful determination of whether the history is consistent with the injury is important.

The humerus is a frequently injured bone in abused children. Such fractures are typically diaphyseal or distal metaphyseal, unlike supracondylar fractures found commonly in nonabusive situations. The mechanism includes pulling, swinging, or jerking the arm, resulting in a range of fractures, including oblique or spiral fractures.

Tibial fractures represent abuse less frequently than other fractures. One must be aware of the "toddler's fracture," a nondisplaced oblique fracture of the distal tibia that can occur with a trivial mechanism in toddlers who are learning to walk (age 9 months to 3 years). However, spiral fractures can signal abuse, so that a careful history must be elicited and correlated with the injury.

Additional fractures related to child abuse are vertebral fractures (occurring after severe hyperflexion, often at the thoracolumbar junction), facial fractures (less than 2% of child abuse injuries), and sternal fractures. Scapular and pelvic fractures, also rare, require a significant amount of force; therefore, the clinician must maintain a high level of suspicion for abuse (50,53).

Bones exhibit varying degrees of healing, depending on the age of the patient. In general, the younger the infant, the more rapidly his or her bones will heal. There are distinct phases of healing. The first phase (induction) occurs immediately after injury and lasts until the appearance of new bone at the fracture site. There is pain and swelling at the area of fracture. If the fracture is nondisplaced, this phase may last only a few days. Appearance on x-ray may only be that of soft-tissue swelling. The fracture itself may not appear until bone resorption occurs. The second phase (soft-callus stage) begins with periosteal new bone formation. A callus forms at the fracture site. This can occur 7 to 10 days after a fracture in infants and 10 to 14 days after a fracture in older children. The third phase (hard-callus stage) occurs when periosteal/endosteal bone converts to lamellar bone and progresses to a callus. This is seen at 14 to 21 days for infants and at 21 to 42 days for older children. The final stage (remodeling) reflects the gradual resorption of bone to yield new bony configuration and correction of deformity. This may appear up to 12 weeks after injury and peaks up to 2 years later. Given this information, healing rib fractures noted on x-ray of a 6-month-old infant are likely 2 to 4 weeks old.

The skeletal survey is an important part of the workup of child abuse. They should be routinely ordered in all children younger than 2 years in whom child abuse is suspected. This may include patients with head injury or other injuries associated with abuse as well as their siblings, who are also at risk. After age 3 years, a skeletal survey should be considered depending on the case, but this is unlikely to be helpful in an asymptomatic child (34). A follow-up skeletal survey may aid in dating injuries and will help to detect healing fractures not visualized on initial films, when suspected (56).

## MUNCHAUSEN SYNDROME BY PROXY

Asher described Munchausen syndrome in 1951 to depict a series of patients whose fanciful descriptions of their fictitious illnesses and medical histories led to numerous surgeries and hospitalizations (57). In 1977, Meadow introduced the term Munchausen syndrome by proxy (MSBP) in pediatrics for cases where a child presents with unfathomable illnesses that require extensive diagnostic evaluations, including invasive tests, surgeries, or hospitalizations (58). MSBP is relatively uncommon and is estimated to occur at a rate of 0.5 per 100,000 (59). MSBP is represented throughout the world, and boys and girls are equally affected with a wide spectrum of severity. Frequently, the caregiver responsible for the deception is the child's mother. Less commonly, men are the perpetrators. There is no specific psychiatric profile of the MSBP perpetrator, although depression and personality disorders may be present (60). MSBP is classified as a factitious disorder in the *Diagnostic and Statistical Manual of Mental Disorders,* 4th edition (61), even though the mother may or may not have a history of Munchausen syndrome. A child is used as a means to obtain attention, often to the point of enforcing the child's invalidism to increase the degree of instability, and therefore the amount of medical attention paid to her. Other characteristics of the caregiver in MSBP are that they have some medical background, such as nursing or emergency medical training, or work in a medical office setting. They are able to describe symptoms such as apnea, seizures, or bleeding that initiate further medical investigation (7).

Some cases of MSBP can *simulate* illness. For example, Meadow (58) described mothers who submitted false histories of illness in their children and submitted contaminated urine for examination. In general, simulated illness is faked in its description but does not harm the child. Alternatively, persons with MSBP can *produce* illness. For example, in the same report, large amounts of salt were fed to a child, producing hypernatremia. A produced illness is one in which the caregiver inflicts injury on the child in order to create the signs of disease, such as scratching the child to generate a rash or injecting saliva into the intravenous line to cause sepsis (57,58). Both simulated and produced illnesses lead to multiple medical procedures and testing. Since Meadow's description, there have been numerous reports of MSBP, including presentations of the child or reporting by the mother of seizures (62), cystic fibrosis (63), and bleeding (64,65). Rosenberg's review of 117 cases not only includes these presentations but also depicts cases of central nervous system depression, apnea, diarrhea, vomiting, fever, and rash. Suffocation, poisoning, or other mechanisms can bring on actual illness in MSBP. Many types of agents have been used to poison children, including ipecac, laxatives, insulin, and chloral hydrate (66).

Morbidity associated with MSBP may be short term or long term. Long-term morbidity is that which leaves permanent disfigurement; it represents 8% of patients (66). Morbidity associated with MSBP includes failure to thrive, nonaccidental injury, poisoning, neglect, and developmental delay. The mortality associated with MSBP is 9% to 11% (66). Children may die from injury or illness inflicted by a caregiver or from complications resulting from medical investigative procedures and hospitalizations.

MSBP should be suspected based on the bizarre presentation of the illness or symptoms that appear only when the mother is present. The primary diagnosis tends to be a very rare disorder and the laboratory investigation does not concur with the child's appearance. There may be multiple, recurrent serious medical problems and/or a family history of an unexplained sibling death, including sudden infant death syndrome (SIDS). The mother is usually overattentive, has a medical background, and makes friends with the medical staff. The father is often absent. Treatments are often not tolerated (vomiting, intravenous line dislodgment), and the child's symptoms and signs are not present when the mother is absent (58).

The diagnosis of MSBP may be difficult to confirm. Toxicologic screens and assays of blood, gastric contents, and intravenous fluids may be helpful for certain types of MSBP associated with poisoning (66). In some circumstances, court orders can be obtained to videotape the child in a controlled setting. Social workers experienced in MSBP, law enforcement personnel, child protective services, and the hospital legal department can be helpful for advice on how to observe the parents. Medical records of the child from other institutions should be reviewed for documentation of day-to-day observations of staff members (60).

If MSBP is suspected, a court order is needed to separate the parent from the child. This can be diagnostic and therapeutic, as the child will improve when the mother is not present. Moreover, all of the children in the home should be examined and have their medical data reviewed. A pediatric social worker and the hospital child protection team can investigate and evaluate the home setting for all children in the household. The current and future health of the child is the focus in MSBP, as is seeking help for the perpetrator who may have mental illness.

## CONDITIONS THAT MIMIC CHILD ABUSE

Mistakes can occur when reporting cases of child abuse. Although the reporting of suspicions of child abuse is mandatory, one should be reasonably certain that the history, physical examination, and laboratory studies support evidence of abuse while ruling out other causes. An incorrect diagnosis of child abuse may trigger an awkward investigation (67,68). Accidental injuries, cutaneous manifestations, skeletal disorders, cultural and racial factors, and SIDS can be mistaken for child abuse by an untrained eye.

Child abuse can be confused with accidental injury. In distinguishing the two, it is important to consider the nature of the injury, the explanation by the caretaker of how it occurred, and the presence or absence of previous injuries. The child's developmental level should also be assessed to determine if the account of injury is plausible. The child's nutritional status, hygiene, and overall health should also be assessed.

Skin lesions are the most common presenting sign of child abuse. However, certain skin manifestations can be confused with child abuse. Mongolian spots, present from birth, can be mistaken for bruises. They may appear gray–blue in dark-skinned children and may be found over the back and buttocks. Mongolian spots are differentiated from bruising in that they are not tender and fade over months to years. Bruising or persistent bleeding can also be seen secondary to acquired or congenital coagulopathies, such as hemophilia or von Willebrand's disease. Acquired causes of bruising or bleeding include idiopathic thrombocytopenic purpura, neuroblastoma and leukemia, and vitamin K deficiency. In these instances, a complete blood count with platelets, prothrombin (PT) time, partial thromboplastin time, bleeding time, and factor level assays, in conjunction with history and physical examination findings, are necessary for the correct diagnosis (69). A detailed history, physical examination, and selected laboratory evaluation should help distinguish a bleeding disorder from abuse.

Some ingestions can be associated with bruising and bleeding. Salicylate ingestion causes subconjunctival and skin petechiae and purpura from increased platelet capillary permeability and decreased platelet adhesiveness. In addition, there are other clinical manifestations, such as vomiting and hyperventilation, as well as abnormal laboratory studies (anion gap metabolic acidosis and positive salicylates in a toxicology screening). Warfarin-type anticoagulants can cause bruising and bleeding by interfering with vitamin K–dependent clotting factors. PT will be prolonged with significant ingestions of these substances (70).

Easy bruising can also be seen with the Ehlers–Danlos syndrome. This syndrome is a rare autosomal dominant connective tissue disorder characterized by eight subtypes with varying severity. Skin in this syndrome is described as "cigarette paper thin" and is associated with hyperelasticity, bruisability, and fragility. Joint hypermobility, dislocation, and kyphoscoliosis are also seen. Children with Ehlers–Danlos may present with gaping lacerations and a history of poor wound healing (71).

Vasculitis can be associated with bruising and be confused with child abuse. In Henoch–Schönlein purpura, there is bruising of the legs and buttocks; in addition, arthritis, nephritis, and gastrointestinal bleeding may be seen. Erythema multiforme is present on the extensor surfaces of the hands, arms, feet, legs, palms, and soles. Lesions can be macular, papular, nodular, urticarial, or vesicobullous. Intradermal hemorrhage or petechiae may be present. The clinical features of the rash can make the diagnosis (72).

Burns, a common presentation of child abuse, can be confused with pediatric skin disorders where blistering is present. Impetigo is a *superficial* skin infection caused by streptococcal and staphylococcal species. Skin lesions, seen on the trunk, face, and extremities, appear as blisters that can rupture, leaving red circular ulcers resembling cigarette burns (72). Cigarette burns appear as *deep* symmetrical craters (8 mm) with purple crusts found on the dorsum of the hand, foot, or face; they heal slowly and leave a scar.

Phytophotodermatitis is a skin reaction characterized by erythema and bullae that denudate in streaking patterns, resembling a caustic burn. This occurs when the skin is exposed first to limes, lemons, or plants that contain furocoumarins and then to the sun. The furocoumarins act by inducing cross-linking of DNA strands on exposure to ultraviolet light (73). The reaction may be delayed for up to 2 to 3 days; therefore, its cause may not be evident.

The hair tourniquet syndrome occurs when a hair or thread wraps tightly around an infant's digit. Distal to the hair, the digit is edematous, painful, and discolored and may resemble a burn.

Skeletal defects that simulate child abuse may be secondary to congenital, metabolic, or nutritional disorders. They may also be caused by infection or drugs. Osteogenesis imperfecta (OI), also known as brittle bone disease, is a group of rare inherited disorders characterized by frequent fractures, blue sclerae, large fontanel, ex-

cessive joint laxity, easy bruisability, short stature, abnormal dentition, and hearing loss (74). Spiral or transverse fractures through the diaphyses are commonly seen; however, metaphyseal fractures seen with child abuse have been reported (75). The disease is caused by a defect in the synthesis of type I collagen (76). There are four major categories of OI, which result from autosomal dominant inheritance or from a spontaneous mutation. Type I OI is the most common, accounting for 80% of cases, and has an incidence of 1 per 30,000 births. It is less severe than the other forms, with fractures occurring between the ages of 2 and 3 years and again between the ages of 10 and 15 years. Other findings include otosclerosis, dentinogenesis imperfecta, enamel fractures of the frontal incisors, and radiographic evidence of bell-shaped crowns and wide pulp chambers (77). Type II OI is the lethal, perinatal form, which occurs in 1 per 60,000 births. It is characterized by extreme bone fragility, crumpled femurs, blue sclerae, and intrauterine or early infant death (78). Type III OI is similar to type II but less severe. In these cases, sclerae may not be blue, and a progressive bowing deformity is usually noted. Type IV OI is very rare and noted by moderate impaired growth and sclerae, which may be blue in childhood and become white in adulthood (78). Wormian bones of the skull are seen in most patients with type III OI and in one third of patients with types I and IV OI. Osteopenia of the bones of types I and IV OI result from the immobilization used to treat fractures rather than causing the initial fracture (79). If an accurate history and physical examination are done, missing the diagnosis of OI is unlikely. If blue sclerae or progressive deformity are absent, and there is a negative family history, the likelihood of abuse in an infant who presents with a spiral femur fracture attributed to minor trauma is much greater than that of OI (80). Skin fibroblast culture allows for analysis of collagen for questionable cases, but these tests are expensive and time consuming (81).

Copper deficiency can also cause bony deformities similar to those seen with child abuse. This element may be deficient in malnourished infants with chronic diarrhea, severely premature infants with low hepatic stores of copper, or children with Menkes' syndrome, also known as kinky-hair disease, which is an X-linked, inherited disorder characterized by defective intestinal absorption of copper (82). Copper deficiency is also associated with hematologic, neurologic, dermatologic, as well as skeletal anomalies. Sideroblastic anemia, leukopenia, neutropenia, as well as distended weak tortuous vessels may be present secondary to defective production of elastin (83). Neurologic manifestations (more severe with Menkes' syndrome) may include intracranial hemorrhage, hypotonia, psychomotor retardation, seizures, failure to thrive, and progressive neurologic deterioration from vascular insufficiency (84). Dermatologic manifestations include thin, coarse, brittle hair and horizontal eyebrows. The bony changes seen with copper deficiency are secondary to abnormal collagen formation. Osteopenia is seen early, which progresses with metaphyseal sickle-shaped spurs at the ends of long bones as well as periosteal reaction along the diaphyses. Fractures through the metaphyseal bone spurs can be mistaken for the metaphyseal-epiphyseal fractures seen with child abuse.

Vitamins D and C deficiencies can produce bone deformities similar to those seen in child abuse. Vitamin D deficiency causes rickets and is seen in covered infants with little exposure to sunlight and no supplemental vitamin D, or in premature infants on total parenteral nutrition without adequate calcium or phosphorus replacement. It can also be seen in children with seizure disorders who are maintained on chronic phenobarbital or phenytoin (85). In advanced rickets, serum calcium and phosphorus are low, and alkaline phosphatase is elevated. Radiographic findings of bones include cupping, fraying of the metaphyseal bones, separation of the metaphyses from the epiphyses, bone demineralization, and cortical thinning (85). Unlike active rickets, the bone density should be normal, and the metaphyseal fractures will appear frayed, as opposed to child abuse where fractures will be sharply delineated fragments. In healing rickets, noncalcified osteoid between the zone of provisional calcification and the main shaft can be mis-

taken for a metaphyseal fracture. Increased periosteal reaction can be mistaken for a healing shaft fracture.

Vitamin C deficiency, or scurvy, can be seen in breast-fed infants of mothers on vitamin C–deficient diets or in infants who have received boiled juice or milk without vitamin supplementation (86). Vitamin C is needed for collagen formation. Clinical findings of vitamin C deficiency include bleeding, swelling of the extremities from subperiosteal hemorrhage, poor wound healing, recurrent fever, and megaloblastic anemia (87). Radiographic changes seen with vitamin C deficiency include generalized osteopenia; the epiphyses are outlined with dense sclerotic rings, and the zones of provisional calcification become thickened, well-calcified lines adjacent to the radiolucent spongiosa. Fractures may be seen through the zones of provisional calcification and metaphyses. With healing, elevated periosteum may become calcified (86). The complete clinical picture, including dietary history, should help differentiate child abuse from scurvy.

Congenital syphilis is an infection that causes bony changes and may mimic abuse. The clinical constellation of symptoms of syphilis includes acral mucocutaneous rash, snuffles, hepatosplenomegaly, lymphadenopathy, recurrent fever, and failure to thrive. One fourth of children with congenital syphilis will have skeletal changes. Infants with congenital infection will present with pseudoparalysis of an extremity secondary to osteomyelitis. Destructive lesions of osteomyelitis in the metaphyses or diaphyses can vary from small corner separations to large cortical lesions and pathologic fractures. Syphilis can be confirmed with serologic testing (86).

Skeletal reactions similar to those seen in child abuse can occur secondary to side effects of certain medications. Prostaglandin E, sometimes used for treatment of congenital heart disease, may be associated with cortical proliferation along the ribs similar to posttraumatic periostitis. Vitamin A toxicity can produce hard, tender, swollen areas on the extremities that appear as periosteal reaction of the diaphyses without fracture. It can also cause widening of the cranial sutures secondary to increased intracranial pressure (88).

Hereditary sensorineuropathy is a rare autosomal recessive disorder that can be confused with child abuse. Patients are unable to feel pain and temperature, so they present to health care providers with multiple and repeated bruises, burns, lacerations, and skeletal deformities. Skeletal injuries may be undetected and lead to complications such as epiphyseal slips, aseptic necrosis, and chronic metaphyseal osteomyelitis (89). The diagnosis is made with a detailed history, sensory neurologic exam, nerve conduction studies, and nerve biopsy.

Certain cultural practices produce patterned skin lesions that may be mistaken for child abuse. Cupping is a common practice among Mexican and Eastern European immigrants, whereby a small amount of alcohol is placed in a cup and lit. The cup is inverted and placed on the skin. With cooling, a vacuum is created that leaves a circular ecchymotic lesion. Cupping is believed to decrease pain and inflammation by drawing the deep-seated offending agent to the surface (90). Coining (*cao gio*) is practiced in Southeast Asia and Vietnam as a treatment for headache, chills, or fever. The back or chest is initially massaged with mentholated oil; then the edge of a coin is rubbed into the skin until petechiae or purpura are present (91). Lesions are usually self-limited, although a case of renal contusion with microscopic hematuria has been reported (92). Spooning (*quat cha*) is similar to coining and practiced in China to relieve headache or fever. Water or saline is applied to the neck, back, shoulder, chest, or forehead, which is then pinched or massaged until it becomes reddened. It is then scratched with a porcelain spoon until ecchymotic lesions appear. It is believed that this practice helps rid the body of "bad winds causing illness" (93). Moxibustion is a form of acupuncture that is practiced in Southeast Asia. The moxa herb is burned on the skin with a piece of yarn, incense, or a cigarette near the area of pain to draw out the illness. Consequently, partial- or full-thickness burns are seen as discrete circular lesions (94). *Maquas* is a practice of Bedouins, Arabs, Druses, Russians, and Oriental Jews, whereby hot metal spits are used to produce burns near the region of disease or pain. It is believed that when pus oozes from the burn, the primary disease drains out (95). Salting is an ancient Asian custom, whereby the skin is salted in the neonatal period to produce healthier skin. However, in one instance, the salt was absorbed through denuded skin leading to hypernatremia and intracranial hemorrhage (96). A sunken fontanel (*mollera caida*) is believed in some Mexican American communities to be the cause of vomiting, diarrhea, and lethargy. Treatment of mollera caida may include shaking the baby upside down, which can lead to retinal and intracranial hemorrhage. When cultural practices injure a child it is important to analyze the context of the therapy before accusing the caretaker of abuse.

It is important to realize that many conditions can, at first, mimic abuse. Although a detailed history and physical can diagnose most of these mimickers, the degree of investigation required can sometimes be difficult in the emergency department. Early involvement of your pediatrician or child abuse expert is essential.

SIDS is a controversial topic because it can mimic abuse. The American Academy of Pediatrics statement on SIDS and child abuse fatalities estimates that fewer than 5% of apparent SIDS deaths are due to abuse (97). Emery in England reports on the danger of accepting SIDS as the cause of unexpected deaths, stating that 10% to 20% of "SIDS" cases are not natural deaths (98). Investigation of all unexpected deaths among children should include a thorough death scene investigation, a complete forensic autopsy, a review of all medical records, and a review of the case by a child-death review team (99). Therefore, referral to the medical examiner and child protective services is appropriate in all unexplained infant deaths.

## NEGLECT

Child neglect can present in many ways, some overt and some subtle. Neglect is the most common form of child abuse. Four hundred forty-one thousand cases were reported in 1997 (100). This may represent only the tip of the iceberg because signs and symptoms are not usually as flagrant as those seen in physical or sexual abuse. Child neglect remains underdiagnosed and underreported, despite statutes that mandate reporting. Unless neglect leads to threatening medical problems or death, it is seldom addressed directly by health care practitioners. The emergency department has become the primary source of health care for many impoverished families. Neglect may be overlooked during an emergency department evaluation because of more severe, acute medical conditions.

The definition of neglect may include all instances in which the major needs of children are not met (101). The major needs of children include food, shelter, protection, clothing, health care, education, and emotional support. Neglect can be physical, social, or emotional. Indications of neglect could include poor hygiene (severe diaper rash), inappropriate clothing for the weather, fatigue, listlessness, consistent hunger, obvious medical/physical problems that have been unattended (missed appointments, absence of appropriate dental care, absence of necessary health aids such as eyeglasses or hearing aid), and failure to thrive.

Neglect can also lead to mental health problems. If children are not stimulated and early lapses in language skills or hearing deficits are missed, additional developmental delay may compound social problems and difficulties in school. Lack of emotional support and developmental stimulation constitute a common cause of neglect and may be associated with depression, anxiety, sleep disturbances, aggressive behavior, and impaired peer group and interpersonal relationships (102).

Determining if a child is at risk for *potential* harm is also included in the assessment of neglect. For example, a small child who is unsupervised for any length of time is at risk for injury from trauma or toxic substance ingestion. Most cases are not clear-cut, and experience and reason may help practitioners determine whether neglect is present. The occasional missed pediatric office visit or clinic visit may simply be noncompliance, but refusal to provide formal health care, ensure that immunizations are up-to-date, and seek rapid medical attention for significant injuries are more consistent with neglect

and abuse. Neglect may manifest as a pattern of omissions or as behavior that repeatedly subjects a child to harm or to potential harm.

Maternal depression or drug or alcohol abuse may contribute to neglect and abuse of children. Family dysfunction, domestic violence, and poverty are other risk factors. Poverty is frequently associated with chaotic and high-risk conditions in neighborhoods where use of drugs, guns, and violence are widespread. Even well-meaning parents may have inferior child rearing techniques. There may only be one parent in such households and he or she may be working several jobs to make ends meet, so the child rearing may fall to someone outside the household. These factors, coupled with poor education and lack of societal resources, foster neglect and abuse.

The evaluation of neglect begins with the patient's medical history, the family history for potential sibling abuse, and whether or not the child has had the standard "medical upkeep" (i.e., meeting developmental milestones, receiving immunizations as recommended, and having regular checkups). Trends can be charted, such as the child's height and growth progress, cognitive development, and any evidence of failure to thrive. The patient's social development, including how he or she is progressing in school, is also an important element to investigate. A careful physical examination can assess physical development, hydration and nutrition status, as well as overt or subtle marks of abuse. Laboratory tests should be performed if failure to thrive may be of organic etiology. If simple problems are noted (such as poor dental hygiene or diaper rash), counseling the parents may prevent further problems. Referral to outside agencies may be of benefit for parenting skills, diet, and so forth. Social work referral may be necessary to apply for Medicaid or state benefits for children.

## CONCLUSION

Once child abuse or neglect is suspected, steps must be taken to protect the child from further abuse. Although not required, it is usually recommended that the family be informed before a report is filed. This helps to maintain a positive and constructive relationship with the family, even if they are the perpetrators. Remind them that you have the child's best interest and safety in mind. If the child is discharged, it must be to a safe environment pending investigation, which could include placement with other family members or emergency foster or shelter care. Child protective services will decide on appropriate placement. Other children in the household are also at risk for abuse and neglect and require timely assessment.

Many state laws require any person who suspects that a child has been subject to abuse or neglect to make a report to child protective services or local law enforcement. Mandated reporters (health practitioners, police officers, educators, and human service workers) who knowingly fail to make a required notification of abuse may be subject to professional sanctions.

Emergency physicians *must* consider child abuse or neglect as a potential source of injury or illness and make appropriate referrals when necessary. The determination of child abuse or neglect will be based on a number of factors, including investigations by child protective services, a hospital child protection team, social workers, and police. The burden of responsibility for the diagnosis does not rest on the emergency physician alone. Although the diagnosis of child abuse can be difficult, especially in the emergency department setting, the emergency clinician may be the only person who can intervene and save a child from a life-threatening situation.

## REFERENCES

1. Caffey J. Multiple fractures in long bones in infants suffering from chronic subdural hematoma. *AJR Am J Roentgenol* 1946;56(2):163–173.
2. Kempe CH, Silverman FN, Still B, et al. The battered-child syndrome. *JAMA* 1962;181(1):105–112.
3. Administration of Children, Youth and Families. *Child maltreatment 1998. Reports from the states to the National Child Abuse and Neglect Data System.* U.S. Department of Health and Human Services, 2000.
4. Duhaime AC, Christian CW, Rorke LB, et al. Current concepts: nonaccidental head injury in infants: the "shaken baby syndrome." *N Engl J Med* 1998;338 (25):1822–1829.
5. Conway EE. Nonaccidental head injury in infants: the shaken baby syndrome revisited. *Pediatr Ann* 1998;27 (10):677–690.
6. Jenny C, Hymel KP, Ritzen A, et al. Analysis of missed cases of abusive head trauma. *JAMA* 1999;28(7): 621–626.
7. Lancon JA, Haines DE, Parent AD. Anatomy of the shaken baby syndrome. *New Anatomist* 1998;253: 13–18.
8. American Academy of Pediatrics Committee on Child Abuse and Neglect. Shaken baby syndrome: inflicted cerebral trauma. *Pediatrics* 1993;92(6):872–875.
9. Duhaime AC, Gennerallie TA, Thibault LE, et al. The shaken baby syndrome: a clinical, pathological, and biomechanical study. *J Neurosurg* 1987;66:409–415.
10. Hymel KP, Bandak FA, Partington MD, et al. Abusive head trauma? A biomechanics-based approach. *Child Maltreat* 1998;3(2):116–128.
11. Tarantino C, Dowd D, Mudock T. Short vertical falls in infants. *Pediatr Emerg Care* 1999;15(1):5–8.
12. Root E. Head injuries from short distance falls. *Am J Forensic Med Pathol* 1992;13(1):85–87.
13. Duhaime AC, Alario AJ, Lewander WJ, et al. Head injury in very young children: mechanisms, injury types, and ophthalmologic findings in 100 hospitalized patients younger than 2 years of age. *Pediatrics* 1992; 90(2)179–185.
14. Reece RM, Sege R. Childhood head injuries: accidental or inflicted? *Arch Pediatr Adol Med* 2000;154: 11–16.
15. Tzioumi D, Oates RK. Subdural hematomas in children under 2 years: accidental or infected? A 10-year experience. *Child Abuse Negl* 1998;22(11):1105–1112.
16. Krous HF, Bayard R. Shaken infant syndrome: selected controversies. *Pediatr Dev Pathol* 1999;2:497–498.
17. Hadley MN, Sonntag VK, Rekate H, et al. The infant whiplash-shake injury syndrome: a clinical and pathological study. *Neurosurgery* 1989;24(4):536–540.
18. Kanter RK. Retinal hemorrhages after cardiopulmonary resuscitation and child abuse. *Pediatr* 1986: 108(3):430–432.
19. Johnson DL, Braun D, Friendly D. Accidental head trauma and retinal hemorrhage. *Neurosurgery* 1993;33 (2):231–235.
20. Block RW. Child abuse—controversies and imposters. *Curr Probl Pediatr* 1999;29:253–272.
21. Odom A, Christ E, Kerr N, et al. Prevalence of retinal hemorrhages in pediatric patients after in-hospital cardiopulmonary resuscitation: a prospective study. *Pediatrics* 1997;99(6):E3.
22. Swenson J, Levitt C. Shaken baby syndrome: diagnosis and prevention. *Minn Med Public Health Rep* 1997;80:41–44.
23. Gilliland MG. Interval between injury and severe symptoms in non-accidental head trauma in infants and young children. *J Forensic Sci* 1998;43(3):723–725.
24. Starling SP, Holden JR, Jenny C. Abusive head trauma: the relationship of perpetrators to their victims. *Pediatrics* 1995;98:259–262.
25. Willman KY, Bank DE, Senac M, et al. Restricting the time of injury in fatal inflicted head injuries. *Child Abuse Negl* 1998;22(10):943–946.
26. The Third National Conference on Shaken Baby Syndrome. Salt Lake City, September 2000.
27. Cameron CM, Lazoritz S, Calhoun A. Blunt abdominal injury: simultaneously occurring liver and pancreatic injury in child abuse. *Pediatr Emerg Care* 1997;13(4)334–336.

28. Coant PN, Kornberg AE, Brody A. Markers for occult liver injury in cases of physical abuse in children. *Pediatrics* 1992;89(2):274–278.

29. Spitz L, Platt M. The battered child and adolescent. In: Spitz WU, Fischer RS, eds. *Medicolegal investigation of death*, 3rd ed. Springfield, IL: Charles C. Thomas, 1993.

30. Kini WJ, Brady S, Lazoritz N. Evaluating child sexual abuse in the emergency department: clinical and behavioral indicators. *Acad Emerg Med* 1996;3: 966–976.

31. American College of Emergency Physicians. Evaluation and management of the sexually assaulted or sexually abused patient, June 1999, Dallas, Texas.

32. Frasier LD. Genital warts in children. *APSAC Advisor* 1998;11:9–10.

33. Smock WS. The forensic aspects of caring for victims of domestic assault: identification of pattern injury. *Physicians for a Violence-Free Society Action Notes* 1997:24.

34. Jenny C, Hay TC. In: *The visual diagnosis of child physical abuse*. The American Academy of Pediatrics and the C. Henry Kempe National Center for the Prevention and Treatment of Child Abuse and Neglect, University of Colorado School of Medicine and Health Sciences Center, 1994.

35. Spitz W. Blunt force injury, sharp force injury, thermal injury. In: Spitz WU, Fischer RS, eds. *Medicolegal investigation of death*, 3rd ed. Springfield, IL: Charles C. Thomas, 1993.

36. Schwartz AJ, Ricci LR. How accurately can bruises be aged in abused children? Literature review and synthesis. *Pediatrics* 1996;97(2):254–257.

37. Wallen E, Crowley KM, Evans RJ, et al. Aging of cutaneous bruises using spectrophotometry. *Proc Am Acad Forensic Sci* 1999.

38. Nelson G, Paletta FX. Burns in children. *Surg Gynecol Obstet* 1969;128:518–522.

39. Purdue GS, Hunt JL, Prescott PR. Child abuse by burning: an index of suspicion. *J Trauma* 1988;28(2):221–224.

40. Lenoski EF, Hunter KA. Specific patterns of inflicted burn injuries. *J Trauma* 1977;17(11):842–846.

41. Hight DW, Bakalar HR, Lloyd JR. Inflicted burns in children: recognition and treatment. *JAMA* 1979;242 (6):517–520.

42. Lenoski EF, Hunter KA. Specific patterns of inflicted burn injuries. *J Trauma* 1977;17(11):842–846.

43. Chadwick D. The diagnosis of inflicted injury in infants and young children. *Del Med J* 1997;69(7): 345–354.

44. Feldman K, Schaller R, Feldman JA, et al. Tap water scalded burns in children. *Pediatrics* 1978;62(1):1–7.

45. Keen JH, Lendrun J, Wolman B. Inflicted burns and scalds in children. *Br Med J* 1975;4:268–269.

46. Stone NH, Rinaldo L, Humphrey CR, Brown RH. Child abuse by burning. *Surg Clin N Am* 1970; 50(6):1419–1424.

47. Ayoub C, Pfeifer D. Burns as a manifestation of child abuse and neglect. *Am J Dis Child* 1979;133: 910–914.

48. Rosenberg NM, Marino D. Frequency of suspected abuse/neglect in burn patients. *Pediatr Emerg Care* 1989;54(4):219–221.

49. Donly K, Nowak AJ. Maxillofacial, neck, and dental lesions in child abuse. In: Reece RM, ed. *Child abuse: medical diagnosis and management*. Baltimore: Williams & Wilkins, 1994:150–166.

50. Sopher IM. Forensic odontology. In: Spitz WU, Fischer RS, eds. *Medicolegal investigation of death*, 3rd ed. Springfield, IL: Charles C. Thomas, 1993.

51. Monteleone JA, Brodeur AE. Identifying, interpreting, and reporting injuries. In: Monteleone JA, Brodeur AE, eds. *Child maltreatment: a clinical guide and reference*, 2nd ed. St. Louis: G. W. Medical Publishing, 1998.

52. U.S. Department of Health and Human Services. Centers for Disease Control and Prevention. 1998 Guidelines for Treatment of Sexually Transmitted Diseases. Morbidity and Mortality Weekly Report, 1998;47 (No. RR-1):108–114.

53. Kleinman PK, Nimkin K, Spevak M, et al. Followup skeletal surveys in suspected child abuse. *Am J Radiol* 1996;167:893–896.

54. Rao P, Carty H. Non-accidental injury: review of the radiology. *Clin Radiol* 1999;54:11–24.

55. Leventhal JM, Thomas S, Rosenfield NS, et al. Fractures in young children: distinguishing child abuse from unintentional injuries. *Am J Dis Child* 1993; 147:87–92.

56. Worlock P, Stower M, Barbor P. Patterns of fractures in accidental and non-accidental injury in children: a comparative study. *Br Med J* 1986;293:100–102.

57. Asher R. Munchausen's syndrome. *Lancet* 1951;1: 339–341.

58. Meadow R. Munchausen syndrome by proxy: the hinterland of child abuse. *Lancet* 1977;2:343–345.

59. McClure RJ, Davis PM, Meadow SR, et al. Epidemiology of Munchausen syndrome by proxy. *Arch Dis Child* 1996;75:57–61.

60. Rosenberg DA. Munchausen syndrome by proxy. In: Reece RM, ed. *Child abuse: medical diagnosis and management*. Baltimore: Williams & Wilkins, 1994: 266–278.

61. American Psychiatric Association. Factitious disorder by proxy. In: *Diagnostic and statistical manual of mental disorders*, 4th ed. Washington, DC, 1994.

62. Guandolfo VL. Munchausen syndrome by proxy. An outpatient challenge. *Pediatrics* 1985;75(3):526.

63. Orenstein DM, Wasserman AL. Munchausen syndrome by proxy simulating cystic fibrosis. *Pediatrics* 1986;78:621–624.

64. Matatack JJ, Weiner ES, Gartner JC Jr, et al. Munchausen syndrome by proxy: a new complication of central vein catheterization. *Pediatrics* 1985;75: 523–525.

65. Clark GD, Key JD, Rutherford P, et al. Munchausen syndrome by proxy (child abuse) presenting as apparent autoerythrocyte sensitization syndrome: an unusual presentation of Polle syndrome. *Pediatrics* 1984;74: 1100–1102.

66. Rosenberg DA. Web of deceit: a literature review of Munchausen syndrome by proxy. *Child Abuse Negl* 1987;11:547–563.

67. Meadow L. Unnatural sudden infant death. *Arch Dis Child* 199;80:7–14.

68. Christoffel K, Zieserl E, Chiaroamonte J. Should child abuse and neglect be considered when a child dies unexpectedly? *Am J Dis Child* 1985;139:876–880.

69. Bays J. Conditions mistaken for child abuse. In: Reece R, ed. *Child abuse: medical diagnosis and management*. Philadelphia: Lea & Febiger, 1994:358–385.

70. Haddad LM, Winchester JF, eds. *Clinical management of poisoning and drug overdose*. Philadelphia: WB Saunders, 1990:914–915, 1125.

71. Owen S, Durst RD. Ehlers–Danlos syndrome simulating child abuse. *Arch Dermatol* 1984;120:97–101.

72. Cohen BA, ed. *Pediatric dermatology*. St. Louis: Mosby, 1999;101,105–108,165,218.

73. Coffman K, Boyce WT, Hansen R. Phytodermatitis simulating child abuse. *Am J Dis Child* 1985;139:239–240.

74. Carty H. Brittle or battered. *Arch Dis Child* 1988; 63:350–352.

75. Astley R. Metaphyseal fractures in osteogenesis imperfecta. *Br J Radiol* 1979;52:441–443.

76. Edwards MJ, Graham JM. Studies of type I collagenin osteogenesis imperfecta. *J Pediatr* 1990;117:67–72.

77. Wright JT, Thornton JB. Osteogenesis imperfecta with dentinogenesis imperfecta: a mistaken case of child abuse. *Pediatrics* 1983;5:207–209.

78. Gahagan S, Rimza ME. Child abuse or osteogenesis imperfecta: how can we tell? *Pediatrics* 1991;88:987–992.

79. Patterson CR, McAllion SJ. Osteogenesis imperfecta: the differential diagnosis of child abuse. *Br Med J* 1989;299:1451–1454.

80. Taitz LS. Child abuse and osteogenesis imperfecta. *Br Med J* 1987;295:1082–1083.

81. Reece RM. *Child abuse: medical diagnosis and management*. Philadelphia: Lea & Febiger, 1994:23.

82. Danks MD, Campbell PE, Stevens BJ, et al. Menkes' kinky hair syndrome: an inherited defect in copper absorption with widespread effects. *Pediatrics* 1972;50:188–201.

83. Ashkenazi A, Levin S, Djaldetti M, et al. The syndrome of neonatal copper deficiency. *Pediatrics* 1973;52:525–533.

84. Levy Y, Zcharia A, Grunebaum M, et al. Copper deficiency in infants fed cow milk. *J Pediatr* 1985;106:786–788.

85. Zeiss J, Wycliffe ND, Cullen BJ, et al. Radiological case of the month. *Am J Dis Child* 1988;142:1367–1368.

86. Brill PW, Winchester P. Differential diagnosis of child abuse. In: Kleinman P, ed. *Diagnostic imaging of child abuse*. Baltimore: Williams & Wilkins, 1987:221–224.

87. Stewart GM, Rosenberg NM. Conditions mistaken for child abuse: Part I. *Pediatr Emerg Care* 1996;12:116–121.

88. Radowski MA. The battered child syndrome: pitfalls in radiologic diagnosis. *Pediatr Ann* 1983;12:894–903.

89. Spencer JA, Grieve DK. Congenital indifference to pain mistaken for non-accidental injury. *Br J Radiol* 1990;63:308–310.

90. Asnes RS, Wisotsky DH. Cupping lesions simulating child abuse. *J Pediatr* 1981;99:267–268.

91. Yeatman FW, Shaw C, Marlow MJ, et al. Pseudobattering in Vietnamese children. *Pediatrics* 1976;58:616–618.

92. Longmire AW, Broom LA. Vietnamese coin rubbing. *Ann Emerg Med* 1987;16:602.

93. Leung AKC. Ecchymoses from spoon scratching simulating child abuse. *Clin Pediatr* 1986;25:98.

94. Feldman KW. Pseudoabusive burns in Asian refugees. *Am J Dis Child* 1984;138:768–769.

95. Rosenberg L, Sagi A, Stahl N, et al. Maqua (therapeutic burn) as an indicator of underlying disease. *Plast Reconstr Surg* 1988;82:277–280.

96. Yercen N, Caglayan S, Yucel N, et al. Fatal hypernatremia in an infant due to salting of the skin. *Am J Dis Child* 1993;147:716–717.

97. AAP Committee on Child Abuse and Neglect. Distinguishing sudden infant death syndrome from child abuse fatalities. *Pediatrics* 1994;94:124–127.

98. Emery J. Child abuse, sudden infant death syndrome, and unexpected infant death. *Am J Dis Child* 1993;147:1097–1100.

99. Reece RM. Fatal child abuse and sudden infant death syndrome: a critical diagnostic decision *Pediatrics* 1993;91:423–429.

100. Administration of Children, Youth and Families. *Child maltreatment 1997*. Reports from the states to the National Child Abuse and Neglect Data System. U.S. Department of Health and Human Services, 1999.

101. Dubowitz H, Black M. Child neglect. In: Reece RM, ed. *Child abuse: medical diagnosis and management*. Baltimore: Williams & Wilkins, 1994:279–297.

102. Cichetti D. How research or child maltreatment has informed the study of child development: perspectives from developmental psychopathology. In: Cichetti D, Carlson V, eds. *Child maltreatment*. New York: Cambridge University Press, 1984.

# 8

# Elder Abuse

Adam J. Geroff and Jonathan S. Olshaker

When I was a laddie
I lived with my granny
And many a hiding ma granny di'ed me.
Now I am a man
And I live with my granny
And do to ma granny
What she did to me.
*Anonymous traditional rhyme* (1)

The abuse or mistreatment of an elderly person constitutes actions that many consider as heinous as abuse of a child. Indeed, state and federal laws exist specifically to protect elder Americans from such activity just as child abuse statutes protect our youth. Great strides have been made over the past three decades in the more widely popularized areas of domestic violence—child abuse and spousal or partner abuse—in terms of research, education, intervention, and overall funding. However, elder abuse, though present in society for centuries, has only recently received attention in the medical literature. Despite the appearance of an increasing number of studies, articles, and books on the subject, there are few national authorities and a relative paucity of research in comparison with other forms of domestic violence. The research that does exist is inconsistent with regard to form, methods, and even definition of simple terms. Certain authors include forms of abuse, such as self-neglect or financial abuse, that others do not. This situation makes a review and comparison of the literature difficult and confusing at times. It parallels the clinical aspect of this problem: many providers simply can't recognize, won't report, and don't intervene appropriately in cases of elder abuse or mistreatment.

Elder maltreatment is a problem that crosses all lines and knows no boundaries. Senior citizens of all races, ethnic, and socioeconomic groups can be victims. Their abusers, while most commonly a close family member such as a spouse or adult child, may also be professional caregivers in a domestic or institutionalized setting. There have been risk factors identified that can stratify those elders at greatest risk for abuse or neglect. However, these individuals are often the hardest to reach and most difficult to evaluate due to isolation, impairment, or dependence. This chapter will delineate the salient features of elder abuse and mistreatment. These points include history, definition of terminology, epidemiologic factors, and a review of specific types of abuse and neglect. Characteristics of abusers and victims will be examined and risk factors elucidated. Clinical aspects will also be discussed, including the varied presentations to health care providers, reporting obligations and issues, and intervention techniques and recommendations. In addition, a review of some of the legal terminology and medicolegal and ethical aspects of elder abuse and maltreatment will be presented.

Ultimately, using this guide as a tool, awareness of this problem can be heightened among providers to identify this type of domestic violence. Once this first step of recognition is achieved, continuing education in this field should follow. This will allow these providers to approach victims of elder abuse or mistreatment in a specialized manner, utilizing appropriate hospital, community, and government resources in a multidisciplined, coordinated effort to achieve positive results for elders, their families, and their caregivers.

## HISTORY

Elder abuse and mistreatment, like all other types of domestic violence, has been an unfortunate part of human existence since ancient times. Greek mythology and literature relate stories of the slaying of parents, called parricide, in order to gain power (2). Some primitive societal customs have involved the killing, abandonment, or have even encouraged the ritual suicide of the less productive tribal elderly to promote the common welfare of the group in times of scarcity (2). In early American history, witch-hunt victims who were tortured or burned at the stake were often postmenopausal women (3). Elder mistreatment, like all forms of family violence, was traditionally regarded as a private matter and was historically deemed excused from outside scrutiny (2,4). Despite the incidence of elder abuse throughout history, it wasn't until 1975 that this subject, called "granny battering," was introduced in two British journals published 1 month apart (5,6). Sporadic reports appeared in the United States soon after, and before the end of the decade the U.S. Senate Special Committee on Aging reported on mistreatments in nursing homes (7) and on domestic parental battering (8). Since this time, there has been more extensive research worldwide (9–17). Research has led to provider awareness, dedication of resources, and appropriation of funds.

In the United States, congressional hearings on this issue first took place in the late 1970s and early 1980s. As a result, in 1987 the amendments to the Older Americans Act sought to define terms for purposes of problem recognition. Following these, the Department of Health and Human Services established an Elder Abuse Task Force in 1990 to expand the scope of federal involvement in elder mistreatment. In so doing, the federal government identified elders in the community as well as residents of institutions as victims in need of aid. A year later, the Elder Care Campaign undertaken by the U.S. Administration on Aging created a National Aging Resource Center on Elder Abuse (NARCEA),

currently called the National Center on Elder Abuse (NCEA). At about the same time, the Joint Commission on Accreditation of Healthcare Organizations (JCAHO) included elder abuse among other forms of domestic violence in its mandate for improvements in the recognition and management of these maladies (7,8,18). Since then, more states have jumped on the bandwagon to pass legislation regarding elder abuse and mistreatment. The relative explosion of interest and preliminary research that arose where virtually none had existed before has prompted some experts to designate the 1980s the decade devoted to eradicating elder abuse (19). Slowly, health care providers, politicians, and other advocates are becoming more aware of this health issue as it is revealed from behind the closed doors that until relatively recently obscured our awareness of child abuse, sexual assault, and domestic-partner battering.

As a tangible approach to this goal, President William J. Clinton's first legislative action was to sign the Family Medical Leave Act in 1993, which, in part, provided families with an easier means to care for their elder relatives. His administration also expanded Medicare benefits to help older Americans and cracked down on fraud. Most recently in 1998, the NCEA received a $1 million grant designed to expand the agency and its services. Hopefully, future leaders will be as supportive of elder care. Indeed, astute elected officials will take this position not only for humanitarian reasons but for electoral reasons as well: as the country ages and today's adult baby boomers become tomorrow's senior citizens, candidates will need elders' support for election.

## THE AGING POPULATION

Despite improvements in elder care during the past 20 years, health care providers can expect to see more cases of elder abuse and mistreatment in the coming decades simply because the American population is aging. Better and more accessible health care, advanced technology, less invasive procedures, and pharmacologic advances are keeping older Americans alive and in many cases healthier than ever before. The introduction of Medicare in the mid-1960s was a major step toward this goal. The emphasis on primary care introduced in the 1980s and its role in disease prevention, risk reduction, cancer screening, and promotion of healthier lifestyles for both young and old has undoubtedly contributed to the "graying of America" (2,18).

Population statistics and projections are indeed staggering. Life expectancy has increased dramatically in this century alone. The U.S. Census Bureau projects the life expectancy for an American child born in 1990 to be more than 75 years, compared with an average life span of 47 years for a child born in 1900 (20). A person who reached age 65 in 1990 could expect to live for an additional 17.2 years (20). These data represent a marked increase over the 12 additional years expected in 1900 and even a significant increase over the 15.2 additional years anticipated by a 65-year-old in 1970 (2,20). The fastest growing segment of the elderly population is the "old-old," that is, age over 75. Often this age group is further divided into the "very old," between ages 75 and 84, and the "oldest-old," age 85 and over. This growth is demonstrated by recent population statistics, which reported a 38% increase in the number of Americans 85 or older from 1980 to 1990. Similarly, the number of centenarians doubled in these 10 years (2,20).

Elderly persons represent an ever-increasing percentage of all Americans. In 1980, there were 25.5 million people older than 65 in the United States, representing 11.3% of the population (21). U.S. Census Bureau projections for the year 2000 estimate that this number will swell to more than 35 million people, or more than 13% of America's population (11–13). Twelve million of these senior citizens will be in the very old age group, and an additional 5 million will be 85 or over when they welcome the new millennium (22). By the year 2020, more than 52 million Americans will be 65 or older (23).

This "elder boom" will bring even more interactions between the elderly and the health care system. It should come as no surprise that elderly people utilize health care resources more often and with disproportionate frequency than the population at large. This applies for both routine care and emergency services. Recent statistics from a 1994 report generated by the American Association of Retired Persons (AARP) showed that patients 65 and older accounted for 35% of all hospital stays and 46% of all inpatient care days (24). Seniors' outpatient visits also outnumber the general population's by nearly 2:1 (2). There will be particular stress placed on emergency physicians and emergency services providers (25). Several studies have demonstrated, as one might expect, that elderly people use emergency services more frequently than the general population (21,26–29). This amounts to an estimated 13.6 million visits to emergency departments nationally in 1990 (21). The elderly also are more likely to require a comprehensive level of emergency care. They are more frequently admitted, and they need an intensive care unit more often than younger patients (21). These trends imply what another group of authors has concluded based on actual data: elder use of emergency services is in fact more efficient than that of young people (29). Perhaps cases of elder abuse and mistreatment will increase in proportion to the projected population growth. Perhaps its incidence and prevalence will drop as elders, their caregivers, and their health care providers become better educated and more cognizant of available resources. Those involved in the care of elders hope for the latter.

## DEFINITIONS AND TERMINOLOGY

Definitions of what comprises elder abuse and mistreatment vary substantially. This variance has been a major barrier to understanding the true prevalence of abused or mistreated elders. Indeed, the terms "abuse" and "mistreatment" may be used synonymously or synchronously with one another depending on which authors are read. The different types of maltreatment are also subject to different definitions. Extensive literature reviews performed for this book and by other authors (17,30) have found no generally accepted meanings for these expressions. Furthermore, what constitutes abuse, mistreatment, or any other act in the opinion of one clinician, social worker, or layperson may not for another. Many authorities, including the American Medical

Association (AMA) (31), prefer the term "mistreatment" to include both abuse and neglect (13,18,32). "Inadequate care" has also been proposed as a more universal phrase (33). In addition, clinical or commonsense criteria for abuse may not be consistent with specific legal definitions. There is even discrepancy with regard to who is considered an elder. Most writers use the age of 65 as the accepted cutoff, but a few studies have included patients as young as 60 (1,11,34,35). One can become very confused. It is best to keep in perspective that the ultimate goal is the safety and welfare of the elderly. Rather than add a new author's interpretation into the mix, the reader should consider the relevant terminology and some of their existing definitions. The following practical definitions have already been published:

A broad definition of elder abuse or mistreatment is any adverse act of omission or commission against an elderly person (36). There is no consideration for intent in this most basic meaning. Other researchers restrict abuse to acts of commission with the intent to cause harm or injury (2). A Connecticut-based group that since 1982 has compiled significant data includes intent in its working definition of abuse: the willful infliction of physical pain, injury, or mental anguish, or the willful deprivation by a caretaker of services necessary to maintain physical and mental health (37). The U.S. Congress in 1985 introduced the Elder Abuse Prevention, Identification and Treatment Act, which sought in part to clarify terminology (Table 8-1) (38). Its definition of abuse is similar to that of the aforementioned group. In 1992, the AMA published a comprehensive and sensible set of terms and classifications (31) This listing (Table 8-2) was an improvement and foreshadowed what will likely become the gold standard for all those involved in the care of the elderly: the National Elder Abuse Incidence Study (NEAIS) of 1996. (39). This project, undertaken by the NCEA through the U.S. Department of Health and Human Services Administration on Aging, empowered a panel of experts to define terms prior to the study of domestic elder abuse. After a pilot testing period of definitions, the final versions were selected and utilized (Table 8-3).

**TABLE 8-1.** *U.S. Congress definitions*

| | |
|---|---|
| **Abuse:** | Willful infliction of injury, unreasonable confinement, intimidation, or cruel punishment with resulting physical harm, pain, or mental anguish; or the willful deprivation by a caretaker of goods or services that are necessary to avoid physical harm, mental anguish, or mental illness |
| **Physical harm:** | Bodily pain, injury, impairment, or disease |
| **Exploitation:** | Illegal or improper act of a caretaker using the resources of an elder for monetary or personal benefit, profit, or gain |
| **Neglect:** | Failure of a caretaker to provide the goods or services that are necessary to avoid physical harm, mental anguish, or mental illness |

Adapted from Jones J, Dougherty J, Schelble D, et al. Emergency department protocol for the diagnosis and evoluation of geriatric abuse, *Am Emerg Med* 1988;17:1006–1015.

"Neglect" is a term that is even more nebulous than "abuse." Some authors consider neglect less serious than abuse with regard to intent (40). Others pointedly remark that neglect,

**TABLE 8-2.** *AMA definitions*

| | |
|---|---|
| **Physical abuse:** | Acts of violence that may result in pain, injury, impairment, or disease |
| **Physical neglect:** | Failure of the caregiver to provide the goods or services that are necessary for optimal functioning or avoidance of the older adult |
| **Psychological abuse:** | Conduct that causes mental anguish in an older person |
| **Psychological neglect:** | Failure to provide a dependent elderly individual with social stimulation |
| **Financial or material abuse:** | Misuse of the elderly person's income or resources for the financial or personal gain of a caretaker or advisor |
| **Financial or material neglect:** | Failure to use available funds and resources necessary to sustain or restore the health and well-being of the older adult |
| **Violation of personal rights:** | Caretakers or providers ignoring the older person's rights and capability to make decisions for himself or herself |

Adapted from Aravanis SC, Adelman RD, Breckman R, et al. *Diagnostic and treatment guidelines on elder abuse.* Chicago: American Medical Association, 1992.

**TABLE 8-3.** *NEAIS definitions*

| | |
|---|---|
| **Physical abuse:** | The use of physical force that may result in bodily injury, physical pain, or impairment |
| **Sexual abuse:** | Nonconsensual sexual contact of any kind with an elderly person |
| **Emotional or psycholo- gical abuse:** | The infliction of anguish, emotional pain, or distress |
| **Neglect:** | The refusal or failure to fulfill any part of a person's obligations or duties to an elder |
| **Abandonment:** | The desertion of an elderly person by an individual who has as- sumed responsibility for provid- ing care or by a person with physical custody of an elder |
| **Financial or material exploitation:** | The illegal or improper use of an elder's funds, property, or assets |
| **Self-neglect:** | The behaviors of an elderly per- son that threaten his or her own health or safety |

Adapted from U.S. Department of Health and Human Services Administration on Aging and the Administration for Children and Families. *The National Elder Abuse Incidence Study.* Washington, DC: NCEA, 1998.

though conceptually different, should not be deemed a lesser form of abuse and can be just as harmful (41). The Connecticut researchers define neglect as the failure of a designated or responsible caregiver to meet a dependent elder's needs, or the inability of an elderly person without a caregiver to provide himself or herself with the means to maintain physical and mental health (37,42). Some experts specifically designate this latter situation as self-neglect (41). Interestingly, neither Congress's nor the AMA's framework addresses the concept of self-neglect. Abandonment is defined as the desertion of an elderly person by an individual or group responsible for providing care or by an individual with physical custody of an elderly person (39).

This jargon can confuse even an experienced provider. The clinician should learn these terms and become familiar with working definitions so as to recognize examples of elder mistreatment and to communicate effectively with the appropriate authorities. Even though various medical organizations, legislative bodies, and government agencies may all adopt seemingly crisp definitions, an individual form of elder mistreatment or abuse does not occur in a vacuum;

a victim of one type of mistreatment too often suffers multiple abuses (18). The bottom line for the emergency provider is still to recognize when an elderly patient has suffered adverse physical or emotional health consequences as a result of abuse or neglect.

## TYPES OF ABUSE/MALTREATMENT

Initial studies in different countries classified elder abuse into three or four categories: abuse, split often into physical and emotional/psychological; financial exploitation; and neglect (11, 37,42,43). Tatara's report for NARCEA in 1990 further expanded the scope of abuse and mistreatment to include three additional types: self-neglect, sexual abuse, and miscellaneous (44). The miscellaneous category was designated for "all other types" of abuse, such as abandonment (perhaps the extreme form of neglect) and violations of a citizen's rights. Furthermore, certain abuses and most incidences of neglect could be either active (committed willfully) or passive (committed without intent) (41).

Physical abuse involves willful infliction of force that results in bodily harm, injury, impairment, or pain. Examples include hitting, slapping, striking with an object, pinching, kicking, pushing, shaking, burning, and rough handling (45,46). The most common instrument used by an abuser to inflict damage, pain, force, or punishment is his or her own hand. A less commonly recognized type of physical abuse is force-feeding. Other abusive behaviors include improper and perhaps unindicated use of physical restraints, intentional withholding of medication, or overmedicating, such as with an anxiolytic or other mood-altering drug.

Physical neglect involves physical harm brought to an elder as a result of a caregiver's failure to provide the means for well-being. Examples may include inadequate feeding or hydration, not enough physical exercise or therapy, unsanitary living conditions, and poor personal hygiene care. Other neglectful behaviors include failing to provide or maintain basic assistive devices, such as eyeglasses, hearing aids, dentures, commodes, canes, walkers, and wheelchairs. The absence or inadequacy of safety precautions, such as bathroom handrails or bed side rails, also qualifies as physical neglect. Some authors specify that neglect is unintentional by definition (45), whereas others subdivide neglect into active and passive forms with regard to intent (41). An example of passive neglect would be an overburdened caregiver simply not having the time or resources to provide the level of care needed by an elder. If that same caregiver intentionally withheld basic items for that elder's quality of life, the neglect would be active.

Intent to cause harm is difficult to evaluate and even more difficult to prove. It is probably beyond the scope of the clinician to delve deeply into the issue of intent. The health care provider should be most concerned with damage control and safe disposition. An even more complex dilemma may arise in the area of self-neglect. Although the term is self-explanatory, self-neglect raises ethical issues and requires value judgments. An elderly person with moderate dementia, for example, who lives alone and cannot provide self-care, who presents with signs of physical neglect represents a case of passive self-neglect. A patient like this is probably incompetent and needs to be cared for, if necessary, against his or her will. Conversely, active self-neglect might involve a homeless adult who chooses not to utilize available community resources for the indigent and chooses a standard of living and personal hygiene below the socially expected norms (41). Other authors dismiss the notion of active self-neglect and specifically exclude this type of conscious and voluntary situation from elder abuse (39).

Psychological abuse is the infliction of mental or emotional anguish by threat, humiliation, or other nonverbal abusive conduct. It may be willful (45). Examples include verbal harassment, yelling, intimidation, and berating. Threatening an elder with punishment, physical abuse, or deprivation of basic needs also constitutes psychological abuse. Infantilization of a competent senior citizen is perhaps the most brazen of emotional abuses. A frustrated caregiver may be unaware of hurtful words hurled at a needy elder in moments of stress. Such negative remarks contribute to feelings of low self-esteem in any age group, particularly in the elderly who may

already harbor feelings of uselessness (47). Clinical depression already is highly prevalent among senior citizens (48); one's interactions at home should not fuel the fire.

Psychological neglect involves unintentional conduct that deprives an elder of good mental health. Examples include inadequate social stimulation caused by ignoring the victim, lack of companionship, or leaving the elder alone for inappropriately long periods of time (18). For instance, a caregiver might provide a dependent elder with adequate food, medical care, and housing but may not interact with that elder much at all. Such a caregiver may be supervising several seniors or may have other responsibilities that preclude him or her from providing even minimal social activity for an individual elder (47). Even facilitating a brief visit from a friend or giving assistance with a phone call to a relative might seem like undue effort for a harried provider.

Financial or material mistreatment may be abusive or neglectful. Directly exploitative behaviors include theft of an elder's money or property, or coercing an elder to change a will, make purchases, or sign any agreement against his or her will. Many elderly people have their checks cashed by others without proper authority. Likewise, elders can fall victim to slick confidence scams perpetrated by professional con men. Many instances of financial abuse involve senior citizens who possess substantial assets. However, even small incomes from government checks can become incentive for an abusive caregiver to exploit an elder, especially when that money may be a household's only regular source of income (47). An exploiter with some official control over an elder's decisions, such as a chosen or appointed guardian, conservator, or someone with power of attorney, may abuse this authority. Financial or material neglect occurs when the elder or the caregiver fails to utilize immediately available funds or resources to meet the elder's needs.

Sexual abuse of an elder involves any nonconsensual sexual conduct or contact between an elder and an abuser. Examples include unwanted touching, fondling, and rape. Other kinds of sexual abuse may be less direct but just as unseemly: coerced nudity, explicit photography, indecent exposure, and lewd talk. Some people mistakenly believe that any sexual activity involving the elderly, even between consenting adults, is somehow inappropriate. This notion is clearly outdated and wrong. There is no reason for an elderly person to stop exploring sexuality on the sole basis of his or her age. Discouraging, restricting, or prohibiting consensual sexual relations between competent persons may be considered abusive. However, some elders may be incapable of consenting to sexual activity. One must be particularly cognizant not to dismiss the possibility that a senior citizen could be sexually assaulted or harassed. This subject is rarely addressed in studies of elder maltreatment, and there are not many data on the sexual abuse of elders. On a positive note, perhaps a contributing factor for the absence of data is infrequency of sexual abuse of elderly persons. One study reports that sexual abuse accounts for less than 1% of all elder mistreatment (49). This study notes that sexual abuse is particularly uncommon in a domestic environment; its usual setting is institutional.

The deprivation of an elder's rights represents a miscellaneous form of mistreatment. These rights may include an elder's right to privacy and his or her right to make decisions. These decisions for a competent elderly person may include medical, financial, or personal choices. Forcing an elder from a private residence without due process or placement of a competent elder in a nursing home against his or her will also fits this category. Medical professionals may unknowingly participate in elder rights violations with regard to reimbursements for certain hospitalizations. It has been suggested that the funding of hospital care based on diagnosis-related groups (DRGs) discriminates against the elderly by potentially denying them the longer hospital course that is often necessary to achieve recovery than younger patients with similar diagnoses (50). DRG coding, with its emphasis on standardization of naturally varied and heterogeneous disease processes, does not account for age and its contribution to morbidity. There is no appreciation of the unique needs and characteristics of the elderly, such as slower recovery, comorbid illness, and possible inferior baseline function. That is not to suggest that all elders require longer hospital stays. Rather, assessment of any patient's level of functioning and the provision for reimbursement, at least in part, on the basis of function-related groups might eliminate this underrecognized iatrogenic mistreatment.

Besides grouping mistreatments by specific types of actions or inactions, elder abuse may also be classified by its setting. Abuse or neglect may occur at the elder's home or at the home of a caregiver. The caregiver would have some special relationship with the elder, such as spouse, sibling, child, other relative, or friend. This is referred to as domestic mistreatment (34,39). Institutional mistreatment takes place outside a private dwelling, as in a nursing home, assisted living facility, group home, or in elder foster care. The perpetrators of this type of maltreatment have some professional or contractual obligation to care for the elder. Abusers and neglecters can include nurses, aides, and licensed private elder care providers. In addition, administrators of facilities can exploit elders with regard to financial or material abuses without ever meeting that elder face to face.

## EPIDEMIOLOGIC FACTORS

The true incidence or true prevalence of elder abuse can only be estimated, but these approximations are frighteningly high for an enlightened and productive modern society. One must remember that the only cases of elder abuse that can be studied directly are those that have been reported. Thousands of cases go unreported each year, so data are skewed at best. Many studies that have attempted to enumerate these statistics have design flaws. There have been considerable discrepancies with regard to term definition, research methodology, data acquisition, sample size, and study goals. This situation makes any meta-analysis at this time impossible. Some studies attempt to extrapolate information using general population statistics to estimate national rates, whereas others confine the conclusions they draw to their data only. In addition, certain research groups have only reported on domestic elder mistreatment. Some other papers fail to include neglect as maltreatment. Sources of information also vary widely. Some focus on a small geographic area, whereas other studies compile data from nationally representative sites. Some studies directly sample cohorts of elderly patients in a community; some rely on previously collected information by protective services agencies; others retrospectively review hospital charts of elders, looking for evidence for or documented suspicion of mistreatment. The following text will review some of the more pertinent epidemiologic studies to date.

One of the earliest surveys by Block and Sinnott in 1979 utilized both primary sources (actual community elders) and secondary sources (medical and elder care professionals) to acquire prevalence data. They found that 4.1% of elders who replied as primary respondents reported at least one incident of abuse (1). The U.S. House of Representatives Select Committee on Aging in 1981 reported a similar prevalence of 4% based on secondary data obtained from state agencies. This prevalence translates into an estimated 1 million abused seniors yearly (39). Other studies estimate the prevalence as high as 2.5 million (51).

The first somewhat large-scale survey was conducted in Boston in the mid-1980s by Pillemer and Finkelhor who interviewed more than 2,000 elders and reported a prevalence of 3.2% (17). This study was one of the first to use clearly defined parameters for the mistreatments sought: physical abuse, psychological abuse, and neglect. These authors modified a previously validated scale popular in the family violence literature called the Conflict Tactics Scale to the specifics of elder abuse. This instrument consists of a brief series of questions designed to elicit evidence and frequency of actions or verbal assaults that might have occurred during a conflict with a relative, friend, or caretaker. Just one reported case of physical violence was sufficient for a positive response to physical abuse. The guidelines for psychological abuse were different. This maltreatment was limited to verbal forms of abuses, and at least ten instances in a person's life after age 65 were required for a positive case of psychological elder abuse. The damaging effects of verbal emotional abuse appear to lie in the chronic nature of repeated infliction, not just once or twice, which explains why fewer instances of verbal assaults were not considered abusive. The assessment of neglect used a different sociological instrument called the Older Americans Resources and Services (OARS) test, which evaluated ten activities of daily living to ascertain whether or not any aid was withheld. Once again, ten aspects of neglect were needed for a positive result. At these rates, the national estimate of abused elder Americans ranged from just over 700,000 to nearly 1.1 million. Because of narrowly defined terms, this study may have actually underestimated this problem's prevalence (51). In addition, an elder who reported fewer than ten separate incidents of verbal attacks or neglectful occurrences would have been excluded from the victim groups. European surveys of similar sample sizes reported comparable rates of abuse in the early 1990s, which showed that elder abuse is a global problem (11). These studies inquired additionally about financial or material exploitation as a type of mistreatment. Prevalence data are summarized in Table 8-4.

The NCEA conducted the most comprehensive study on elder abuse to date in 1996, the NEAIS. The U.S. Department of Health and Human Services published its results in 1998. The study's fundamental goal was to determine the incidence of domestic elder abuse and neglect in the United States. Its design was quite elegant and its conclusions well supported. The NEAIS estimated about 450,000 (range 211,000 to 689,000) cases of domestic elder abuse and/or neglect during the study year. This figure does not include incidents of self-neglect and rises to

**TABLE 8-4.** *Prevalence of elder mistreatment (%)*

| Mistreatment | Pillemer | Ogg | Comijs | Lau/ Kosberg |
|---|---|---|---|---|
| All types | 3.2 | 8.8 | 5.6 | 9.6 |
| Physical violence | 2.0 | 1.7 | 1.2 | 7.1 |
| Psychological | 1.1 | 5.6 | 3.2 | 5.0 |
| Neglect | 0.4 | N/A | 0.2 | N/A |
| Financial/ material | N/A | 1.5 | 1.4 | 5.2 |

approximately 551,000 (range 315,000 to 787,000) when all cases are totaled. Alarmingly, adult protective services (APS) could have expected notification on a mere 20% of these cases. The NEAIS concluded that nearly 450,000 elders suffered domestic abuse or neglect in 1996. Of this sum, only 16% of cases were reported to APS offices. That leaves 84% of victims below the tip of the iceberg and unidentified by APS. In other words, there are more than five times as many new instances of elder abuse and neglect occurring in domestic settings than those about which APS already knows. The figures improve slightly when self-neglect cases are included in the calculations, but they are still dismal. Seventy-nine percent of elder sufferers of all mistreatments, including self-neglect, remain unknown to an APS agency. It is worthwhile to examine this study in depth. For a thorough review, refer to the Appendix at the end of this chapter.

## VICTIM AND PERPETRATOR CHARACTERISTICS

The NEAIS and other data collectors have compiled demographic information about the victims of abuse as well as the perpetrators in order to better characterize both groups of people. Drawing definite conclusions is difficult due to the many differences in study design, but some patterns emerge upon examination of the literature. The available data suggest that victims of domestic elder abuse and neglect are more typically older than 75 or 80 years, depressed, and to some degree unable to provide self-care. Perpetrators in general are more likely male and closely related to the victim. Abusers also had a high rate of alcoholism and substance abuse.

Age has been shown as a risk factor for mistreatment. NEAIS results show that seniors in the over-80 group are abused or neglected two to three times beyond their proportion in the general population (39). APS agencies reported that this group held wide majorities in all categories of maltreatment except for abandonment. Earlier studies have also suggested this on the basis that the most elderly may have the most overall heath problems and be the most dependent and susceptible to maltreatment (2,12, 17,36). Although some recent studies have not found a direct link between frailty or dependency and the likelihood of abuse (13,43,52), it seems reasonable that an elder's overall physical infirmity and dependence may increase susceptibility to mistreatment (42). With regard to gender, the NEAIS data strongly demonstrated a female majority among victims in proportional excess to population differences (39). Similar to age, this predominance was shown for all categories except for abandonment reported by APS agencies. Whether or not gender truly is a risk factor is still in question. Some studies demonstrate statistical significance of a female majority (52), whereas others simply reflect a trend (13,43) toward this predominance. Others reveal the opposite: that more men than women suffer reported mistreatments (17). For some time, geriatrics authorities have felt that the mental health of an elder was an important risk factor for maltreatment (36). NEAIS researchers compiled data for both depression and dementia in abused elders. Both disorders were significantly prevalent among victims. Approximately 45% of NEAIS entrants were judged to be moderately or severely depressed, whereas more than 50% of them were at least "sometimes confused," if not "very confused" or completely disoriented (39). These numbers greatly exceed the prevalence of these mental illnesses in the general population (53,54).

It may surprise some people to learn that the most common perpetrator of mistreatment against elders is a very close relative, either the victim's own child (2,36,39) or spouse (17,52). Table 8-5 summarizes NEAIS data with regard to the perpetrators. A poor premorbid relationship between them or a history of prior violence may contribute to future mistreatment (12). One characteristic that particularly stands out among abusers is substance abuse (42). Some experts assert that a history of substance abuse, most commonly alcoholism, in a care provider is the single most reliable predictor of elder abuse and neglect (36). Such a care provider would have impaired ability to make care decisions, may be unable to control his or her behavior, and might

**TABLE 8-5.** *NEAIS data: perpetrators of elder mistreatment (%)*

| Perpetrator | APS Data | Sentinel Data |
|---|---|---|
| **Adult child** | **47.3** | **30.8** |
| Spouse | 19.3 | 30.3 |
| Friend/neighbor | 6.2 | 5.7 |
| Grandchild | 8.6 | 4.2 |
| Service provider | 4.2 | 4.2 |
| Other family member | 8.8 | 24.0 |

be motivated to exploit an elder's material resources to support the addiction. A history of psychiatric illness in the perpetrator also predisposes that caregiver to abuse an elder. One study documented that 35% of abusers have an addiction problem or psychiatric ailment (55). Although sources differ, an additional circumstance that may characterize a person responsible for abuse involves how much the perpetrator depends on the victim (42). There often exists a significant degree of dependency with regard to money, housing, or even emotional issues that can predispose a relationship toward abuse or neglect.

While some authors focus on victim assessment and others on perpetrator evaluation to elucidate a handy chart of risk factors for elder abuse, one must bear in mind two important points. First, the care-giving relationship comprises very complex emotional and physical interactions between the elder and the provider. Many so-called risk factors that affect one person also invariably affect the other. For instance, some authors identify external stressors on a relationship as influential factors for mistreatment. Such stress may involve financial woes, bereavement, and illness that may afflict any family member. Second, there is enough controversy in the literature to make any conclusions drawn speculative at best. Unlike coronary artery disease, whose reliable risk factors have been well studied among many thousands of patients, elder abuse may occur with few or no identifiable risk factors. The practitioner must approach every senior citizen who may be a victim of domestic violence with the same level of suspicion regardless of age, background, or comorbidity.

## ASSESSMENT/SIGNS AND SYMPTOMS

Elders who have been neglected or abused may present daunting diagnostic challenges to the clinician. Some mistreated elders might display obvious physical findings that will arouse a provider's suspicion. Others' presentations will be subtle and may indeed be indistinguishable from or confused with sequelae of normal aging (56), disease processes, or accidental injury patterns. The vigilant clinician should always entertain the possibility of abuse or mistreatment in any elder who presents for care. Equal attention must be paid to institutionalized seniors. Asking a few additional questions in an inoffensive and caring manner regarding an elder's welfare as part of a routine history may elicit a discovery that would warrant additional inquiry. Knowledge of the risk factors for elder abuse and neglect as discussed above should help direct the practitioner's approach to an elderly patient. Home health care providers are in a unique position to assess an elder's condition in the very setting where the mistreatment may be occurring.

An appropriate assessment requires time commitment. Although a busy emergency clinician may not be the person performing the entire assessment, this provider should have enough knowledge to perform adequate screening to determine which patients may benefit from additional evaluation. The thought of an additional responsibility should not be discouraging. It is not the role of the emergency provider to do the complete appraisal. As a parallel, think of a patient who arrives with chest pain and a clinical presentation suggestive of unstable angina. The emergency physician treats the patient and in so doing accumulates enough data to reach a decision of whether or not additional evaluation (i.e., telemetry or cardiac care unit admission or cardiology consult) is indicated. Then an inpatient provider takes over. Similarly, resources for elder assessment should be available. Every practitioner needs to be familiar with the resources accessible at his or her site. Emergency departments should develop and enact written protocols or clinical pathways for elder abuse, as many have done for other forms of domestic violence. Unfortunately, few have.

Taking a medical history from a senior citizen in general is a complex and elaborate process. Adding the burden of evaluating for elder abuse can make this task even more difficult. As a starting point, the AMA has proposed a series of screening questions that can be employed by any health care provider (Table 8-6). Although this guide has yet to be validated as formally effective, it may be employed in an initial attempt to uncover mistreatment. Some authors recommend screening for all elderly hospital patients, with particular urgent attention afforded those with cognitive or functional impairment (18). Indeed, it has been noted that such diminished capacity will not necessarily discredit an elderly victim's ability to report or describe abuse or neglect (7,31). The AMA encourages the questioning of all senior citizens regarding domestic violence regardless of whether signs and symptoms of mistreatment are present (31).

Certain points illustrating interviewing technique should be employed when screening an elder. First, it is important to interview any potential victim alone. The salient descriptions of maltreatment should be documented in the victim's own words. Specific and direct inquiries with regard to the frequency, type, and severity of maltreatment must be asked. Afterward, interviewing the caregiver (if available) separately may expose important discrepancies that might suggest a problem. All experts recommend that the elder be questioned and examined before interviewing the caregiver or suspected perpetrator. If nothing else, this method may in some small way reassure the elder that his or her story, in his or her own words, told in confidence, is of utmost importance to the clinician. The tone of the encounter should be nonjudgmental to elicit the most useful information. Although one's initial natural reaction to any abusive situation might be disgust and contempt, the health-care provider must temper this reaction and approach the case in a non-confrontational manner. Such a measured and calm approach has been shown to yield more data (2). The examiner should incorporate screening and other direct questioning in such a way as to make these seem like a routine part of the assessment. This may help a patient feel more secure. Focusing on the elder as a whole patient, not simply as a victim, and approaching the problem as one of unmet patient needs may provide for a less intimidating interview process. Indeed, the first encounter by an emergency provider may be the most spontaneous and useful source for information if conducted properly. It may pave the way for subsequent revelations during a social work or APS evaluation, especially because such formal consultations may seem very threatening to an elderly victim (18). General guidelines for the clinician during a patient encounter are presented in Table 8-7 (57).

General observations that are suggestive but by no means diagnostic of elder mistreatment include delays in getting medical attention, missed

**TABLE 8-6.** *AMA screening questions*

1. Has anyone ever touched you without your consent?
2. Has anyone ever made you do things you didn't want to do?
3. Has anyone taken anything that was yours without asking?
4. Has anyone ever hurt you?
5. Has anyone ever scolded or threatened you?
6. Have you ever signed any documents you didn't understand?
7. Are you afraid of anyone at home?
8. Are you alone a lot?
9. Has anyone ever failed to help you take care of yourself when you needed help?

Adapted from Aravanis SC, Adelman RD, Breckman R, et al. *Diagnostic and treatment guidelines on elder abuse*. Chicago: American Medical Association, 1992.

**TABLE 8-7.** *Guidelines for the encounter*

1. Express concern
2. Validate patient concerns
3. Assess and treat medical problems
4. Assess cognitive and functional status
5. Document findings and preserve evidence and chain of custody
6. Assess psychosocial needs and safety
7. Involve appropriate consultants
8. Ensure safe disposition
9. File report

Adapted from Ramsey-Klawsnik H. Assessing physical and sexual abuse in health care settings. In: Baumhover LA, Beall SC, eds. *Abuse, neglect and exploitation of older persons: strategies for assessment and intervention*. Baltimore: Health Professions Press, 1996:67–87.

appointments, doctor or ER "hopping," and any physical abnormality that is inconsistent with the explanation provided by either the elder or the caregiver. There may be suspicious inconsistencies between two given histories. Also, noting how an elder interacts with the caregiver may prove invaluable. Inappropriate or abusive behavior may be observed directly. An absent caregiver may suggest neglect or abandonment. The elder may appear afraid of the care provider or act very docile and obedient. Spontaneous and inappropriate crying may occur. More examples of historical revelations and physical findings are detailed in Table 8-8. This list is by no means all-inclusive and may not help at all in many cases. Some studies demonstrate that typical physical signs of elder abuse correlated poorly with reports (12). Nevertheless, the emergency care provider must maintain a high index of sus-

picion and take appropriate steps to ensuring the safety and well-being of the elder. Such measures may be extremely varied to meet the individual needs of each patient relative to the resources available to the provider. Communication with a reliable primary care physician to convey possible concerns and ensure follow-up may suffice in some cases. Hospital admission is always an option to guarantee (hopefully) a safe environment and adequate care. The involvement of a geriatrics consult team, if available, may be appropriate, as may consultation with a hospital social worker or direct referral to an APS agency.

The physical examination and diagnostic workup in the ED likewise must be tailored to meet the individual patient's needs. A guideline with regard to elder care in general is to err on the side of conservative practice. If a test

**TABLE 8-8.** *Pertinent findings on history and physical examination*

**Physical abuse and neglect**
Patterned injuries: Slap marks, fingertip pressure bruises, rope or ligature marks on wrists/ankles, bite marks, immersion line
Bruises: Especially on areas of the body not over bony prominences, multiple ages
Wounds: Laceration, abrasion, puncture, especially if untreated or in various stages of healing, decubiti
Head injury: Traumatic alopecia, scalp swelling
Burns: Cigarette marks, scald burns with an immersion line, absent satellite splash burns
Fractures: Spiral/oblique orientation without a given twisting mechanism, multiple fractures of different ages, mechanism not consistent with history
Subdural hematoma: From violent shaking with cerebral atrophy as well as direct blow
Nutrition: Dehydration, cachexia, weight loss, electrolyte abnormalities, fecal impaction
Drug levels: Sub-therapeutic or toxic, or presence of a drug not prescribed
Disease patterns: Untreated chronic disorders, excessive exacerbations of chronic disease
Poor hygiene: Filth, soiled with excrement, infestation, dental caries
Personal effects: Inadequate clothing, shoes, glasses, hearing aid, dentures
Living conditions: Fire hazard; infestation; inadequate heating, air conditioning, or plumbing
**Psychological abuse and neglect**
Communication: Ambivalence, withdrawal, poor eye contact, cowering, noncommunicative
Mood/affect: Agitation, depression, passivity, anxiety, hopelessness
Behavior: Fear, apprehensiveness, shame, paranoia, infantile behavior
Motor: Involuntary movement, rocking, sucking, trembling
Psychosomatic: Poor appetite, disturbed sleep patterns, posttraumatic stress disorder (may result from physical abuse as well)
Interactions: Caregiver insists on remaining with patient at all times, elder fearful of caregiver
**Sexual abuse**
Wounds: Located over breasts or genitalia
Infection: New sexually transmitted disease without reported sexual activity
Bleeding: Unexplained vaginal or anal bleeding
Pain/tenderness: On pelvic or rectal exam
**Abandonment**
Institutional desertion: Leaving an elder at a hospital without means of return
Public desertion: Leaving an elder at a public location to be picked up by police or emergency medical service
Homelessness
**Self-neglect**
Many of the above

or procedure is considered as possibly being indicated in the first place, then it should be ordered. So-called cost-effective strategies and evidence-based medicine are often not in the best interests of the elderly. All practitioners should become patient advocates when treating the aged, especially when the possibility of abuse or neglect arises. The evaluation of the elderly at a minimum involves a head-to-toe physical exam in a hospital gown, on a stretcher or a bed. Trying to examine a frail senior citizen with a physical or mental handicap who is fully or partially clothed and seated in a wheelchair will only do the patient a disservice. It may seem time consuming or inconvenient to perform this simple task, but only a meticulous examination will uncover occult findings that may be consistent with maltreatment. Ancillary data may include baseline laboratory tests, such as complete blood count (CBC), basic chemistry profile (CHEM-7, albumin), coagulation panel, urinalysis, and toxicology screen with drug levels if indicated. These tests may provide clues to aid in the evaluation of bruises, altered mental status, dehydration, and malnutrition. Radiographic evaluation of the elderly should also be liberally utilized. Unlike the abused pediatric population, no constellation or types of fracture patterns have been elucidated for abused elders (58). However, senior citizens are more likely to sustain fractures on the basis of bone demineralization, osteoporosis, or metastatic disease. Any significant bony tenderness or unexplained soft-tissue swelling should be considered a fracture until proven otherwise. Similarly, age-related cerebral atrophy and vein fragility contribute to the development of a subdural hematoma from even relatively mild head trauma (59). For this reason, a computed tomogram scan of the brain should be an important part of the diagnostic workup in cases of suspected or possible elder abuse. Any history or evidence of sexual assault should be fully assessed by a trained forensic examiner specializing in this field by colposcopy, evidence collection, and venereal culturing. The neurologic evaluation should include an assessment of cognitive status. This can be administered through tools such as Fol-

stein's Mini Mental State Examination (60) or the Short Portable Mental Status Questionnaire (61).

Even experienced providers can be fooled by findings that may mimic abuse. Skin bruises, for instance, may represent senile purpura (Fig. 8-1) or may develop secondary to thrombocytopenia or coagulopathy. Fractures that appear traumatic may actually be pathologic as a result of underlying disease. A senior with poor visual acuity may not be able to maintain good hygiene. Cachexia or weight loss can result from underlying malignancy. Certain cultural practices, such as spooning, coining, or moxibustion, endured willingly, leave wounds that mimic physical abuse (62).

Even if suspicious or questionable findings are present, the diagnosis of elder abuse or neglect may require more time than is practical for an emergency care provider. The primary goals of this provider are (a) to treat any active medical issues and (b) secure a safe environment

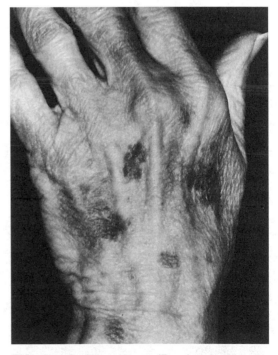

**FIG. 8-1.** Senile purpura. (Reprinted with permission from: Habif TP. Light-related diseases and disorders of pigmentation. In: Habif TP, ed. *Clinical dermatology: a color guide to diagnosis and therapy.* St. Louis: Mosby–Year Book, 1999:601.)

for the elder until all issues can be addressed. If this safe environment is an acute care hospital bed at 10 p.m. on a Friday because no family is present or reliable or because the hospital's resources are unavailable, then this must be the disposition. The emergency provider must stand firm and act as the patient's advocate in this scenario, which may be met with resistance from administrators or gatekeepers.

Comprehensive evaluation includes the following:

- Patient demographics: name, age, social security number, address, phone number
- Physical health: medical history, medications, advance directive
- Functional status: limitations, normal activities of daily living
- Cognitive status: confusion, dementia
- Mental health: psychosis, depression
- Personal hygiene: cleanliness, appropriateness of clothing, continence
- Support system: family/friends with contact numbers
- Current care providers: names, relationship, and contact numbers
- Financial resources: income amount and sources
- Social situation: type of dwelling, living alone, isolated
- History of violence: domestic violence in past or currently
- Physical examination
- Ancillary tests: radiography, laboratory studies
- Documentation of injuries/lesions: sketch and photographs
- Legal contacts: next of kin, power of attorney, conservator, and guarantor
- Safety in current living arrangement

Naturally, this information must be documented accurately. A descriptive narrative should be supplemented with sketches or diagrams of physical lesions. Photographs provide an excellent means of documentation. These must be labeled properly and should have some reference to scale in view as well as the means to positively identify the subject, such as an initial picture showing the victim from the waist up.

## REASONS FOR ABUSE

The reasons for elder maltreatment are as varied as the individual elders themselves. They encapsulate a broad and complex range of physical, sociological, psychological, and cultural factors. Certainly, no single or simple explanation can account for such a complicated process. Many purported causes focus on sociological theories, which are of lesser importance to the practicing clinician, especially an emergency care provider. A thorough understanding is not necessary for the clinician to recognize, diagnose, treat, and refer cases of elder abuse or mistreatment; however, an overview is helpful. Many authors have examined the issue of why people mistreat their elders; no consensus has been reached.

Some theories focus on the impairment and the dependency of the elder. Such a person would become more vulnerable to mistreatment by another. The perpetrator may be able to take advantage of the elder with less risk of being caught. Furthermore, a dependent elder may not report or corroborate an abusive situation because he or she might lose the caregiver. Some abusive family members report that a lack of gratitude in return for care given to an impaired victim has led to maltreatment (63). Perhaps more common is the following situation: An elderly person's impairments worsen over time, and eventually that person's needs exceed the caregiver's capacity to provide adequate care. The caregiver may simply ignore or neglect the situation, or directly lash out at the elder. A more recent study found the opposite: that abused victims were not more likely to be functionally impaired than nonabused controls (64) Conversely, the more important aspect of the abuser–victim relationship was the perpetrator's dependence on the victim. In many cases, a caregiver may be financially or emotionally dependent on the elder. This could precipitate a dangerous situation in which a caregiver materially exploits an elder or attempts to assert authority over the victim to preserve a sense of power or dominance. Some authors offer evidence to dispute the notion that abused elders are frailer than their nonabused counterparts (12,45,64–66).

Other characteristics of the abuser have led to psychoanalytic theory of abuse and neglect. Some authorities propose that psychopathology of a perpetrator alone may be enough to precipitate mistreatment, particularly physical abuse (18). When the perpetrator is a child of the elder, an additional factor may be an unresolved filial crisis. This theory proposes that the child's relationship with his or her parent never advanced beyond the parent–child discord of adolescence. A mature relationship between adults was never cultivated as the child aged, and unresolved conflict that should have been settled as the adolescent developed contributes to later abuses (66). Additional theories focus on transgenerational family violence. These hypotheses pose that violence toward family members is a learned phenomenon that becomes a normative behavioral pattern among children who are exposed to it repeatedly while growing up. Some perpetrators actually report overt retaliation for past victimization as reasons to abuse or neglect elderly parents (8).

Another theory focuses on generalized discrimination against the elderly, known as ageism. Common myths held by many people that fuel ageism include senior citizens being unproductive and resistant to change. Often abusers and mistreaters correlate age with functional impairment and assume that all elderly individuals suffer from or will succumb to Alzheimer's Disease. Nothing could be further from the truth. Although the cause of this debilitating form of dementia has yet to be fully elucidated, it is clear that age is only one of many factors (2). Unfortunately, many laypersons are not enlightened to the potential contributions and value of senior citizens and discriminate against them, either willfully or unknowingly.

The typical studies that attempt to understand "why" are small series of relatively few patients. Though interesting to behavioral scientists or sociological theorists, such conceptual models do not translate well into practical terms. It is easy for the clinician to become lost in a sea of social or behavioral hypotheses when attempting to understand elder abuse and neglect. Perhaps this is because elder mistreatment should not have a solid foundation in explanations, or reasons, or causes. Too much explaining may lead to rationalization of these despicable acts, for which society should, under no circumstances, accept any justification.

## REPORTING

The reporting of elder abuse and neglect is the cornerstone to intervention, treatment, and prevention. Most states have statutes that cover mandatory reporting of suspected elder abuse. Table 8-9 lists by state the contact phone numbers for reporting suspected elder mistreatment. Reporting will also aid in the understanding of this problem by providing additional databases for analysis. The source of any report to authorities may be the elder person; however, more commonly it is another person. That person could be someone with frequent and close contact, such as a family member or friend, or could be a professional with an episodic connection to the victim, such as a home health-care provider, social worker, financial manager, nurse, or physician. The last group represents persons particularly accessible to improving their ability to detect elder mistreatment through awareness and education efforts. Unfortunately, physicians report elder abuse infrequently (51,67,68) despite the standpoint taken by the AMA that they "are in an ideal position to recognize, manage and prevent elder mistreatment" (31). One facet of elder mistreatment that this mandate overlooks is provider awareness. Physicians are indeed in an ideal position to intervene, but only by first becoming better educated about this problem. The AMA's first step, recognition, can only be achieved through better physician education. Studies suggest that the latter steps, improved management and prevention, should naturally follow when clinicians have an appropriate knowledge base (69). Unfortunately, formal training appears inadequate, with only 25% of residency-trained emergency physicians receiving any education in this area during their residencies.

Fortunately, overall reporting has increased. NCEA data indicate that in 1986 a total of 117,000 reports of elder mistreatment were

**TABLE 8-9.** *State reporting contacts*

| State | Domestic Elder Abuse | Institutional Elder Abuse |
|---|---|---|
| Alabama | 800-458-7214 | 800-458-7214 |
| Alaska | 800-478-9996 | 800-478-9996 |
|  | 907-269-3666 | 907-269-3666 |
| Arizona | 877-767-2385 | 877-767-2385 |
| Arkansas | 800-482-8049 | 800-582-4887 |
| California | None available | 800-231-4024 |
| Colorado | 800-773-1366 | 800-238-1376 |
| Connecticut | 888-385-4225 | 860-424-5200 |
| Delaware | 800-223-9074 | 800-223-9074 |
| District of Columbia | 202-727-2345 | 202-434-2140 |
| Florida | 800-962-2873 | 800-962-2873 |
| Georgia | 800-677-1116 | 404-657-5726 |
|  |  | 404-657-4076 |
| Guam | 671-475-0268 | 671-475-0268 |
| Hawaii | 808-832-5115 | 808-832-5115 |
|  | 808-243-5151 | 808-243-5151 |
|  | 808-241-3432 | 808-241-3432 |
|  | 808-933-8820 | 808-933-8820 |
|  | 808-327-6280 | 808-327-6280 |
| Idaho | 208-334-2220 | None available |
| Illinois | 800-252-8966 | 800-252-4343 |
| Indiana | 800-992-6978 | 800-992-6978 |
| Iowa | 800-362-2178 | 515-281-4115 |
| Kansas | 800-922-5330 | 800-842-0078 |
|  | 785-296-0044 |  |
| Kentucky | 800-752-6200 | 800-752-6200 |
| Louisiana | 800-259-4990 | 800-259-4990 |
| Maine | 800-624-8404 | 800-624-8404 |
| Maryland | 800-91-PREVENT | 800-91-PREVENT |
|  | (1-800-917-7383) | (1-800-917-7383) |
| Massachusetts | 800-922-2275 | 300-462-5540 |
| Michigan | 800-996-6228 | 800-882-6006 |
| Minnesota | 800-333-2433 | 800-333-2433 |
| Mississippi | 800-222-8000 | 800-227-7308 |
| Missouri | 800-392-0210 | 800-392-0210 |
| Montana | 800-332-2272 | None available |
| Nebraska | 800-652-1999 | 800-652-1999 |
| Nevada | 800-992-5757 | 800-992-5757 |
| New Hampshire | 800-949-0470 | 800-442-5640 |
|  | 603-271-4386 | 603-271-4396 |
| New Jersey | 800-792-8820 | 800-792-8820 |
| New Mexico | 800-797-3260 | 800-797-3260 |
|  | 505-841-6100 | 505-841-6100 |
| New York | 800-342-9871 | None available |
| North Carolina | 800-662-7030 | 800-662-7030 |
| North Dakota | 800-755-8521 | 800-755-8521 |
| Ohio | None available | 800-282-1206 |
| Oklahoma | 800-522-3511 | 800-522-3511 |
| Oregon | 800-232-3020 | 800-232-3020 |
| Pennsylvania | 800-490-8505 | 1-800-254-5164 |
| Puerto Rico | 787-725-9788 |  |
|  | 787-721-8225 |  |
| Rhode Island | 401-222-2858, x321 | 401-222-2858, x321 |
| South Carolina | 800-868-9095 | 800-868-9095 |
| South Dakota | 605-773-3656 | 605-773-3656 |
| Tennessee | 888-277-8366 | 888-277-8366 |
| Texas | 512-834-3784 | 512-438-2633 |
|  | 800-252-5400 | 800-458-9858 |
| Utah | 801-264-7669 | 801-264-7669 |
|  | 800-371-7897 | 800-371-7897 |
| Vermont | 800-564-1612 | 800-564-1612 |

**TABLE 8-9.** *Continued.*

| State | Domestic Elder Abuse | Institutional Elder Abuse |
|---|---|---|
| Virgin Islands | None available | None available |
| Virginia | 888-832-3858 | 888-832-3858 |
|  | 804-371-0896 | 804-371-0896 |
| Washington | 800-422-3263 | 800-562-6078 |
| West Virginia | 800-352-6513 | 800-352-6513 |
| Wisconsin | 608-266-2536 | 800-815-0015 |
|  |  | 608-266-8944 |
| Wyoming | 307-777-6137 | 307-777-7123 |

Adapted from U.S. Department of Health and Human Services Administration on Aging and the Administration for Children and Families. *The National Elder Abuse Incidence Study,* Washington, DC: NCEA, 1998.

received by state APS agencies. Each year thereafter for the next decade a steady rise in the number of reports occurred (70) such that by 1996, the year of the NEAIS, this sum had grown to 293,000 nationwide (39). This remarkable increase of 150% may be attributed in part to increased awareness and dedication of resources as well as to mandatory reporting laws. Of note, over this time period the total elder population increased by only 10% (39). NEAIS data with regard to reporting of elder mistreatment are presented in Tables 8-10 and 8-11. Notable are the different distributions of reporters of self-neglect compared with those who report non–self-inflicted domestic abuse and neglect. The population projection estimates calculated by NCEA researchers concluded that more than five times as many events of mistreatment were unreported than were reported to authorities. Previously published data indicated that anywhere from 1 in 5 to as few as 1 in 14 cases were reported to APS agencies (7,31,68).

The NEAIS did not differentiate among specific health-care providers in its category "Hospitals." Therefore, these data cannot provide insight into physician reporting. Other statewide studies addressed this question specifically, with embarrassing results. A Michigan group sought to characterize reporting patterns among physicians by examining all reported cases of suspected elder abuse in Michigan from 1989 to 1993. In this state, more than 17,000 total cases were reported, with physicians supplying only 2% of the reports. Nonphysician health-care providers performed more admirably, accounting for 26% of the total, and 25% of reports originated with social workers or mental health workers. Interestingly, the largest overall reporting body was the community at large (41%) (68). This may suggest that cases of elder mistreatment that went unreported in the community may be the most difficult to detect, even for physicians. The authors acknowledge that some extraneous factors may contribute to physicians' low representation, such as delegation of reporting

**TABLE 8-10.** *NEAIS data: reporters of elder abuse and neglect*

| | |
|---|---|
| Family | 20% |
| Hospitals | 17.3% |
| Law enforcement | 11.3% |
| In-home service providers | 9.6% |
| Friend/neighbor | 9.1% |
| Physician/nurse/medical clinic | 8.4% |
| Out-of-home service providers | 5.2% |
| Bank official | 0.4% |
| Public health officials | 0.1% |
| Victim | 8.8% |
| Other | 5.1% |

**TABLE 8-11.** *NEAIS data: reporters of self-neglect*

| | |
|---|---|
| Hospitals | 19.8% |
| Friend/neighbor | 19.1% |
| In-home service providers | 12.3% |
| Law enforcement | 11.7% |
| Physician/nurse/medical clinic | 11.5% |
| Out-of-home service providers | 7.8% |
| Family | 6.5% |
| Bank official | 0.4% |
| Public health officials | 0.0% |
| Victim | 1.4% |
| Other | 26.5% |

duties to other staff or electing not to report suspected cases. However, common sense dictates that major barriers exist in physician reporting of suspected elder abuse and neglect.

There is a myriad of reasons why elderly victims do not report an abusive situation. Traditionally, there have been considerable obstacles to the detection and reporting of elder mistreatment. This situation is not dissimilar from other forms of domestic violence, which until recently have been considered private matters exempt from public or government inquiry (2). Often victims do not come forward in order to keep the mistreatment a private affair. Hopefully, these ingrained beliefs will break down as society recognizes with increasing fervor its role in acknowledging elder abuse as a form of domestic violence. Some seniors, having been victims of ageism in the past, do not believe that they will be considered trustworthy and honest historians when reporting abuse or mistreatment. Some, due to physical or emotional handicap, may have great difficulty communicating about this sensitive topic. Others hope that it will simply go away by itself. Some even learn to put up with abuse or neglect as part of their lives, perhaps becoming convinced by a perpetrator that it is deserved. An elderly person may feel ashamed at reporting maltreatment, especially if he or she was duped, or if the perpetrator is a friend or family member. The victim may fear repercussions, such as further or worsening abuse by a perpetrator if a report is made. He or she may fear separation from family or the loss of individual freedoms if the abuse is revealed. Alternatively, a victim may try to protect an abuser if the abuser is a friend or relative or the victim's only caregiver. Perhaps the most frightening prospect is the acceptance of maltreatment simply because of a pattern of victimization. This has been proposed to relate to elder abuse in a similar way to its application in the understanding of battered women, that is, some adult battered women show a pattern of repeated sexual assault as children. It is possible that this model extends into old age and contributes to abuse (2).

Differences in the perception of abusive situations among the elderly of various ethnic groups have recently been examined by two professors of social work using a sample of 90 elderly women (71). This approach is a novel and important one for gaining insight into the victims of elder mistreatment. All previous authorities from the diverse backgrounds of professionals who participate in elder care (medicine, nursing, social work, psychology) have focused on their skilled perceptions of what constitutes abuse of the elderly. Naturally, their definitions and classifications are based on formal education and training. Despite their good intentions, few of these authorities are senior citizens themselves, so a "grass roots" perspective is lacking. This survey examined lay seniors' views and acknowledged that these perceptions may not be entirely consistent with practitioners' judgments. Furthermore, certain significant cultural patterns of what would be defined as abuse and what would trigger help-seeking behavior were found among the three ethnic groups queried. Analysis of such behaviors and further studies should help professionals develop new and effective operational definitions and practical strategies for intervention.

There are obvious reasons of protecting one's own interests that perpetrators do not report mistreatment. However, studies of abusers show that they tend to rationalize their actions and minimize or deny the harm inflicted. Often perpetrators believe their actions to be justified because the victim was deserving of those consequences. They may feel provoked by an elderly person's behavior or demeanor to mistreat that person and not recognize that mistreatment is indeed occurring. Mentally ill or substance-abusing care providers may use their illness as an excuse for abusive or neglectful behavior, or their impairment may truly prevent them from knowing what they are doing. Even if an abuser expresses remorse after an incident, one study shows that this remorse is transient and the victim is eventually subjected to more and worsening abuses (2,72).

Barriers to reporting also exist within the medical community. Confusion over what constitutes abuse or neglect and over their varying definitions contributes. Other commonly cited reasons for poor physician reporting include fear of legal entanglements; unfamiliarity or ignorance of reporting statutes and procedures; fear of making a situation worse; and confidentiality issues and preserving the relationship with the patient (18,67,68,73,74). A national survey of more than 700 practicing emergency physicians performed in 1996 sought to gain insight into physician awareness and perceptions of this problem (75). This study revealed some startling results. Nearly one third of respondents characterized elder maltreatment as a rare occurrence, and more than 80% of physicians reported that they rarely asked elderly patients in the emergency department direct questions about mistreatment. This data correlate with an earlier survey of Alabama ED personnel done in 1988. In Alabama, more than 22% of ED physicians believed that "very few" senior citizens were victims of abuse (76). A Connecticut-based research group found similar results when they reviewed over 500 ED charts (77). These collectors used local APS data to compile a list of substantiated cases of community-based elder abuse. They then researched these elders' visits to local EDs in the 5 years prior to their initial identification by an APS agency as an abuse victim. Their trained reviewers retrospectively found that more than 37% of these visits were related with high probability to abuse based on the findings reported in the ED chart. Yet only 9% of these encounters resulted in an APS referral. Alarmingly, even in those cases of an obvious injury, physicians inquired about family violence less than 14% of the time. Table 8-12 lists the most commonly reported reasons for failure to report suspected elder mistreatment. This list reflects all of the inadequacies in the system that must be addressed on a local, state, and national level by government agencies, private organizations, and professional societies in order to provide for the welfare of the abused and neglected elderly. To compound matters, the Policy Statement on the Management of Elder Abuse and Neglect published in 1998 by the American College of Emergency Physicians (ACEP) places the emergency physician in direct conflict with the mandatory reporting laws that exist in most states in America (78). In this statement, ACEP opposes mandatory reporting of elder abuse and neglect when a patient is mentally competent. This mandate recognizes the "autonomy of the competent elder and the confi-

**TABLE 8-12.** *Reasons elder mistreatment is not reported*

| Reasons | % |
| --- | --- |
| Minor injuries or subtle signs only | 41 |
| Victim denial | 27 |
| Unfamiliarity with reporting procedure | 26 |
| Unclear about definitions | 19 |
| Failure to recognize the mistreatment | 19 |
| Ignorance of reporting laws | 18 |
| Inadequate community resources to respond | 17 |
| Patient confidentiality concerns | 4 |
| Incident already reported | 4 |
| Patient was admitted | 4 |
| Fear of legal involvement | 2 |
| Liability risks | 2 |
| Belief that it is the victim's responsibility to report | 2 |

Adapted from Jones JS, Veenstra TR, Seamon JP, et al. Elder mistreatment: national survey of emergency physicians. *Ann Emerg Med* 1997;30:473–479.

dentiality of the relationship" with the patient. It does encourage the recognition and management of this problem and reporting events "when appropriate," in accordance with patient wishes. Certainly, many clinicians will encounter this ethical and legal dilemma as they become more familiar with elder abuse and treat its victims.

An important question to consider with a competent elder is how much weight should be given to that victim's assessment of the situation and what he or she desires as a plan of action (71). What may seem to a practitioner as a clear-cut case in which an elder would benefit from involvement of social services and/or law enforcement may not be perceived as such by the victim, perhaps with good reason. The clinician must not practice in a vacuum; one must be aware of hospital resources, local agencies, and state laws. There must be an open dialogue between the clinician and the elder that involves family or caregivers, if appropriate. The provider must listen to the patient and understand any hesitation to seek help, but the provider must also take the time to explain his or her point of view. A sincere approach with free exchange may convince a reluctant patient that filing a report is the right thing to do. This way both provider and patient are in agreement on the course of action. The quick solution would be to fall back on a mandatory reporting statute and to state that there is no choice in the matter. However, this could impose another unwelcome circumstance on an already victimized senior citizen and prove to be counterproductive. It is advisable to sit down (literally) and earnestly try to persuade a competent elderly victim that help is available. Above all, any practitioner must act in what he or she believes is in the best interests of the patient. Remember, the old man or old woman underneath the bed sheet is somebody's grandparent, just as the doctor or nurse behind the starched white coat is somebody's grandchild.

The genuine value of mandatory reporting was demonstrated by a study of the events reported in California in 1984, shortly after mandatory reporting was instituted in this state. A dramatic increase in total number of reports occurred in that year. Nearly 85% of victims willingly accepted help that was offered as a result of the report (79). Presumably, many of these elders would have declined to file a report on a voluntary basis, thus being cast adrift until the next abusive or neglectful experience. The profound implications of this finding are difficult to dispute. Clearly, mandatory reporting serves to capture a group of vulnerable senior citizens and administer to them the service and care to which they are entitled.

## INSTITUTIONAL ABUSE

The expected growth of the elderly population will contribute to a dramatic rise in the number of senior citizens living in nursing homes or other institutions that provide all types and levels of care. Federal and state governments oversee and monitor almost all such facilities in this country. Their agencies estimate that by the year 2030 3.5 million elderly will occupy such institutions nationwide (80). This will expose millions of elders to the possibility of institutional mistreatment. The types of abuse that occur in a residential or nursing facility are not particularly different from what has already been described with regard to domestic elder abuse and neglect. All of the previously mentioned forms of maltreatment can occur in an institutionalized setting. The perpetrator may be a staff member, as is most commonly the case, or the abuser may be a fellow resident/patient or an intruder. One form of mistreatment that is unique to a nursing facility is failure to establish and follow a long-term plan of care or rehabilitation for a patient (7,51). This can result in profound physical and emotional distress for an isolated and infirm senior citizen. Experienced practitioners who evaluate and treat nursing home patients on emergency or chronic bases need only remember the multitude of patients whose problem lists include the diagnosis "failure to thrive" in order to understand the potential scope of this problem. In addition, many disorders common to institutionalized patients, such as pressure sores, dehydration, and urinary tract infections, could likely be avoided with more attentive care.

Institutionalized elders are placed at risk by their vulnerable physical and cognitive states as well as by the inexperience and inadequate training of staff (7,31). The most likely staff perpetrators of this form of mistreatment are nurses' aides (2,81). These persons have the most contact with the patients but have the least training and the lowest educational status among professional care providers. Many nursing homes suffer from understaffing, insufficient funding, and high employee turnover (7,31). Often their employees receive no specific instruction in the care of the elderly and perform their duties without proper supervision. With these inadequacies, the results of a large survey of nursing facility care providers ($N = 577$) may not be terribly shocking: More than 20% of those interviewed reported having witnessed physical abuse committed by another staff member, and a full 70% reported having witnessed psychological abuse (14). Furthermore, 10% confessed that they themselves had committed an act of physical abuse, and 40% admitted guilt with regard to the infliction of psychological abuse (14). Naturally, such a survey would likely underreport the true number of abusive situations based on reporter bias, which makes these data even more striking. Of note, more than 60% of these employees were nursing aides, and fewer than 50% of the total had any training beyond high school.

The vast range in levels of care at different types of facilities contributes to the difficulty in monitoring for abuses. Facilities that provide skilled nursing services or some level of medical care are required to uphold certain standards of care. Such sites are typically more actively regulated than a boarding facility for the elderly with mild cognitive impairments who do not need nursing supervision (31). Since the 1990s, there has been tremendous political effort to settle on a "Patient's Bill of Rights" for all Americans. Nursing home residents have been fortunate to have this agenda legislated since 1987 as the Nursing Home Reform Act. This law set national standards of care for nursing facilities and provided specific rights to which each resident is entitled. Such rights protect patients from all forms of abuse, inappropriate use of restraints, and Medicaid discrimination. This law guarantees access to advocates such as a personal physician and an ombudsman. Although the mere existence of such a law does not necessarily mean that it is being obeyed, it provides for investigation and supervision by the federal Office of the Inspector General and stiff penalties for violations. It is an important step to ensuring proper care for institutionalized senior citizens.

## THE PHYSICIAN, THE LAW, AND ETHICS

It is of paramount importance that clinicians familiarize themselves with the laws regarding elder abuse in the state(s) in which they practice. The federal Older Americans Act, while providing definitions and funding research and training in elder mistreatment, is much more limited in its scope than current federal laws covering child abuse and domestic violence. Therefore, individual states' laws are even more pertinent to the everyday practical management of this problem. The first statutes appeared in 1977, and as of mid-1999 all 50 states plus the District of Columbia have specific statutes that address elder abuse and neglect. In general, each jurisdiction has statutes that cover three categories of elder care: APS, institutional abuse, and a long-term care ombudsman program (LT-COP) (82).

It is not possible or practical in this chapter to detail each state's specific codes. Rather, the clinician should be aware that wide variation exists with regard to each individual state's requirements and specifications. For instance, many states have no separate law for institutionalized elders. Those that do define "institution" or "long-term care facility" differently. Furthermore, some states include mental health sites under the umbrella of "institutional," whereas others specifically do not. In general, all state laws will define abuse, provide social services for victims, delineate eligibility for services, and institute a means for reporting and investigation. Here again one encounters the problem of jurisdictional variability. Definitions and terminology differ from state to state, as do the ages and circumstances around which a victim may receive help from APS. Some states include both acts of commission and acts of omission as prohibited conduct, whereas others do not. In many states, it is not enough merely to be a mistreated or neglected senior citizen; there must also exist some defined statutory disability or impairment in order to apply a state APS law. Specific types of abuse, such as sexual assault, may be separately categorized. Most states do require reporting of suspected elder abuse or neglect to appropriate authorities. However, some jurisdictions allow for reporting on a voluntary basis.

The LTCOP exists specifically to provide an advocate for residents of a long-term care facility. The role and authority of the ombudsman varies from state to state, but in general this person acts to ensure that residents' rights under federal laws are being protected and not violated. He or she interacts with law enforcement and local or state APS as appropriate if an inquiry leads to suspected abuse or criminal activity. Certainly much of what is considered elder maltreatment is criminal. A perpetrator may be prosecuted under criminal laws that pertain to the nature of the abuse, such as assault, theft, and rape. Some states have enacted specific criminal laws that provide for crimes against the elderly, often with stiffer penalties (82). These jurisdictions may classify forms of elder mistreatment as felonies, misdemeanors, or either, depending on legal specifications.

Some states specifically provide for reclassification of a crime to a higher offense when the victim is a senior citizen (83). Often the age of a victim is used as an aggravating factor at a sentencing proceeding. Although this subject is very daunting, the busy practitioner need not be an expert in the law to manage these victims. He or she must have an overall familiarity with the laws that pertain in his or her jurisdiction. More importantly, the clinician must acknowledge this lack of expertise and utilize appropriate services and agencies in order to provide optimal care in an unfortunate situation.

Mandatory reporting clauses have triggered a volatile debate among providers. Currently, all but eight states have legislated mandatory reporting of suspected elder mistreatment. The so-called voluntary states are Colorado, Illinois, New Jersey, New York, North Dakota, Pennsylvania, South Dakota, and Wisconsin (83). Even within this narrowed sphere of reference, jurisdictional variability persists: each state has designated different professionals as mandatory reporters. In general, persons such as physicians, nurses, and mental health or social workers are almost always included among those required by statute to report. Some states specifically include others, such as attorneys, dentists, clergy members, and even ambulance personnel (83). As previously discussed, such laws may place a practitioner at odds with a patient's wishes and with ACEP's policy statement. With regard to the latter, a closer examination of this policy reveals that it opposes mandatory reporting specifically to the criminal justice system. Notably absent is a mention of reporting to a social services agency or to a hospital social worker. Depending on individual state laws, a report made to APS may or may not automatically trigger notification of law enforcement. Most practicing clinicians will not know this unless they are intimately familiar with their state's provisions. Furthermore, even if a report is made, some statutes specifically enable the elder to refuse an investigation. If the mental competency of an elder is in question, ACEP's policy implies no opposition to mandatory reporting. Certainly, clinicians would agree with this on all levels. It is the situation of a competent elderly person refusing intervention that presents a legal and ethical dilemma. The legal predicament is fairly concrete: A law may mandate the practitioner to act specifically against a patient's wishes. If push comes to shove, the provider has a statutory requirement to report suspected elder abuse in those jurisdictions. Most states with such laws include provisions for reporter immunity from any liability associated with compliance.

The ethical predicament of filing an unwelcome report, either for legal reasons or because the clinician truly believes that doing so is in the patient's best interests, is one that may be more disturbing to practitioners. Such a quandary deserves a forum for dialogue and discussion. There is a paucity of information available in the medical literature that addresses this ethical issue, yet this is the concern that may place the greatest emotional burden on both the elder and the clinician. Our enlightened society champions the potential contributions of senior citizens and encourages them to act as independently thinking, productive members. However, a case of elder mistreatment may force a practitioner to usurp a person's most basic societal liberty: the freedom to choose how to manage his or her life. A provider, naturally, should always strive for what is in a patient's best interests. It is highly likely that reporting a case of elder abuse to an appropriate APS agency or hospital social work department would benefit an elder. The likelihood is low that harm will be done. Even an uncooperative victim of abuse or neglect at the very least becomes known to APS. This way, periodic checks can be made and the elder becomes aware of available services. These small steps toward making initial contact may avert a disastrous future event.

Opponents to mandatory reporting clauses commonly cite four distinct reasons. First is the violation of the elder's right to self-determination. Elderly people are presumed competent, unless examination suggests otherwise, and critics maintain that taking this decision away from them perpetuates ageism. Second, detractors allude to patient–physician confidentiality and the need for the clinician to establish a relationship based on trust. Another potential shortcoming is that mandatory reporting may discourage self-reporting and may deter an elder from seeking help on his or her own. Lastly, some opponents fear that mandatory reporting will overwhelm already overburdened social services with many reports that lack validity. These concerns should be considered. Likewise, strong arguments exist for mandatory reporting. The most important considerations and the central themes that the clinician must always revisit are the safety and welfare of the elder. This may supersede confidentiality or self-determination interests. Legally, the inclusion of immunity clauses for mandatory reporters legislates that indeed the duty to disclose and report outweighs other factors such as confidentiality. Some language goes as far to specifically waive patient–physician privilege (84). Furthermore, a senior citizen may already feel deterred from self-reporting and may not have the benefit of adequate support in order to choose freely whether or not to file a report. Another consideration is that there may be a public good served by reporting elder abuse. If the maltreatment constitutes criminal activity, then the public at large, in addition to the victim, stands to benefit from reporting and prosecution.

A practitioner who is subject to mandatory reporting may be held criminally or civilly liable for failing to comply with a statutory requirement. Most statutes designate that a willful act of noncompliance is a criminal offense. Fortunately for practicing clinicians, the enforcement of such clauses is very rare (83). Of more concern to practitioners should be civil liability. The civil courts have traditionally been used to hold medical providers accountable, and this circumstance does not change with regard to elder abuse. Most laws stipulate that a reporter need only have a reasonable level of suspicion that maltreatment exists in order to initiate a report. A provider is expected to uphold this standard and potentially be held liable if failure to report results in damages to a victim. A new twist on civil liability has emerged recently. A California physician was sued in civil court for both malpractice and elder abuse for allegedly undertreating pain in a hospice patient. The use of elder abuse statutory violations in this case places the defendant at greater risk. There are no restrictions placed on pain and suffering awards based on elder abuse claims, whereas damages claimed in traditional malpractice cases in California are limited to $250,000. The medical community awaits the outcome of this trial watchfully (85).

Other legal issues clinicians encounter frequently when treating elderly patients involve decision making power. A competent elder is presumed capable of making decisions. Furthermore, such a competent person may revoke or change any previous agreement that was entered voluntarily. All states have laws that enable a senior citizen to grant someone else power of attorney. Statutes vary, but essentially such an agreement must be entered voluntarily and while the granter is competent. The term "durable" refers to a clause that specifically permits the power of attorney to continue after the granter becomes incompetent and thus incapable of revoking this power. Of note, not all power-of-attorney agreements contain a durable clause. Typically, such power is specifically classified into two separate areas: health care/medical decision making and financial matters. The specifics of different agreements vary: one person may hold joint power of attorney in both areas, or different people may hold power in each area. Likewise, an elder may appoint a financial manager but not specifically a medical attorney. Sometimes state courts will appoint a person to have power of attorney when an elder is unable to perform this duty. This appointee is called a guardian or conservator.

Practitioners should be familiar with the terminology that applies in their jurisdiction in order to meet the needs of the elderly patient. One must also be wary that guardians, conservators, and attorneys are not exempt from perpetrating abuse against those whose interests they have agreed to serve.

## CONCLUSION

Unfortunately, the specter of elder abuse is alarmingly prevalent among senior citizens today. It is a difficult problem to understand and study, with a multitude of causative factors. Therefore, a simple solution is lacking. Fortunately, however, elder mistreatment has become more visible through interdisciplinary recognition of patterns of abuse and neglect, resource availability, and legislative action. As shocked as medical professionals and members of the community at large should be at such transgressions, we must not stand still with mouths agape. Medical professionals especially should hail the opportunity to impact the life of an elderly person so profoundly. We are familiar with helping the elderly through many trying times: an acute disease process, new limitations set by a debilitating condition, and the illness or death of a spouse or loved one, to name a few. All clinicians have taken specific action toward the healing of the bodies and the minds of elders stricken with many conditions: heart failure, stroke, Parkinson's disease, dementia, and many others. We must add elder mistreatment to the list of common diseases of the elderly and always be on our guard to diagnose, treat, and intervene on behalf of a victim. A critical point for the emergency provider is that any suspected case of elder mistreatment should be reported. It is not necessary for the provider to be the accuser, the judge, or the jury. Indeed, the provider must shun these roles and remain an objective observer, all the while being an advocate for the patient without being judgmental. The provider must simply recognize that a situation deleterious to the patient may be occurring. In many cases, such a situation will be neglect due to a caretaker's being overwhelmed or uneducated about proper care for the elder in his or her charge. Often a caregiver welcomes outside involvement that assists in providing better overall physical and emotional care for an elderly individual.

A proactive approach can help: hospitals and communities need to provide adequate resources that are easily accessible to clinicians and potential victims. Legislative bodies must allocate more funds for research, treatment, and intervention. The elderly must be sought out, reminded of their rights, and informed that people and resources are willing and able to help them. Hospital protocols should be developed in advance and all personnel well versed in their application. To do any less, or to ignore a po-

tential abusive or neglectful situation, can only result in more harm to a potential victim. Clinicians universally are instructed to "do no harm," yet many may not realize the damaging consequences of passive acquiescence. Through such vigilance, the physical, emotional, and financial welfare of our senior citizens can be preserved, protected, and cultivated as we await their next contribution to our lives.

## APPENDIX: THE NEAIS

The NEAIS primarily sought to answer one question: what is the incidence of domestic elder abuse and neglect in the United States? The study employed rigorous definitions and methodology to collect and interpret data. Its figures were utilized to calculate an estimate of national elder abuse incidence within a 95% confidence interval. NEAIS was designed to limit its scope to cases of domestic, not institutional, elder mistreatment because of legislative directive. Specifically, the Family Violence Prevention and Services Act of 1996 (P.L. 102-295) mandated that the abuse, neglect, and exploitation of elderly Americans be studied so as to prevent family violence in the domestic setting. Therefore, elderly residents of nursing homes, group homes, assisted-living facilities, acute or subacute care hospitals, or any institution were not included. If the above incidence data seem lower than expected, consider that many thousands of cases of elder abuse do occur in such establishments (14). Cases of self-neglect were reported separately. The congressional legislation provided for funding of this study through the Administration for Children and Families and the Administration on Aging, both under the auspices of the U.S. Department of Health and Human Services. The NCEA performed the research through both the American Public Welfare Association and a private survey research company with experience in domestic violence survey techniques. Data were collected from a nationally representative sample of 20 different counties in 15 states over 8-week-long blocks of time in 1996. The study periods in different counties were staggered throughout 1996 to account for any seasonal variation. Researchers classified elder mistreatment into the seven types of maltreatment listed in Table 8-3. They defined their terms explicitly, and one instance of any kind of mistreatment was sufficient to include an elder as a victim. Standardized definitions were drafted for NEAIS by a panel of experts after an analysis of states' nomenclature, local discussions, and consensus meetings. NEAIS used two sets of sources in each selected county to acquire data: social services agencies and designated community sentinels. Local APS or Area Agency on Aging (AAA) organizations contributed the reports that came to the database during the study weeks. These reports may or may not have been substantiated by that agency, and only substantiated reports were considered positive. Details with regard to the nature of the abuse, the characteristics of both the victim and the perpetrator, and the original informant were also collected.

Sampling local APS offices is a useful means for gaining insight into elder abuse. However, one of its inherent flaws is that for a case of elder abuse or neglect to be recorded, it must be recognized and reported to that agency. As with all types of domestic violence, many incidents go unreported. This reality has been described as the "iceberg theory" (Fig. 8-2). Only a small

portion of an iceberg is visible above the water line. The larger submerged segment cannot be seen and its true dimensions remain unknown. Similarly, the unreported elder mistreatment cases lurk below the tip of the iceberg and somewhere beyond any APS agency's outreach program. In order to capture elder abuse cases not initially reported, a sentinel approach was also used. This approach had already been developed as an alternative to general population studies. It has been used in large national incidence studies of child abuse (86). The sentinels were people in the community who had frequent contact with the elderly but were not APS case workers. More than 1,100 law enforcement officers, hospital workers, elder care providers, home nurses, bank employees, and other citizens of the study areas were independently selected to perform this duty. They received specialized training to recognize signs and symptoms of all forms of elder mistreatment. Since sentinels directly observed cases of elder abuse, neglect, or self-neglect, these cases were presumed substantiated. Sentinels reported any instances directly to NEAIS; some also reported their cases to the appropriate APS agency. Investigators accounted for this circumstance by eliminating any duplication of a reported case from the database.

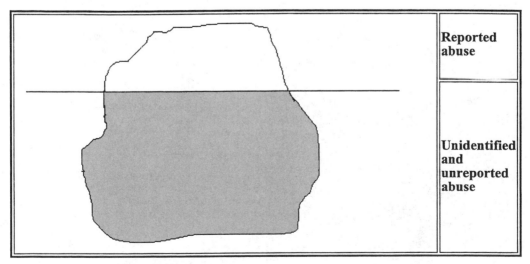

**FIG. 8-2.** Iceberg theory of elder abuse. (Reproduced from the National Elder Abuse Incidence Study.)

Likewise, a single elder was only included once in the study, even if he or she was the victim of more than one episode of maltreatment during the study period. In this manner, incidence, not prevalence, could be determined.

APS sources contributed 1,466 cases of elder abuse, neglect, and self-neglect to NEAIS prior to their substantiation. Sentinels contributed 140 cases, bringing the total number of unduplicated cases for study to 1,606. NEAIS investigators incorporated a sophisticated system of weighting and adjustment to their data and used population statistics to calculate an estimated national number of case reports of domestic elder mistreatment. By the APS figures, this study estimated that in 1996 there were more than 236,000 unduplicated reports of domestic elder maltreatment (abuse, neglect, or self-neglect) filed in the United States. This estimated number is comparable to the actual total number of case reports received by all state APS agencies that year, 290,314. The gap between these numbers would close when one considers that the latter figure does not account for duplication of cases or repeatedly victimized elders. Indeed, before NEAIS statisticians adjusted for duplication, the estimated number of national APS reports was more than 286,000. The difference between this unadjusted estimate and the actual total is less than 1.5%, demonstrating the accuracy of the NEAIS estimate. Of these reports, nearly half are substantiated. This percentage figure actually underestimated the number of truly abusive or neglectful circumstances because nonsubstantiation of a report does not guarantee that such a situation is absent. Rather, an unsubstantiated report of elder mistreatment might mean that levels of proof or other statutory requirements were not met but a dangerous condition might still exist. Also, some cases still remained under active investigation when researchers compiled data. Other investigations were terminated because the alleged victim declined to cooperate, died, moved, or otherwise was lost to follow-up. Surely some of these reported events would have achieved substantiation. Figure 8-3 depicts the outcomes of APS investigations.

It is unclear why NEAIS researchers selected age greater than 60 years for their definition of elderly; most previous studies on elder abuse and elder utilization of services utilize age greater than 65 years (13,17,21,25,26,37,43,52, 77,87,88). A limitation of the sentinel method involves an inherent underestimation of abused or neglected elders. The sole basis for use of

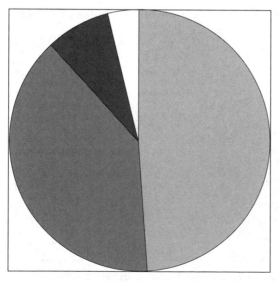
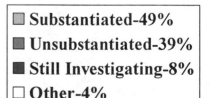

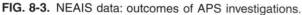
**FIG. 8-3.** NEAIS data: outcomes of APS investigations.

sentinels is that they will have contact with the elderly in the community. However, unlike child abuse where school represents a universal community institution where all children must congregate, no such place exists for the elderly. Thus, the most isolated seniors, who may be at the greatest risk, rarely leave home to interact with a community member. Additionally, the NEAIS investigators acknowledge that many of their data have wide confidence intervals because of a small sample size. More resources dedicated to expanding the sample size and lengthening the study time could limit the confidence intervals and provide more accurate and precise statistical estimates. One additional criticism not identified by the authors regards reporting by the sentinels. The presumption of NEAIS is that victims reported to the study by sentinels would have gone unnoted by APS. This is not necessarily true. Perhaps the sentinel, even without specific training for the purposes of this study, would have recognized a possible case of abuse, neglect, or exploitation and reported it to APS or other authorities. After all, the sentinel did by definition have contact with the elder. Many were trained observers, such as police officers, nurses, and physicians, whose skills may have enabled them to detect a suspicious situation prior to NEAIS training. Despite its flaws, this study represents the most comprehensive effort to date and shall serve as a foundation for continued research and awareness well into the 21st century.

NEAIS indicated that the most common form of domestic maltreatment involved neglect. Self-neglect was the most common type overall, uncovered in 38% of all substantiated APS and sentinel reports. When self-neglect cases were excluded, neglect still represented the most common mistreatment of the remaining incidents, nearly 50%. Table 8-13 lists the percentage of types of maltreatment discovered in all the substantiated cases. This analysis is consistent with an earlier NARCEA survey that found that more than half of all cases of domestic maltreatment reported to APS agencies in 1990 and 1991 involved self-neglect (18). The distribution of harm types for the remaining cases demonstrated that the most prevalent form of non–self-perpetrated

**TABLE 8-13.** *NEAIS data: analysis of substantiated cases with distribution of harm types*

| | |
|---|---|
| Physical | 25.6% |
| Psychological | 35.4% |
| Financial/material | 30.2% |
| **Neglect** | **48.7%** |
| Abandonment | 3.6% |
| Sexual | 0.3% |
| Other | 1.4% |

mistreatment was still neglect. Table 8-13 summarizes this information. Self-neglect and neglect were also the most common aberrant behaviors among a cohort of elders living in New Haven, Connecticut who were longitudinally studied for more than 10 years (87). Other researchers with more narrow inclusion criteria for neglect have published prevalence data showing neglect to be much less common than other forms (Table 8-4). Neglect may be the most difficult type of harm to prove. This is suggested by the substantiation rates found in NEAIS, which are shown in Table 8-14. Only about half of all cases reported to APS in 1996 met validation requirements. As one might expect, physical abuse was the type of maltreatment most frequently verified. APS workers in the individual New Haven area were able to substantiate all forms of neglect with greater frequency than the rate reported by NEAIS's national compilation of agencies (87). Their data show verification rates of 78% for self-neglect, 71% for neglect, and 75% for abuses. Variance from state to state would be expected because of differences in individual statutes and availability of resources. In any case, all types of abuse and neglect are sufficiently prevalent to warrant concern among health-care providers.

**TABLE 8-14.** *NEAIS data: substantiation rates for APS reports*

| | |
|---|---|
| Total | 48.7% |
| Physical | 61.9% |
| Psychological | 54.1% |
| Financial/material | 44.5% |
| Neglect | 41.0% |
| Abandonment | 56.0% |
| Sexual | N/A |

## REFERENCES

1. Davidson JL. Elder abuse. In: Block MR, Sinnott JD, eds. *The battered elder syndrome: an exploratory study.* College Park: University of Maryland, 1979: 49–66.
2. Quinn MJ, Tomita SK. *Elder abuse and neglect,* 2nd ed. New York: Springer Publishers, 1997:9–10.
3. Stearns PN. Old age conflict: the perspective of the past. In: Wolf R, Pillemer K, eds. *Elder abuse: conflict in the family.* Dover: Auburn House, 1986:3–29.
4. Attorney General's Task Force on Family Violence. Final report. Washington: US Government Printing Office, 1984.
5. Burston GR. Granny-battering. *Br Med J* 1975;3:592.
6. Baker AA. Granny battering. *Mod Geriatr* 1975;5: 20–24.
7. Aravanis SC, Adelman RD, Breckman R, et al. Diagnostic and treatment guidelines on elder abuse and neglect. *Arch Family Med* 1993;2:371–381.
8. Wolf RS. Elder abuse: ten years later. *J Am Geriatr Soc* 1988;36:758–762.
9. Kurrle SE, Sadler PM, Cameron ID. Elder abuse: an Australian case series. *Med J Aust* 1991;155:150–153.
10 Kurrle S. Abuse of the elderly: a hidden problem. *Aust Family Phys* 1992;21:1742–1748.
11. Ogg J, Bennett G. Elder abuse in Britain. *Br Med J* 1992;305:998–999.
12. Homer AC, Gilleard C. Abuse of elderly people by their careers. *BMJ* 1990;301:1359–1362.
13. Lachs MS, Berkman L, Fulmer T, Horwitz RI. A prospective community-based pilot study of risk factors for the investigation of elder mistreatment. *J Am Geriatr Soc* 1994;42:169–173.
14. Pillemer K, Moore DW. Abuse of patients in nursing homes: findings from a survey of staff. *Gerontologist* 1989;29:314–320.
15. Coyne AC, Reichman WE, Berbig LJ. The relationship between dementia and elder abuse. *Am J Psychiatry* 1993;150:643–646.
16. Reis M, Nahmiash D. Validation of the Indicators of Abuse (IOA) screen. *Gerontologist* 1998;38:471–480.
17. Pillemer K, Finkelhor D. The prevalence of elder abuse: a random sample survey. *Gerontologist* 1988; 29:51–57.
18. Rosenblatt DE. Elder mistreatment. *Crit Care Nurs Clin N Am* 1997;9:183–192.
19. Kosberg JI. Preventing elder abuse: identification of high risk factors prior to placement decisions. *Gerontologist* 1988;28:43–50.
20. U.S. Bureau of the Census. Sixty-five plus in America. *Curr Popul Rep (Special Studies),* Series 1023–178, 1992.
21. Strange GR, Chen EH, Sanders AB. Use of emergency departments by elderly patients: projections from a multicenter data base. *Ann Emerg Med* 1992;21:819– 824.
22. U.S. Senate Special Committee on Aging. Aging America: trends and projections. Washington, 1988.
23. Schneider EL, Guralnik, JM. The aging of America: impact on health care costs. *JAMA* 1990;263:2335–2340.
24. American Association of Retired Persons. *A profile of older Americans.* Washington, 1994.
25. McNamara RM, Rousseau E, Sanders AB. Geriatric emergency medicine: a survey of practicing emergency physicians. *Ann Emerg Med* 1992;21:796–801.

26. Lowenstein SR, Crescenzi CA, Kern DC, Knight S. Care of the elderly in the emergency department. *Ann Emerg Med* 1986;15:529–535.
27. Baum SA, Rubenstein LZ. Old people in the emergency room: age-related differences in emergency department use and care. *J Am Geriatr Soc* 1987;35:398–404.
28. Gerson LW, Skvarch L. Emergency medical service utilization by the elderly. *Ann Emerg Med* 1982;11:610–612.
29. Spaite DW, Cris EA, Valenzuela TD, et al. Geriatric injury: an analysis of prehospital demographics, mechanisms, and patterns. *Ann Emerg Med* 1990;19:1418–1421.
30. Tatara T. *Elder abuse in the United States: an issue paper.* Washington: NARCEA, 1990.
31. Aravanis SC, Adelman RD, Breckman R, et al. *Diagnostic and treatment guidelines on elder abuse.* Chicago: American Medical Association, 1992.
32. Hudson MF. Elder mistreatment: its relevance to older women. *J Am Med Women's Assoc* 1997;52:142–146.
33. Fulmer TT, O'Malley TA. *Inadequate care of the elderly: a health perspective on abuse and neglect.* New York: Springer Publishers, 1987.
34. Tatara T. *NARCEA's suggested state guidelines for gathering and reporting domestic elder abuse statistics for compiling national data.* Washington: NARCEA, 1990.
35. Lau EE, Kosberg JI. Abuse of the elderly by informal care providers. *Proceedings of the annual meeting of the Gerontological Society,* Dallas, 1978:10–15.
36. Kosberg JI, Nahmiash D. Characteristics of victims and perpetrators and milieus of abuse and neglect. In: Baumhover LA, Beall SC, eds. *Abuse, neglect, and exploitation of older persons: strategies for assessment and intervention.* Baltimore: Health Professions Press, 1996:31–49.
37. Lachs MS, Williams MA, O'Brien S, et al. The mortality of elder mistreatment. *JAMA* 1998;280:428–432.
38. Jones J, Dougherty J, Schelble D, Cunningham W. Emergency department protocol for the diagnosis and evaluation of geriatric abuse. *Ann Emerg Med* 1988;17: 1006–1015.
39. US Department of Health and Human Services Administration on Aging and the Administration for Children and Families. The National Elder Abuse Incidence Study. Washington: NCEA, 1998.
40. Johnson T. Critical issues in the definition of elder mistreatment. In: Pillemer K, Wolf R, eds. *Elder abuse: conflict in the family.* Dover: Auburn House, 1986:167–196.
41. Fulmer TT, Gould ES. Assessing neglect. In: Baumhover LA, Beall SC, eds. *Abuse, neglect, and exploitation of older persons: strategies for assessment and intervention.* Baltimore: Health Professions Press, 1996:89–103.
42. Lachs MS, Pillemer K. Abuse and neglect of elderly persons. *N Engl J Med* 1995;332:437–443.
43. Lachs MS, Williams C, O'Brien S, et al. Risk factors for reported elder abuse and neglect: a nine-year observational cohort study. *Gerontologist* 1997;37:469– 474.
44. Tatara T. *Suggested state guidelines for gathering and reporting domestic elder abuse statistics for compiling national data.* Washington: National Aging Resource Center on Elder Abuse, 1990.

45. McCreadie C. Introduction: the issues, practice and policy. In: Eastman M, ed. *Old age abuse: a new perspective*. London: Chapman & Hall, 1994:3–22.

46. O'Malley TA, O'Malley HC, Everitt DE, et al. Categories of family mediated abuse and neglect of elderly persons. *J Am Geriatr Soc* 1984;32:362–369.

47. Sengstock MC, Steiner SC. Assessing nonphysical abuse. In: Baumhover LA, Beall SC, eds. *Abuse, neglect, and exploitation of older persons: strategies for assessment and intervention*. Baltimore: Health Professions Press, 1996:105–122.

48. Blazer DG. The epidemiology of psychiatric disorders in late life. In: Busse EU, Blazer DG, eds. *Geriatric psychiatry* Washington: American Psychiatric Press, 1989: 235–262.

49. Tatara T. Understanding the nature and scope of domestic elder abuse with the use of state aggregate data: summaries of the key findings of a national survey of state APS and aging agencies. *J Elder Abuse Negl* 1993; 5:35–57.

50. Wilkinson TJ, Sainsbury R. Diagnosis related groups based funding and medical care of the elderly: a form of elder abuse? *N Z Med J* 1995;108:63–65.

51. Kleinschmidt KC. Elder abuse: a review. *Ann Emerg Med* 1997;30:463–472.

52. Paveza GJ, Cohen D, Eisdorfer C, et al. Severe family violence and Alzheimer's disease: prevalence and risk factors. *Gerontologist* 1992;32:493–497.

53. German PS, Shapiro S, Skinner EA, et al. Detection and management of mental health problems of older patients by primary care providers. *JAMA* 1987;257:489–493.

54. Jolley S, Jolley D. Psychiatry. In: Pathy MSJ, ed. *Principles and practice of geriatric medicine,* 3rd ed. London: John Wiley and Sons, 1998:1031–1053.

55. Steiner RP, Vansickle K, Lippmann SB. Domestic violence: do you know when and how to intervene? *Domestic Violence* 1996;100:103–116.

56. O'Brien JG. Screening: a primary care clinician's perspective. In: Baumhover LA, Beall SC, eds. *Abuse, neglect, and exploitation of older persons: strategies for assessment and intervention*. Baltimore: Health Professions Press, 1996:51–64.

57. Ramsey-Klawsnik H. Assessing physical and sexual abuse in health care settings, In: Baumhover LA, Beall SC, eds. *Abuse, neglect, and exploitation of older persons: strategies for assessment and intervention*. Baltimore: Health Professions Press, 1996:67–87.

58. Lachs MS, Fulmer T. Recognizing elder abuse and neglect. *Geriatr Emerg Care* 1993;9:665–681.

59. Levy DB, Hanlon DP, Townsend RN. Geriatric trauma. *Geriatr Emerg Care* 1993;9:601–620.

60. Folstein MF, Folstein SE, McHugh PR. Mini-mental state: a practical method of grading the cognitive state of residents for the clinician. *J Psychiatr Res* 1975;2: 189–198.

61. Pfeiffer E. A short portable mental status questionnaire for the assessment of organic brain deficit in elderly patients. *J Am Geriatr Soc* 1975;23:433–441.

62. Look KM, Look RM. Skin scraping, cupping, and moxibustion that may mimic physical abuse. *J Forensic Sci* 1997;42:103–105.

63. Ansello E. Causes and theories. In: Baumhover LA, Beall SC, eds. *Abuse, neglect, and exploitation of older persons: strategies for assessment and intervention* . Baltimore: Health Professions Press, 1996:9–29.

64. Pillemer KA. Risk factors in elder abuse: results from a case control study. In: Pillemer KA, Wolf RS, eds. *Elder abuse: conflict in the family*. Dover: Auburn House, 1986:239–263.

65. Korbin JE, Anetzberger G, Thomasson R, et al. Abused elders who seek legal recourse against their adult offspring. *J Elder Abuse Negl* 1991;3:1–18.

66. O'Connor F. "Granny-bashing": abuse of the elderly. In: Hutchins N, ed. *The violent family: victimization of women, children and elders*. New York: Human Sciences Press, 1988:104–114.

67. Bird PE, Harrington DT, Barillo DJ, et al. Elder abuse: a call to action. *J Burn Care Rehab* 1998;19:522–527.

68. Rosenblatt DE, Cho K, Durance PW. Reporting mistreatment of older adults: the role of physicians. *J Am Geriatr Soc* 1996;44:65–70.

69. Tilden VP, Schmidt TA, Limandri BJ, et al. Factors that influence clinicians' assessment and management of family violence. *Am J Public Health* 1994;84:628–633.

70. Tatara T, Kuzmeskus L. *Types of elder abuse in domestic settings*. Washington: NCEA, 1998.

71. Moon A, Williams O. Perceptions of elder abuse and help-seeking patterns among African-American, Caucasian American, and Korean-American elderly women. *Gerontologist* 1993;33:386–395.

72. Sonkin DJ, Durphy M. *Learning to live without violence*. San Francisco: Volcano Press, 1982.

73. Brewer RA, Jones JS. Reporting elder abuse: limitations of statutes. *Ann Emerg Med* 1989;18:1217–1221.

74. Jones JS. Elder abuse and neglect: responding to a national problem. *Ann Emerg Med* 1994;23:845–848.

75. Jones JS, Veenstra TR, Seamon JP, Krohmer J. Elder mistreatment: national survey of emergency physicians. *Ann Emerg Med* 1997;30:473–479.

76. Clark-Daniels CL, Daniels RS, Baumhover LA. Abuse and neglect of the elderly: are emergency department personnel aware of mandatory reporting laws? *Ann Emerg Med* 1990;19:970 977.

77. Lachs MS, Williams CS, O'Brien S, et al. ED use by older victims of family violence. *Ann Emerg Med* 1997; 30:448–454.

78. American College of Emergency Physicians. Policy statement: management of elder abuse and neglect. *Ann Emerg Med* 1998;31:149–150.

79. Garfield AS. Elder abuse and the states' adult protective services response: time for a change in California. *Hastings Law J* 1991;42:809–932.

80. Kusserow RP. *Resident abuse in nursing homes*. Washington: US Government Printing Office, 1990.

81. Payne B, Cikovic R. An empirical examination of the characteristics, consequences, and causes of elder abuse in nursing homes. *J Elder Abuse Negl* 1996;7: 61–74.

82. Goldstein MZ. Elder neglect, abuse, and exploitation. In: Dickstein LJ, Nadelson CC, eds. *Family violence: emerging issues of a national crisis*. Washington: American Psychiatric Press, 1989:101–124.

83. Moskowitz S. Saving granny from the wolf: elder abuse and neglect—the legal framework. *Conn Law Rev* 1998: 31:77–204.

84. Velick MD. Mandatory reporting statutes: a necessary yet underutilized response to elder abuse. *Elder Law J* 1995;3:165–190.

85. Foubister V. Doctor faces charges for allegedly undertreating pain. *Am Med News* 2000;43.
86. Sedlak AJ, Broadhurst DD. *The Third National Incidence Study of Child Abuse and Neglect (NIS-3).* Washington: United States Department of Health and Human Services, 1996.
87. Lachs MS, Williams C, O'Brien S, et al. Older adults: an 11-year longitudinal study of adult protective service use. *Arch Intern Med* 1996;156:449–453.
88. Comijs HC, Pot AM, Smit JH, et al. Elder abuse in the community: prevalence and consequences. *J Am Geriatr Soc* 1998;46:885–888.

# 9

# Treating Survivors of Intimate Partner Abuse

## Forensic Identification and Documentation

### Daniel J. Sheridan

Intimate partner abuse has profound physical and psychological health effects on millions of Americans and is now a crime in every state. The objectives of this chapter are to (a) give an overview of the dynamics of domestic abuse; (b) provide a brief legal overview; (c) describe clinical forensic assessments and documentation; (d) identify common domestic violence injuries; and (e) review the principles of forensic photography.

Estimates vary, but each year in the United States at least 4 million women experience ongoing physical, psychological, sexual, and financial abuse from a male intimate partner (1). The numbers of men abused by female intimates is estimated in the tens of thousands (1), and there is growing recognition of abuse occurring in gay and lesbian intimate relationships (2–4).

While there is overlap in assessment and intervention techniques between these varying types of intimate partner abuse, this chapter will focus primarily on women victimized by male intimates.

### ABUSE OF WOMEN

The battered-women's movement originally conceptualized domestic violence as a social, public policy, and criminal justice concern (5–9)— a view still strongly supported by many (10,11). However, early in the battered-women's movement, a few visionaries recognized abuse of women as a major health issue (12–16).

During the past 20 years, as the number of clinical and research articles on the health consequences of abused women has swelled, domestic violence has come to be viewed as a major public health concern. Nevertheless, only a handful of health professionals have examined the health link between abuse, domestic homicide, and the role of clinical forensics, despite growing documentation of the seriousness of physical, psychological, and sexual domestic violence (17–27).

Sequelae from physical abuse of women by male intimates are relatively easy to assess. There are physical findings: bruises, lacerations, sharp injuries, fractures, old and new scars, patterned injuries, and pain and bleeding. Physical injuries from domestic violence can be lavaged, debrided, sutured, x-rayed, scanned, and photographed. However, physical abuse is almost never the first form of abuse experienced by battered women. The first form of domestic violence is a combination of verbal and emotional abuse. These include name calling, public embarrassment, veiled and explicit threats of harm, harassment, lies, "mind games," and other psychological manipulations. Sexual assault of women by current or former male intimates is a common yet underrecognized problem (28–30). Assessing and intervening in situations of domestic financial abuse seldom is viewed as being in the purview of medical treatment; however, this form of abuse is a common power and control tactic and a major barrier to women's leaving abusive relationships (31,32).

For many women, the various forms of abuse may change and escalate when they attempt to leave the abusive relationship. For thousands of battered women, leaving the abusive relationship is marked by increased harassment and danger. Tragically, for more than 2,000 women every year, leaving an abusive relationship results in their death and sometimes in the deaths of their children at the hands of their abusive male partners (20,33,34). Data from three domestic homicide studies (33) found that estrangement from the abusive relationship disproportionately explained the risk of homicide of women, especially between 2 months to a year following separation. These data support the assertion that the first year out of an abusive relationship is the most deadly for battered women. Wilson and Daly concluded that not only was physically leaving an intimate relationship a risk factor for homicide but that beginning the process of leaving was "an important risk factor in uxoricide" (p. 6). Wilson and Daly also stated that countless more women are subjected to near-lethal violence and increased violence, jealousy, coercion, threats, and other control tactics while in the process of leaving relationships.

### "If I Can't Have You, No One Can"

Wilson and Daly (33) prefaced their paper with a quotation from a man who killed his wife after being separated for a month saying that if he could not have her, no one could. That same threat has been echoed in hundreds of the domestic violence histories given to this author in clinical practice. Campbell (20) entitled her discussion of power and control in homicides of female partners "If I Can't Have You, No One Can." Homicide data from police files in Dayton, Ohio from the 1980s demonstrate that more than 64% of the 28 women killed by an intimate or formerly intimate male partner had a history of being physically abused, and in the same percentage of cases the police reports indicated that male jealousy was a primary motive (19). This finding supports arguments that male jealousy connotes male control and ownership (20).

Campbell's (20) further work reviewed domestic homicides against women who had either left the relationship or had expressed an intention to leave. Thirteen (46%) of Campbell's sample of murdered women had actually left the relationship ($n = 11$) or had threatened to leave the relationship ($n = 2$). All four of the male victims of homicide in Campbell's study used violence against their estranged wives just prior to the wives' use of homicide. The police records reported that the murdered men had expressed jealousy toward the women having a new male intimate and were trying to get back together at the time of their deaths. Campbell cited one case in which a man "constantly harassed his ex-wife and returned many times to the house to violently accost her for months after the divorce" (p. 106). On one such occasion, the ex-husband was let into the home by one of his children. The woman locked herself in her bedroom, then shot and killed her ex-husband when he kicked down the bedroom door and came toward her. Despite what appeared to be a case of self-defense, the woman was convicted of voluntary manslaughter and sentenced to 20 years in prison (20).

### THE PROCESS OF LEAVING AN ABUSIVE RELATIONSHIP

Health professionals have been at the forefront of clinical research on the process women go through to leave abusive relationships (35–38).

### Regaining Personal Integrity

While interviewing 18 abused women about their utilization of health care services, Fishwick (35) discovered that a major factor influencing women's help-seeking behavior revolves around a process of maintaining personal integrity. Early in the relationship the woman's goal is to protect her personal integrity by developing and sustaining a successful relationship. When the abuse begins, her personal integrity is threatened and she makes numerous attempts to stop the abuse while keeping the relationship intact. As the abuse continues, there is a further erosion of her personal integrity, and she intensifies her efforts to improve the relationship. However, at this point she begins to acknowledge that the abuse and the relationship process are unjust. In the final phase, the woman acknowledges that she needs to reclaim her personal integrity to have a better life for herself and her children. It is in this phase that she demonstrates more help-seeking behaviors and is more receptive to interventions that facilitate a process of leaving.

### Entrapment and Recovery in Abusive Relationships

Landenburger (36,37) interviewed 30 women who were in abusive relationships or in the process of leaving, and identified a process of entrapment in and recovery from abusive relationships. First in Landenburger's four-phase process is a concept called *binding*. This phase describes the beginnings of the relationship and the onset of abuse. The woman stays very focused on the positive aspects of the relationship and suppresses the negative aspects (abuse) by (a) focusing on her strong desire for a loving relationship, (b) overlooking the warning signals of increasing abuse, (c) working on trying to make the relationship better, and (d) questioning her own behaviors as a possible cause of the abusive treatment. The binding phase transitions over time into the *enduring* phase. During the binding phase the woman's suppression of the abuse is unconscious. However, in the enduring phase, the woman consciously blocks out her abuser's negative behaviors, takes responsibility for his abuse, and knowingly places energy into placating her abuser. She tries to actively hide the abuse from the children, family, neighbors, and police. Although she hopes the relationship can be saved, she struggles with a shrinking sense of self.

In Landenburger's third phase, *disengaging,* the woman begins to recognize that she is not alone in her struggles, that other women are experiencing similar behaviors from male intimates. She may have arrived at this recognition from reading books or the newspaper, watching television, or talking and listening to friends. She cautiously begins to find a support network. She still cares for her abuser but reluctantly begins to think that she must leave the relationship to be safe. She labels herself as abused, actively seeks help, re-recognizes and develops an emerging feeling of self-worth, and often reaches a

breaking point that propels her into the final phase, that of *recovery*.

In recovering, the abused woman struggles with basic survival for herself and her children, grieves the loss of the relationship, searches for meaning about why she endured the relationship, and questions if she will ever be able to enter another relationship. For some women this reflective awareness period occurs as they tell their stories to supportive people, especially as they leave the relationship.

### Termination Readiness

May (38) conceptualized that when a woman is first abused, she struggles with cognitive dissonance. If the level of dissonance produced by the abuse is low, the woman has a low level of readiness to terminate the relationship. She continues to try to improve the relationship until a moderate or severe abusive episode raises the dissonance level to a point where she enters a process labeled termination readiness.

Early in this phase she identifies as a result of advertisements, books, movies, or conversations with friends that she is in an abusive relationship. She validates this identification from social supports and begins rebuilding and strengthening her self-esteem and self-efficacy. From termination readiness, the woman enters the separation phase. She begins rehearsals of leaving, which include cognitive and physical work, such as stashing money, packing bags, hiding car keys, purposefully breaking some of the abuser's rules, and making short attempts at leaving. Once the woman has left and is able to stay out of the relationship, she enters an autonomy phase during which she develops more positive social supports, interacts and relates with more positive role models, and espouses less traditional feminine role behavior (38).

### WHY DOES SHE STAY? VERSUS BARRIERS TO LEAVING!

It is common for providers, while treating a severely abused woman, to wonder why a woman would stay in an abusive relationship. Why would she return time and time again? Why does she stay? When one questions why a woman stays in an abusive relationship, in essence, the health care provider is holding the battered woman accountable for her abuser's behavioral choices. Unfortunately, health care provider's rarely say to the abusive male, "Why do you abuse?" Instead of questioning why she stays, it is better to reframe the question as, "What are her barriers to leaving?"

## Psychological Barriers to Leaving

Several psychological explanations for why women stay in abusive relationships have been developed. They include brainwashing (39), mind control and active recapture techniques (40), the Stockholm syndrome (41,42), and traumatic bonding (43,44).

Sonkin (39) and many others have contrasted psychological abuse in domestic violence with brainwashing of war and political prisoners (45–48). For example, Biderman's chart of coercion, which depicts eight brainwashing techniques that have been used on prisoners of war and political prisoners: isolation, monopolization of perception, induced debility and exhaustion, threats, occasional indulgences, degradation, demonstrating omnipotence, and enforcing trivial demands (49).

Boulette and Andersen (40), based on decades of clinical counseling experience, believe that cult members and battered women experience similar forms of brainwashing and mind control and share many common characteristics. Using parallels from cultic mind control and brainwashing techniques, they hypothesized that women often become trapped in abusive relationships. They describe cultic systems as exerting totalistic and demanding degrees of extreme control over individual freedom through various degrees of psychologically coercive and deceptive behaviors, including social isolation, confusion and guilt, threats of harm, love with strings attached, lying, and distortions of reality.

Battering that includes mind control, according to Boulette and Andersen (40), includes early verbal and/or physical dominance that can begin during or shortly after the courtship phase. Gradually, the batterer emotionally and geographically isolates and sometimes literally im-

prisons the woman, cutting her off from contact with family and friends. During this process, the batterer weakens the woman's access to a support network, minimizes her escape options, and fosters the development of a partner who is more docile and behaviorally malleable. To enforce this process, the abuser uses fear arousal and maintenance techniques that include actual and verbal threats of physical harm, direct threats with weapons, humiliation, public embarrassment, and intimidation by fear (40).

So often are the women blamed for causing the violent and coercive behaviors by their male abusers that the women begin to self-blame. This induction of guilt by the battering male toward the woman is occasionally softened by his contingent expressions of love. If she does not adequately acknowledge his love for her, he continues to degrade, devalue, and malign her until she capitulates (40). The abusive male is often jealous, accusing the woman of infidelity even while blatantly flaunting his own promiscuity. The problems within these violent relationships and dysfunctional families are expected to be kept secret at all costs. To break the family secret has been accompanied by the male abuser's threats of increased or lethal harm (40). To compensate for the cognitive dissonance resulting from experiencing the above behaviors, many battered women develop an enforced loyalty to the abusive male partners, exaggerating the so-cially acceptable behaviors and verbalizing a need to change and rescue the men from their violent actions (42). Women have described this behavioral pattern as cyclic, noting that it leads to feelings of powerlessness and helplessness (9,40), alternating with a sense of hopefulness when the abuser exhibits some positive behaviors. The abusers temporarily modify their behavior so that the women believe there is hope that the violence, threats, manipulations, and isolation will eventually end (40).

The brainwashing of battered women, whether conceptualized as that of a prisoner of war or as a cult member, often occurs insidiously and over an extended period. This gradual process provides a partial explanation for the difficulty some battered women have in objectively assessing the severe levels of abuse and danger and to question their capacity to leave their abusers. However, these techniques are less explanatory for battered women who begin experiencing severe physical, sexual, and psychological abuse very early in the intimate relationship before brainwashing occurs. A frequently asked question is, "Why don't those women just leave?" Two highly related models have been used to explain this phenomenon: the Stockholm syndrome (42) and the traumatic bonding (43,44) models.

### *The Stockholm Syndrome: Bonding with Your Captor*

The Stockholm syndrome represents an attempt to explain the seemingly paradoxical response of some hostages to their captors. First attributed to a hostage situation in a bank in Stockholm, and subsequently identified in multiple hostage and kidnapping situations, hostages sometimes develop a significant fondness and attraction to their captors. The Stockholm syndrome (42) is characterized by four conditions:

1. The captor threatens and has the capacity to kill the captive;
2. The captive cannot safely escape; therefore, he or she is totally dependent on the captor;
3. The captive is isolated from contact with others outside of the hostage situation and is dependent on the captor; and
4. The captor is perceived as showing some degree of kindness or benevolence toward the captive.

When the Stockholm syndrome is applied to battered women, the captive (battered woman) accurately identifies that the aggressor (the abuser) has the power of life and death, and actively identifies with the aggressor via pathologic transference and traumatic psychological infantilism (42). Women in ongoing abusive relationships with male intimates experience varying levels of physical abuse interspersed with transient periods of kindness and benevolence from their abusers. Battered women are sometimes literally held hostage by their abuser at knifepoint or gunpoint. Many home hostage situations that result in police intervention and media coverage involve domestic violence. When battered women say, as they often do, that they feel as if they are prisoners in their own homes, they may be struggling with the dynamics of brainwashing, mind control, and the transference effects of the Stockholm syndrome.

### *Traumatic Bonding: Intermittent Good–Bad Behavior*

Women in abusive relationships frequently minimize the seriousness of the abuse and tend to justify and defend the severe abusive behaviors of their abuser. This seemingly illogical connectedness with the aggressor, especially after severe trauma, has been explained by a model of traumatic bonding. A model of traumatic bonding (43,44) was developed to explain powerful emotional attachments in abusive relationships created by intermittent abuse and power imbalances. Traumatic bonding can quickly solidify as the subjugated person develops a continual lowering of self-esteem and less ability to live independently. At the same time, the abusive person develops an inflated sense of power. The stronger person becomes increasingly dependent on the weaker to maintain the feeling of power, a feeling the abuser does not want to relinquish.

The unpredictability of this intermittent abuse, coupled with periods of reconciliation, feigned (or partially sincere) contrition, and isolation from the reality checks of family and friends, are catalysts that accelerate traumatic bonding and battered women's fantasies of loving partners (44). Traumatic bonding can occur very early in a relationship (43,44); in fact, it appears to occur for some women during the dating relationship (50). Intermittent abuse in which women separated the "good-man image" from the "bad-man image" has been identified (50) in a sample of 90 college students, 43% of whom reported a history that experts interpreted to be psychologically abusive.

### Active Recapture Measures

From their extensive clinical practices, Boulette and Andersen (40) recognized that many battered women struggle with shedding the traumatic bonds that make them feel like prisoners in their own homes. This can be a difficult and, at times immobilizing, process that requires overcoming multiple barriers to leaving, including active recapture techniques described by Boulette and Andersen in their clinical paper on mind control and the battering of women. These recapture behaviors include cocky disbelief, confused searching, bargaining, pleading, threatening, and revenge.

Initially, an abusive man is shocked that his wife or girlfriend would dare to leave him. He is convinced that she cannot exist without him and that soon she will come back to him (40). Sometimes he has so thoroughly convinced her that she cannot make it without him that she does return to him, begging his forgiveness.

If she does not reenter the relationship, he begins a period of anxious and/or panicked searching (40). When he discovers where she is staying, he sends bargaining messages that include promises of changed behavior that highlight future love, fidelity, and kindness (40). Most women, from this researcher's clinical experience, do not want the relationship to end. They want to return to an ideal relationship full of love, fidelity, and kindness. Promises of change can be a very effective recapture technique (9,40), enticing women back into relationships on multiple occasions.

Over time and after multiple broken promises of change by the abuser, the battered woman stops being swayed by his bargaining tactics. The abuser then often activates the recapture technique of pleading, during which time he pleads and begs for another chance, frequently shedding tears and exhibiting physiologic signs of remorse (40). The woman may interpret tears and sobbing as signs of love. She feels sorrow and pity for the man and guilt for precipitating his tears. Men who are successful with the recapture technique of pleading often have brief periods of improved behavior (40), which Walker (9) described as the honeymoon phase. However, when pleading fails to recapture the abused woman, the abusive man can quickly escalate to the recapture techniques of threats and revenge (40). Threats of physical, sexual, and fi-

nancial harm to her, the children, and her family escalate. He may threaten to kidnap the children or have her institutionalized. Interspersed in the threats are instances of physical abuse and destruction of property and/or pets (40). If she persists in her efforts to stay out of the abusive relationship, the batterer plans revenge tactics that could easily culminate in the woman's being severely injured or killed. Johnson (51) described severe threats and serious abuse as patriarchal terroristic control intended to control women and to keep them from leaving the abusive relationship. These recapture and patriarchal terroristic methods help perpetuate the woman's sense of being a prisoner in her home and help facilitate the processes of mind control, brainwashing, and traumatic bonding (40,42,44,51).

## From Fear to Fatigue: Clinically Identified Barriers to Leaving Abusive Relationships

From extensive clinical experience, this author has compiled a practical list of terms that help the provider to better understand a battered woman's barriers to leaving. They are discussed in the following sections.

### Fear

A battered woman stays in an abusive relationship because of fear of being further abused and/or fear of failure. Her abuser has said to her, "If you try to leave me I'll kill you. I'll hurt the kids." He may say, "I know you can hide from me, but I know where your mother lives, where your sister lives. I dare you to leave. If you hide from me, you'll read about your family in the papers." Or maybe he has convinced her she cannot live without him. She is afraid of failure. She is afraid that if she leaves him she will not be able to provide food and shelter for her children.

### Finances

A battered woman stays in an abusive relationship because she cannot afford to leave. Ending a relationship, even a nonabusive relationship, is expensive and usually results in financial loss for both parties. In many abusive relationships, the abuser has so controlled the finances that the woman has little or no access to money.

### Father

A battered woman stays in an abusive relationship because she wants her children to be with their father. She does not want to be a single mother. As long as the man is relatively good to the children, she will stay and endure his abusive behavior toward her. One of the prime motivators for women to begin the process of leaving is when the abuser begins to threaten and/or hurt the children. Another motivator is when the children begin to mimic his abusive language or his abusive physical behavior.

### Faith

A battered woman stays in an abusive relationship because her religion has taught her that marriage is for life, through good times and bad times, until death. Until very recently, religious leaders in the community had little or no training in domestic violence awareness and interventions. It is not uncommon for a battered woman, upon seeking religious counseling, to hear from the clergy, "Be a better wife. Pray harder. Offer it up. Cook better meals." Some untrained clergy may try to do couples counseling, which is contraindicated in most ongoing abusive relationships.

### Forgiveness

A battered woman stays in an abusive relationship because she forgives her abuser when he says he is sorry for hurting her. Most battered women do not want the relationship to end. They want the abuse to end. Most abusive relationships do not begin on the first date. If on her first date with a man he called her a fat pig, broke her nose, and then forced her to have sex with him, undoubtedly the chances for a second date would be slim. However, in most abusive relationships, the woman has seen a side of the man that can be good and caring, tender and loving. She has seen a man who can be quite wonderful and who has the ability to shower her with love, attention, and affection. When he tells her he is sorry for hurting her, often with tears in his eyes, she wants to believe that he will change. She wants to believe it was extenuating stressors that made him hurt her. She wants to believe it was the stress from his job, the stress from the children, the stress from his first wife that made him hurt her. She wants to believe he will change back to the man with whom she fell in love. And she believes she can help change him.

### Fantasy/Fix

A battered woman stays in an abusive relationship because she has a fantasy she can fix her abuser. She believes if she loves him a little harder; does everything he asks of her; limits her activities outside the home; and keeps the children from increasing his stress, then the relationship will improve. She does not understand that she cannot fix him because *he* does not believe anything is wrong with him. He blames her for all their problems. She does not understand that only he can change his own behaviors, only he can change his own attitudes.

### Family

A battered woman stays in an abusive relationship for extended-family reasons. Either her family does not yet know she is in an abusive relationship or her family has become somewhat estranged from her because she keeps returning to the abusive relationship. She may not have easy access to her family support system if she and her abuser moved a great distance away.

### Friends

A battered woman stays in an abusive relationship because she has not been able to maintain many friendships and lacks a social support network. Common among abusers of all ages is social isolation. The more isolated one is emotionally and/or geographically from a support and safety network, the more difficult it is to leave.

### Familiarity

A battered woman stays in an abusive relationship because she was reared in an abusive home and accepts that being beaten by a man is a necessary part of being a woman. She may have witnessed her grandmother being beaten, or maybe her mother was beaten. She knows her older sister is being beaten. This author has had many battered women say to him, "Don't you beat your wife? Don't all men beat women?"

### Full

A battered woman stays in an abusive relationship because she has tried to leave but discovered that the emergency women's shelter was full and all of the beds were occupied. Or perhaps there was space for her in the shelter, but the shelter has a policy of not allowing teenage boys into the home. She stays because she does not want to leave her teenaged son at home without her to protect him.

### Find

A battered woman stays in an abusive relationship because she knows from prior attempts at leaving that her abuser will search for her until he finds her, even if it means searching state by state.

### Fatigue

A battered woman stays in an abusive relationship because she has become too physically and emotionally exhausted to leave. She is so fatigued that she cannot muster the sustained energy needed to develop and implement a safety plan.

## LEGAL OVERVIEW

Physical abuse within intimate relationships is now a crime in every state. As such, medical documentation of domestic violence has potential forensic (pertaining to the law) implications. What the provider writes or does not write in the medical record may be crucial in court. Unfortunately, health care providers tend to under-document domestic violence histories, examinations, and findings (17,25,27). Health care providers need to know if mandatory reporting to police of domestic violence cases is in effect in their community or state. For example, in California not only does the health care provider need to make a telephone report to the police in a timely manner, but the provider must also provide the police a written summary of the battered patient's history. This must be done, even if the patient instructs the provider to keep the information confidential. In Illinois, while the police are routinely called to the medical treatment area when any suspected crime victim or perpetrator presents for treatment, the provider is not obligated to divulge to the police any information gathered during the history or exam. The decision to talk or not talk with the police is entirely up to the victim.

In many communities, the address where the abuse reportedly occurred determines the police agency that needs to be notified of the domestic violence crime. If the victim was abused in one community or county and travels to a health facility in another city or county, the local police may not want to get involved. It is not uncommon for the health-care provider to find herself or himself in the middle of police jurisdiction turf battles. To avoid some of these conflicts, it is helpful for the health-care agency to have developed, *a priori,* networking relationships with all regional law enforcement agencies. In some states, police notification is dependent on the severity of the patient's injuries or if the injury was penetrating with either a knife or a firearm.

Health-care providers who work at institutions at or near state borders often need to become familiar with two states' reporting requirements and two sets of legal terminology. For example, in the State of Oregon, if one person inflicts an injury on another, it is the crime of assault. Assaults can range from misdemeanors to felonies. In the State of Washington, the identical act is called a battery, with the level of battery ranging from misdemeanor to felony.

If legal advocacy is provided to battered patients, the provider must have a working knowledge of the definitions of various violence related crimes. What level of abuse is most probably a misdemeanor? What level is a felony? For what types of violent crimes do the police send only a patrol officer, as opposed to cases in which the police may dispatch a detective and/or an evidence specialist? In rural settings, the level and timeliness of police response may vary significantly from that provided in an urban setting.

Health-care providers need to know if there is mandatory arrest or pro-arrest in their state. It is not uncommon for an abuser to bring his wife or girlfriend to the health-care setting for treatment of the injuries he just inflicted. Often he will wait in the waiting room or hover around the woman in the examination/treatment area. With mandatory arrest of domestic violence perpetrators, the odds go up that the reported abuser will be arrested (on-site) if the police come to the medical facility. In situations where the police are governed by domestic violence pro-arrest statutes, the responding officer(s) have much more discretionary power to decide who does or does not get arrested.

All states have implemented some form of domestic violence civil court remedies either in the form of specialized restraining orders or orders of protection. Health-care providers need to know what form of civil remedy is issued in their state. These protective orders can be quite helpful in several general areas and can be crafted to address unique issues of the victim. In general, restraining/protective orders can give the victim immediate, emergency, temporary custody of the children; can make the reported abuser leave the home; can order the reported abuser to stay 500 feet away from the victim or not come to the victim's workplace or school. This author has often gone to court and obtained restraining or protective orders on behalf of battered women who are going to be hospitalized for more than a couple of days. The appropriate legal forms were completed and signed by the victim and then notarized by a hospital representative (usually from the business office) at the patient's bedside. This author went to court as the victim's proxy. Some judges telephoned the hospital and spoke directly with the patient, whereas others accepted the paperwork without question. In all of these cases, the orders were modified to include a clause that the reported abuser was not to come within 500 feet of the hospital, thus giving the hospital, its staff, and other patients some additional safety and legal protection. Violations of many types of civil restraining/protective orders often result in criminal sanctions and can give local law enforcement the power to arrest simply because the civil order was violated.

## ASSESSMENT AND IDENTIFICATION

Routine screening for domestic violence in all health-care settings has now been recommended as the norm (52). However, for assessment to work, the woman's privacy is paramount. The health-care provider will never elicit a history of abuse if in the examination room with the woman is her husband/boyfriend, any children older than 3 years, his mother, her mother, or other people who may be later "quizzed" by the abuser. Whether it is because of fear of further harm and/or embarrassment, a woman will not share her abuse history in front of an audience. It is best to establish a policy within every health-care institution that all patients will have some period of time in which they will be interviewed and/or examined alone. This author has also found sitting at the same eye level as the patient, when culturally appropriate, to be an effective interviewing technique with women being assessed for battering.

There are many types of routine abuse screens in use within health-care settings. Among the most tested and used is a five-item Abuse Assessment Screen (AAS) developed by Helton (53) and modified by the Nursing Research Consortium on Violence and Abuse (Fig. 9-1) or a shortened three-item version of the AAS (55) (Fig. 9-2). The AAS is as effective at screening for abuse (55) as the 19-item Conflict Tactic Scale (CTS) (56) and the 30-item Index of Spouse Abuse (57). When the AAS was further tested on a large, ethnically stratified cohort of women, it was found to be an extremely effective domestic violence screening tool (58).

However, it is not acceptable to merely routinely screen for the presence or absence of domestic violence. If, during a routine domestic

1. Are you ever afraid of your partner?

2. Do you feel your partner tries to control you?

3. Do you feel emotionally abuse or hurt by your partner?

4. Has your partner ever hit, slapped, kicked, or otherwise physically hurt you?

5. Has your partner ever forced you into sex when you did not want to participate?

**FIG. 9-1.** Five-Item Abuse Assessment Screen. (From Helton A. Protocol of care for the battered women. Houston: Houston Chapter of the March of Dimes, 1986.)

violence screening process, a woman shares that she has been slapped and kicked during the past year and has been forced into sex by her husband/boyfriend when she did not want to participate, additional assessment is required. If a patient told a health care provider that she was experiencing crushing chest pain, shortness of breath, sweating, and pain shooting down her left arm, it is doubtful the provider would move on to assess the patient's bunions. A reasonable provider would ask additional cardiac assessment questions while obtaining physical findings and tests. The symptoms could be nothing more than atypical indigestion or they could be symptomatic of a life-threatening cardiac crisis.

Battered women may be at just as much risk of lethal sequelae as the above fictitious patient. Therefore, if there is a positive history of recent abuse on routine assessment, the next logical clinical step for the prudent provider would be to administer the 23-item HARASS tool (Harassment in Abusive Relationships: A Self-report Scale) (59) (Fig. 9-3) coupled with administration of the 15-item Danger Assessment (DA) (60) (Fig. 9-4). Both tools are self-report scales and take a few minutes to complete.

The HARASS tool was developed for clinical use by women in the process of leaving abusive relationships (59). It was designed to be used in conjunction with Campbell's (60) Danger Assessment to better identify battered women at risk for increased abuse and/or domestic homi-

cide. The items on the HARASS tool were created from qualitative analysis of interviews with women leaving abusive relationships, from the author's extensive clinical experiences, and from interviews with community-based domestic violence expert service providers. The reliability of the HARASS tool was supported by Cronbach's $\alpha$ of 0.93 for the OFTEN scale and 0.92 for the DISTRESS scale. The HARASS tool has preliminary evidence (via factor analysis) for three subscale groupings. These groupings had logical support in the literature and were named as follows: (a) stalking-like behaviors, (b) threatening behaviors, and (c) controlling-his-commodities behaviors that encompass children, property, and forced sex. All of these behaviors have been linked to domestic homicide. The HARASS scale was positively and significantly correlated with the concurrent administration of the DA but was not redundant (59).

Campbell (60) developed the DA to attempt to predict the known link between intimate partner abuse and homicide. From her extensive clinical research experience and from published lists of possible lethal danger signals in abusive intimate partner relationships (61,62), Campbell's DA instrument lists behavioral warning signals that have been clinically associated with domestic homicide. The DA is not a scale for initial domestic violence assessment. Designed for use with women already identified as abused, the DA, in either clinical and/or research settings, is a scale that attempts statistical prediction as opposed to clinical prediction. All of the items

## Abuse Assessment Screen

1. **WITHIN THE LAST YEAR,** have you been hit, slapped, kicked, or
   otherwise physically hurt by someone?                      YES          NO

   If YES, by whom? _____

   Total number of times _____

2. **SINCE YOU'VE BEEN PREGNANT,** have you been hit, slapped,
   kicked, or otherwise physically hurt by someone?           YES          NO

   If YES, by whom? _____

   Total number of times _____

MARK THE AREA OF INJURY ON THE BODY MAP. SCORE EACH INCIDENT
ACCORDING TO THE FOLLOWING SCALE:                                        SCORE

1 = Threats of abuse including use of a weapon

2 = Slapping, pushing; no injuries and/or lasting pain

3 = Punching, kicking, bruises, cuts and/or continuing pain

4 = Beating up, severe contusions, burns, broken bones

5 = Head injury, internal injury, permanent injury

6 = Use of weapon; wound from weapon

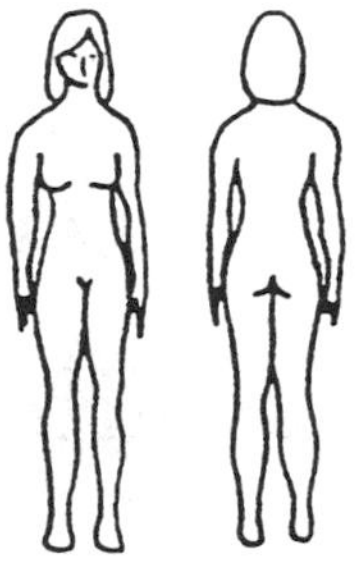

If any of the descriptions for the higher number apply, use the higher number.

3. **WITHIN THE LAST YEAR,** has anyone forced you to have
   sexual activities?                                         YES          NO

   If YES, by whom? _____

   Total number of times _____

Developed by the Nursing Research Consortium on Violence and Abuse.
Readers are encouraged to reproduce and use this assessment tool.

**FIG. 9-2.** Three-Item Abuse Assessment Screen.

on the DA have been established as correlates of homicide, and as such the DA is "best thought of as a statistical risk factor assessment, rather than a (clinical) prediction instrument per se" (60).

Prediction of violent behavior in general, and life-threatening, potentially lethal violence in particular, has been fraught with inaccuracy (63). Campbell (60) and Sheridan (59) recommend that the DA and the HARASS tools be used with caution and as part of clinical discussions with women involved in abusive relationships as an informal predictor of potential homicide. The data obtained from the additional

*H* arassment in

*A* busive

*R* elationships:

*A*

*S* elf-report

*S* cale

Many women are harassed in relationships with their abusive partners, especially if the women are trying to end the relationships. You may be experiencing harassment. This instrument is designed to measure harassment of women who are in abusive relationships or are in the process of leaving abusive relationships. By completing this questionnaire, you may better understand harassment in your life. If you have any questions, please talk with the service provider who gave you this tool.

*Harassment is defined as a persistent pattern of behavior by an intimate partner that is intended to bother, annoy, trap, emotionally wear down, threaten, frighten, terrify and/or coerce a woman with the overall intent to control her choices and behavior about leaving the abusive relationship.*

There are no right or wrong answers. Do not put your name on the form. The instrument takes about 10 minutes to complete.

**FIG. 9-3.** HARASS scale. (Permission to use the HARASS tool in clinical settings has been universally granted by its creator. Dr. Sheridan would appreciate notification if the HARASS tool is used in formal research studies.)

assessment questions can help guide the healthcare provider and the patient to develop better safety plans.

## DOCUMENTATION OF DOMESTIC VIOLENCE

Historically, documentation of histories of abuse has been both sparse and forensically useless. It is common to read poorly written medical histories, such as:

43-year-old female presenting with history of multiple facial trauma, struck by known assailant.

A much more forensically useful entry would be:

43-year-old female presenting with history of multiple facial trauma, states she was struck four times to the right face with a closed fist and kicked one time to the left ear by her hus-

band, James Jones (DOB 4-19-58) at 1130 hours yesterday at the corner of Fourth and Main Street, witnessed by her two children, David, 16, and Nicholas, 13.

Even when medical documentation is not sparse, it is often "sanitized." For example, an abused patient is rushed to the emergency department by paramedics immediately after being beaten. In an "unsanitized" progress/admission note, the provider documents not only the patient's presenting physical trauma but also that the patient is visibly upset and crying. The provider writes that the patient states her boyfriend, George Thomas Doe, knocked her to ground, forced the barrel of handgun into her mouth, and said, "If you ever leave me, bitch, I'll blow your mother ?#%ing head off and drown your &%#ing kids." The "sanitized" entry may read, "Patient reports being knocked to ground by known assailant who then threatened

For each item, circle the number that best describes how often the behavior occurred. Next, rate how distressing the behavior is to you. If the behavior has never occurred, circle 0 (NEVER) and go to the next question. If the question does not apply to you, circle NA (NOT APPLICABLE). If you are still in the relationship please circle below MY PARTNER. If you have left the relationship, please circle below MY FORMER PARTNER.

| THE BEHAVIOR | HOW OFTEN DOES IT OCCUR?<br><br>0 = Never<br>1 = Rarely<br>2 = Occasionally<br>3 = Frequently<br>4 = Very Frequently<br>NA = Not applicable | | | | | | HOW DISTRESSING IS THIS BEHAVIOR TO YOU?<br><br>0 = Not at all distressing<br>1 = Slightly distressing<br>2 = Moderately distressing<br>3 = Very distressing<br>4 = Extremely Distressing<br>NA = Not applicable | | | | | |
|---|---|---|---|---|---|---|---|---|---|---|---|---|
| MY PARTNER/FORMER PARTNER (circle one) | | | | | | | | | | | | |
| 1. Frightens people close to me | 0 | 1 | 2 | 3 | 4 | NA | 0 | 1 | 2 | 3 | 4 | NA |
| 2. Pretends to be someone else in order to get to me | 0 | 1 | 2 | 3 | 4 | NA | 0 | 1 | 2 | 3 | 4 | NA |
| 3. Comes to my home when I don't want him there | 0 | 1 | 2 | 3 | 4 | NA | 0 | 1 | 2 | 3 | 4 | NA |
| 4. Threatens to kill me if I leave or stay away from him | 0 | 1 | 2 | 3 | 4 | NA | 0 | 1 | 2 | 3 | 4 | NA |
| 5. Threatens to harm the kids if I leave or stay away from him | 0 | 1 | 2 | 3 | 4 | NA | 0 | 1 | 2 | 3 | 4 | NA |
| 6. Takes things that belong to me so I have to see him to get them back | 0 | 1 | 2 | 3 | 4 | NA | 0 | 1 | 2 | 3 | 4 | NA |
| 7. Tries getting me fired from my job | 0 | 1 | 2 | 3 | 4 | NA | 0 | 1 | 2 | 3 | 4 | NA |
| 8. Ignores court orders to stay away from me | 0 | 1 | 2 | 3 | 4 | NA | 0 | 1 | 2 | 3 | 4 | NA |
| 9. Keeps showing up wherever I am | 0 | 1 | 2 | 3 | 4 | NA | 0 | 1 | 2 | 3 | 4 | NA |
| 10. Bothers me at work when I don't want to talk with him | 0 | 1 | 2 | 3 | 4 | NA | 0 | 1 | 2 | 3 | 4 | NA |
| 11. Uses the kids as pawns to get me physically close to him | 0 | 1 | 2 | 3 | 4 | NA | 0 | 1 | 2 | 3 | 4 | NA |
| 12. Shows up without warning | 0 | 1 | 2 | 3 | 4 | NA | 0 | 1 | 2 | 3 | 4 | NA |

**FIG. 9-3.** *Continued.*

her and her children." It should be evident the first entry is much more forensically useful than the second. Statements made by the victim in the unsanitized progress note may also be viewed as an "excited utterance." Excited utterances are statements made by a victim or witness immediately or shortly after experiencing some type of traumatic event. Excited utterances are presumed by the courts to be true statements. Courts often allow excited utterances to be introduced as evidence, as exceptions to the hearsay, because the presumption is that the victim was too excited and did not have time to fabricate a lie.

Histories of abuse in the patient record should always be detailed and unsanitized, even if the reported abuse occurred days, weeks, or years ago. When a medical provider documents patient statements made in the routine course of health-care delivery, the statements have been viewed by the courts as truthful and are allowed in court as evidence (*White v Illinois,* 1992). Statements made to and recorded by health professionals are often referred to as "medical exceptions to hearsay."

Realistic constraints on time management of busy health-care providers make it almost impossible to chart, verbatim, the histories provided by abused patients. However, extensive, fact-filled paraphrasing of the presenting history of abuse and a summary of past abuse events is invaluable in court. Verbatim documentation of select, poignant statements made by the abused patient is ideal. If the reported or suspected abuser is present, any statements and/or behaviors by him that are threatening, controlling, and/or in conflict with the patient's history should also be documented, especially

| THE BEHAVIOR | HOW OFTEN DOES IT OCCUR? 0 = Never 1 = Rarely 2 = Occasionally 3 = Frequently 4 = Very Frequently NA = Not applicable | | | | | | HOW DISTRESSING IS THIS BEHAVIOR TO YOU? 0 = Not at all distressing 1 = Slightly distressing 2 = Moderately distressing 3 = Very distressing 4 = Extremely Distressing NA = Not applicable | | | | | |
|---|---|---|---|---|---|---|---|---|---|---|---|---|
| 13. Messes with my property (for example: sells my stuff breaks my furniture, damages my car, steals my things) | 0 | 1 | 2 | 3 | 4 | NA | 0 | 1 | 2 | 3 | 4 | NA |
| 14. Scares me with a weapon | 0 | 1 | 2 | 3 | 4 | NA | 0 | 1 | 2 | 3 | 4 | NA |
| 15. Breaks into my home | 0 | 1 | 2 | 3 | 4 | NA | 0 | 1 | 2 | 3 | 4 | NA |
| 16. Threatens to kill himself if I leave or stay away from him | 0 | 1 | 2 | 3 | 4 | NA | 0 | 1 | 2 | 3 | 4 | NA |
| 17. Makes me feel like he can again force me into sex | 0 | 1 | 2 | 3 | 4 | NA | 0 | 1 | 2 | 3 | 4 | NA |
| 18. Threatens to snatch or have the kids taken away from me | 0 | 1 | 2 | 3 | 4 | NA | 0 | 1 | 2 | 3 | 4 | NA |
| 19. Sits in his car outside my home | 0 | 1 | 2 | 3 | 4 | NA | 0 | 1 | 2 | 3 | 4 | NA |
| 20. Leaves me threatening messages (for example: puts scary notes on the car, sends me threatening letters, sends me threats through family and friends, leaves threatening messages on the telephone answering machine) | 0 | 1 | 2 | 3 | 4 | NA | 0 | 1 | 2 | 3 | 4 | NA |
| 21. Threatens to harm our pet | 0 | 1 | 2 | 3 | 4 | NA | 0 | 1 | 2 | 3 | 4 | NA |
| 22. Calls me on the telephone and hangs up | 0 | 1 | 2 | 3 | 4 | NA | 0 | 1 | 2 | 3 | 4 | NA |
| 23. Reports me to the authorities for taking drugs when I don't | 0 | 1 | 2 | 3 | 4 | NA | 0 | 1 | 2 | 3 | 4 | NA |

**FIG. 9-3.** *Continued.*

if he directly (or indirectly) threatens the patient or staff.

## TYPES OF INJURIES

Unfortunately, health-care providers often misuse common forensic medical definitions. There is a taxonomic system of forensic terminology that should be consistently used in all medical documentation. The following sections are based in part on common preferred forensic definitions (17,64–66) and on the author's extensive clinical experiences:

### Patterned Injuries

Patterned injuries are those in which the provider has reasonable certainty that the presenting injury was caused by an unknown object, a specific object, or a specific mechanism.

### Pattern of Injuries

Pattern of injuries refers to injuries in various stages of healing, including old and new patterned injuries, fractures, and scars.

### Abrasions

An abrasion is the scraping of the skin or mucous membrane usually caused by friction against an object or surface. Most abrasions are superficial; however, the longer a person is dragged against a rough surface, and the rougher the surface, the more extensive the injury. Battered women are often dragged along the ground by the abuser. The ground surface helps determine the type of abrasion. Being dragged (supine) along a carpeted surface by one's feet usually results in "rug burn" abrasions to the woman's lower back and elbows. Being dragged (prone) on a carpet

| Optional:<br><br>List other harassing behaviors that you have experienced.<br>Circle how often and how distressing the behaviors<br>are to you.<br><br>**THE BEHAVIOR** | **HOW OFTEN DOES IT OCCUR?**<br><br><br>0 = Never<br>I = Rarely<br>2 = Occasionally<br>3 = Frequently<br>4 = Very Frequently | **HOW DISTRESSING IS<br>THIS BEHAVIOR TO YOU?**<br><br>0 = Not at all distressing<br>I = Slightly distressing<br>2 = Moderately distressing<br>3 = Very distressing<br>4 = Extremely Distressing |
|---|---|---|
| 24. _____ | 0   I   2   3   4 | 0   I   2   3   4 |
| 25. _____ | 0   I   2   3   4 | 0   I   2   3   4 |
| 26. _____ | 0   I   2   3   4 | 0   I   2   3   4 |

Please answer a few additional questions:


_____ Your age in years

Check the statement that best describes you.

❏  Married, living with an abusive partner.
❏  Single, living with an abusive partner.
❏  Married, living apart from an abusive partner.
❏  Single, living apart from an abusive partner.

How long were you in the above relationship? _____

Are you still in the relationship? ❏ YES  ❏ NO

If you have left the relationship, how long have you been out? _____

What is your approximate annual income? _____

How many years of school have you completed? _____

Check the statement that best describes you.

❏      Asian/Pacific Islander
❏      Black/African American
❏      Caucasian/White
❏      Hispanic
❏      Native American/American Indian
❏      Other_____

**FIG. 9-3.** *Continued.*

by one's feet may result in rug burns to the anterior chest, breasts, abdomen, and/or knees. Being pulled along a carpeted surface could result in rug burns to the posterior or anterior shoulder area depending on how much twisting motion is being applied either by the abuser or by the woman as she tries to break free. Carpet fibers (trace evidence) may be present in or around the wound, and should be documented, photographed, and preserved as evidence.

Being dragged along the pavement (concrete and/or asphalt) via the same mechanisms as above will result in similar, but probably more severe, abrasion injuries that often contain trace evidence such as dirt, cinders, glass, and pebbles. Being dragged along a dirt or grass surface usually produces less severe abrasion injury but an abundance of trace evidence.

During strangulation assaults, the abuser may inflict fingernail scratch abrasions to the battered woman's neck (Figs. 9-5 through 9-7, see Colorplate following page 144). Or while being strangled, the battered woman may try to pry the assailant's hands from her neck and in so doing scratch herself. The assailant may have fingernail scratch abrasions to his face, neck, and arms inflicted by the woman in self-defensive efforts. Being strangled with a rough rope or cord may produce ligature abrasions in a more circular pattern around the neck (Fig. 9-8, see Colorplate following page 144).

Punch injuries by assailants wearing rings can produce a variety of abrasions. Simple wedding bands seldom leave abrasive imprint injury. However, raised rings, especially those with pointed corners, can cause significant

## Danger Assessment

Several risk factors have been associated with homicides (murder) of both batterers and battered women in research that has been conducted after the killings have taken place. We cannot predict what will happen in your case, but we would like you to be aware of the danger of homicide in situations of severe battering and for you to see how many of the risk factors apply to your situation. (The "he" in the question refers to your husband, partner, ex-husband, ex-partner or whoever is currently physically hurting you).

Please check YES or NO for each question below.

| YES | NO | | |
|-----|-----|-----|-----|
| _____ | _____ | 1. | Has the physical violence increased in frequency over the past year? |
| _____ | _____ | 2. | Has the physical violence increased in severity over the past year and/or has a weapon or threat with a weapon been used? |
| _____ | _____ | 3. | Does he ever try to choke you? |
| _____ | _____ | 4. | Is there a gun in the house? |
| _____ | _____ | 5. | Has he ever forced you into sex when you did not wish to do so? |
| _____ | _____ | 6. | Does he use drugs? By drugs I mean "uppers" or amphetamines, speed, angel dust, cocaine, "crack," street drugs, heroin, or mixtures. |
| _____ | _____ | 7. | Does he threaten to kill you and/or do you believe he is capable of killing you? |
| _____ | _____ | 8. | Is he drunk every day or almost every day? (In terms of quantity of alcohol.) |
| _____ | _____ | 9. | Does he control most of all of your daily activities? For instance, does he tell you whom you can be friends with, how much money you can take with you shopping or when you can take the car? (If he tries, but you do not let him, check here_____.) |
| _____ | _____ | 10. | Have you ever been beaten by him while you were pregnant? (If never pregnant by him, check here_____.) |
| _____ | _____ | 11. | Is he violently and constantly jealous of you? (For instance, does he say, "If I can't have you, no one can.") |
| _____ | _____ | 12. | Have you ever threatened or tried to commit suicide? |
| _____ | _____ | 13. | Has he ever threatened or tried to commit suicide? |
| _____ | _____ | 14. | Is he violent outside of the home? |

_____ TOTAL YES ANSWERS

**THANK YOU. PLEASE TALK TO YOUR NURSE, ADVOCATE OR COUNSELOR ABOUT WHAT THE DANGER ASSESSMENT MEANS IN TERMS OF YOUR SITUATION.**

Note: From Campbell, J. (1986). Nursing assessment for risk of homicide with battered women. *Advances in Nursing Science, 8*(4), 36-51.

**FIG. 9-4.** Danger Assessment (DA). (Permission to use the DA tool in clinical settings has been universally granted by its creator. Dr. Campbell requests notification if the DA tool is used in formal research studies.)

abrasion injury or worse (laceration and/or partial or complete avulsion). Often abrasion injuries from rings are linear or curvilinear and centered in the middle of a punch-like contusion (Figs. 9-7 and 9-9, see Colorplate following page 144). The more angled the point of impact, the longer the abrasion. When punched straight on by an assailant wearing a ring with a stone, visible on the victim may be a punch-like contusion with a circular, oval, semicircular, or horse-shoe-shaped abrasion in the center of the injury. Whenever any form of ring-related abrasion is suspected, it would be prudent to secure the suspect's ring. Inside the ring may

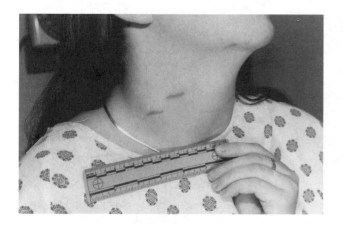

FIG. 9-5. Patterned, fingernail-like scratch abrasions to the left lateral neck and chin from strangulation mechanism of injury.

dence (skin and blood), or the ring pattern may be matched to the injury pattern.

### Avulsion

An avulsion injury is the tearing away of a structure or part. Partial avulsions are more common and can result from blunt force trauma over bony surfaces. Punch injuries to a woman's face can result in complete or partial avulsions to her nose, lips, chin, and forehead (Fig. 9-7, see Colorplate following page 144). Being struck with a solid object with a jagged edge can avulse tissue anywhere on the body.

### Bruise/Contusion

A bruise is the superficial discoloration in the skin or other organ due to hemorrhage from broken

blood vessels from blunt force trauma. A bruise is also called a contusion. More specifically, in a contusion, there is usually swelling, pain, tenderness, and discoloration to injured site. The causes of contusions in domestic violence injuries are almost endless. Any significant blunt force mechanism of injury will cause bruising. However, there are some classic patterned contusions that are frequently seen on battered women.

Fingertip-like blunt force injury often results in dime-sized or nickel-sized, circular contusions most often seen on the victim's arms, especially

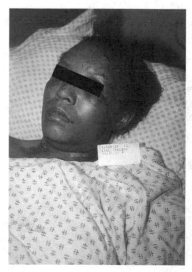

FIG. 9-7. Patterned, punch-like abrasion from a ring with stone to the mid-forehead; sutured partial avulsion injury to the nose; punch-like contusion to the left eye involving the sclera; and strangulation-related abrasions to the neck.

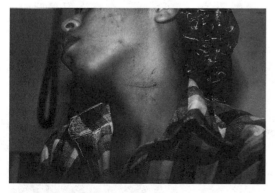

FIG. 9-6. Patterned, fingernail-like scratch abrasions to right lateral neck from strangulation mechanism of injury.

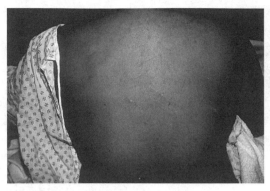

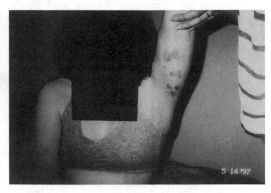

**FIG. 9-8.** Newer, patterned, looped, cord-like contusions to the right upper posterior shoulder and left lower posterior shoulder; patterned, looped, cord-like scar to the right mid-lateral back; patterned, scabbed, cord-like abrasions to the mid-back; patterned, kick/stomp heel-like contusion to the left mid-back; and patterned foot kick/stomp-like, with heel imprint and sole imprint to upper left posterior, superior shoulder.

**FIG. 9-10.** Multiple, patterned, fingertip-like contusions to the left upper arm.

the medial surface of the upper arms (Fig. 9-10, see Colorplate following page 144). The bruises are often in a close, somewhat triangular pattern of two or three (index, middle, and ring fingers) with a distinct, often slightly larger, circular thumb tip imprint bruise opposite the others. Other common locations for fingertip bruising are the neck (bruise is inflicted during strangulation) and the inner, medial knees and thighs (bruise is inflicted during forced sexual assault) (Fig. 9-9, see Colorplate following page 144).

Punch-like contusions to battered women are frequently seen to many areas of the body (Fig. 9-7, see Colorplate following page 144). These contusions are usually oval to circular and with clearly demarcated edges of bruised skin to nonbruised skin (new injuries). Abusers often punch women in the arm, especially the left arm (Fig. 9-11, see Colorplate following page 144). Most people are right-handed. During a face-to-face argument, the abuser will throw a right-handed punch. The right-handed victim will turn away from the punch in a manner that "offers up" the left side to be struck. If the abuser lands a full punch, the contusion is usually well defined to her upper lateral arm.

If she raises her arm to block the punch, she will be bruised to the ulnar surface of the blocking arm (Figs. 9-12 and 9-13, see Colorplate following page 144). These self-defense-

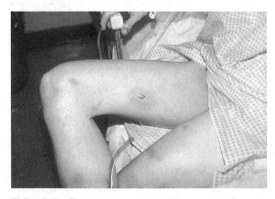

**FIG. 9-9.** Patterned, punch-like contusion to right medial thigh with a patterned imprint abrasion from ring with a stone; patterned, fingertip-like contusions to right medial knee and left anterior medial thigh from a reported marital rape.

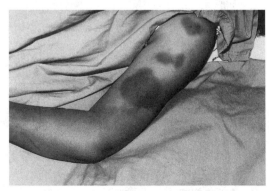

**FIG. 9-11.** Multiple, patterned, punch-like contusions to the left upper arm.

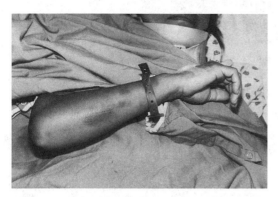

**FIG. 9-12.** Patterned, defensive posture-like contusions to ulnar surface of the left arm.

like contusions to her forearms are usually less defined and can have linear lines of abrasion mixed in with the contusion from the assailant's arm sliding down her arm upon impact. Mid-ulnar bone contusions and fractures can result.

Many battered women report being abused in the car as they drive around with their abusers. Usually the abuser is driving and the battered woman is in the passenger seat. In a full-sized

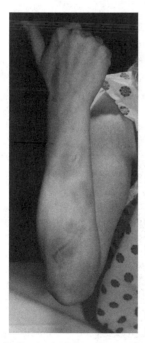

**FIG. 9-13.** Patterned, defensive posture-like contusions to the right lower arm.

vehicle, when he chooses to strike her, he will punch or push with his right arm, making contact to her left arm and left face. This mechanism can also result in right side or right facial/head injury from her striking the passenger door and/or window with the right side of her body. In a small vehicle, he may start the abusive episode by striking her with his left elbow, and as she cowers more to the right side of her seat, he then may begin throwing full punches with his right arm. In this case, she also may have secondary right-sided injuries.

Many battered women examined by this author shared that during abusive episodes in the car the abusers have also tried to push them out of the door of the moving car, or they have tried to intentionally jump out of the moving car to escape the abuse. The women reported that they ended up dangling half in and half out of the car, dragging their hands and arms on the ground. This mechanism of injury usually results in severe "road-burn" abrasions in addition to the blunt force punch and/or elbow trauma. Battered women who totally exit a moving car have usually presented for emergency care with multisystem trauma with multiple types of injuries, external and internal.

Punch-like contusions to a battered woman's abdomen, chest, and back are common hidden injuries (Fig. 9-14, see Colorplate following page 144). While painful, these patterned contusions would not keep the woman from leaving the home because they would not be seen in the normal course of her day. However, if the

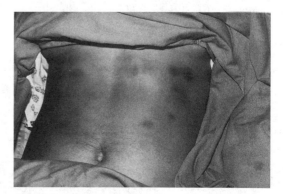

**FIG. 9-14.** Patterned, hidden, punch-like contusions to the upper abdomen, lower anterior chest.

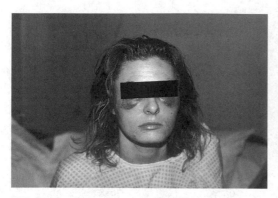

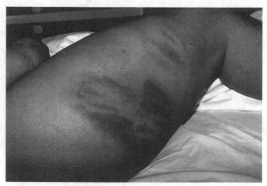

**FIG. 9-15.** Bilateral, periorbital contusions from a single punch to the midface/forehead (raccoon eyes).

**FIG. 9-16.** Patterned, foot kick/stomp-like contusion to the right, superior lateral thigh pushing blood outward from the point of impact and patterned, foot kick/stomp-like contusion to the right inferior lateral thigh.

abuser wants to further isolate the woman, he will punch her in the face. Battered women with facial injuries often seclude themselves in their homes until the facial trauma injury has healed. When punched directly in the mid-face, battered women often develop bilateral, periorbital contusions. Bilateral, periorbital contusions are also caused by certain nasal surgeries and as a sequela to basilar skull fractures (Fig. 9-15). Some health professionals erroneously describe these injuries as bilateral periorbital ecchymoses.

### Ecchymoses

*Ecchymoses* are not the same as contusions and bruises. Ecchymoses are hemorrhagic spots, larger than petechiae, that are nonelevated and usually painless. Contusions are caused by blunt force trauma and involve swelling and pain. Ecchymotic spots are caused by bleeding of a medical, hematologic nature, not trauma.

Battered women are frequently kicked or stomped by their abusers. This mechanism of injury can produce very distinct patterns of injury. When stomped by a foot with a heeled boot or shoe, a distinct pattern is seen (Figs. 9-8 and 9-16, see Colorplate following page 144). A full-impact kick with heeled shoe or boot will leave the heel imprint and a bruise imprint from the sole of the shoe. A kick with a gym shoe may leave the distinct pattern from the bottom of the

gym shoe. These types of patterned kick injuries are most visible on the back, buttocks, and thighs. Kick bruising to a woman's shins is most consistent with defensive posture injury. During the beating, the woman will curl up on the ground in a fetal-like position to protect her face, chest, and abdomen.

### Lacerations

In addition to the contusions, blunt force trauma results in *lacerations,* which are wounds caused by the tearing of tissue, usually over bony prominences. Lacerations are not sharp injuries like cuts or incisions. Unfortunately, many health care providers have developed an erroneous habit of calling any break in the skin from any cause a laceration. Lacerations are distinguished from sharp cutting injuries in a number of ways. Lacerations are usually jagged at the skin edges. When the wound is spread apart, lacerations do not have smooth edges, and have varying depth. Lacerations are often accompanied by bruising that involves the split area of skin.

### Cuts/Incisions

*Cuts or incisions* produce openings in the skin that are usually very straight. When spread apart, the tissue along the sides of sharp injuries is smooth and the depth is more consistent. If upon examination or from the patient's history the health-care provider cannot determine if a break in the skin is a laceration or an incised, sharp injury, then document what it looks like and refer to it as a "wound."

### Petechiae

With a strangulation mechanism of injury, the battered woman may develop facial petechiae, which are minute, pinpoint, nonraised, perfectly round, purplish–red spots caused by intradermal or submucous hemorrhage. The petechiae can also be seen in the conjunctiva of the eye. Occasionally, facial and eye petechiae can be caused by nonabusive activities, such as child birth, severe vomiting, or very strenuous physical activity such as weight lifting.

### Traumatic Alopecia

Battered women report that their abusers often pull them or drag them by the hair. Not only is this form of abuse acutely painful, it can result in traumatic alopecia. Unless a segment of the scalp has literally been torn away in a scalping manner, traumatic alopecia can be very difficult to photograph. To document traumatic alopecia photographically, this author has carefully pulled a comb through the battered patient's hair and photographed the copious loose hairs removed by the comb.

### Slap Injuries

Slap and/or punch injuries to the patient's ears can produce enough force to rupture the battered woman's ear drum(s). Unless there are other more severe injuries, this author has observed that battered women with ruptured traumatized membranes tend to have delays in seeking treatment. In general, any woman with injuries who has delayed seeking medical attention should be more assertively screened for domestic violence. Slap injuries to flat areas of the body, such as the back, face, buttocks, or shoulders, can initially produce a patterned, erythemic outline of the hand.

Within 24 hours the slap injury could show two to four linear bruises in parallel. The bruises are thin and represent broken vessels in the victim's tissue to the sides of the slapping fingers of the abuser (17).

### Firearm Injuries

Battered women with firearm injuries are usually in need of emergency care. Evidence collection and preservation may be secondary to life-saving interventions. However, it is crucial that one member of the trauma/resuscitation team be delegated the task of evidence collection and preservation. All cut and removed clothing must be placed in separate paper bags, sealed, labeled, and secured in a locked, ventilated cabinet. Any trace evidence (e.g., soil, grass, glass) must be preserved and accurately labeled. All bullets and/or fragments must be wrapped in a protective gauze, such as Telfa, and placed in a clean, dry, plastic container. Multiple bullets or bullet fragments should never be placed in the same container and allowed to bounce off each other. This motion destroys microscopic riflings and may prevent ballistics experts in the police crime lab from making a positive identification of the weapon. Health professionals, in most cases, are not adequately trained to determine which bullet hole is the exit or entrance wound. In fact, Randall found health professionals to be accurate in determining bullet entrance and exit wounds only half of the time (67). Health professionals should never make any written opinions as to the caliber of the bullet used in the shooting.

### Bite Marks

During domestic abuse, battered women are often subjected to biting, with the bites being frequently to sexual areas. Vale and Noguchi found that women were bitten most frequently on the breasts, followed by the arms and legs (68). Bite injuries often result in unique patterned injuries that can be successfully matched to the assailant's teeth (69). Protocols for the photographic documentation of bite injuries have been developed by the American Board of Forensic Odontology and include close-up photography at both a 90-degree angle to the wound and at what appears to be angle of the bite, if present (70). The photographs should also include shots that include a right-angled ruler.

### Sexual Assault

Sheridan (59) and Campbell (28) found that sexual abuse of woman by intimate male partners occurred in nearly half of their cases, with forced sex often occurring after the women had left the abusive relationship. Therefore, every woman who has been identified as battered needs to be assessed for a possible forensic sexual assault examination. If the reported sexual assault occurred within the previous 72 hours, offering the victim a sexual assault exam has been considered standard. Most sexual assault examiners have been taught that after 72 hours there is no longer enough evidence in or on the victim to justify subjecting her to the trauma of a sexual assault exam. However, the 72-hour "rule" is not an absolute, only a guideline. There may be numerous circumstances, based on victims' histories, to perform a forensic sexual assault exam beyond 72 hours. For example, consider doing an exam beyond 72 hours with victims who have not bathed or showered and/or are still wearing the same clothing worn during or immediately after an assault.

## PHOTOGRAPHS AND BODY MAPS

Although detailed written histories of domestic abuse are essential components of thorough forensic exams, taking photographs of all battered women's injuries, new and old, is even more critical. Even though these photographs are taken for the medical documentation of observed and treated injuries, the photographs can be invaluable in criminal and/or civil court proceedings. The most important criterion for a "good picture" is that it be a true and accurate representation of what the health-care provider examined and treated on the day of the exam. Most forensically trained abuse examiners prefer using 35mm cameras with print film. How-

ever, prints from Polaroid and digital cameras are also effective in court. All photographic documentation systems have advantages and disadvantages.

Photographs should be taken after signed consent has been obtained. If the victim is unconscious, the photographs should be taken immediately and consent obtained when the patient's condition improves. Photographs of wounds should be taken before and after the wound is cleaned. Photographing the "dirty" wound may corroborate the victim's history as a result of the presence of trace evidence in the wound. All patterned injuries and pattern of injuries should be photographed. In fact, some patterned injuries become more apparent over time. Therefore, every abuse patient should be offered follow-up photography 1 and 2 days after initial treatment. Every series of photographs (no matter the camera style) should start with a full-frame identification picture of the victim. Then, for each wound on the victim, the patient should be photographed initially from several feet away, with each subsequent photo coming in closer and closer (Fig. 9-17, see Colorplate following page 144). The final photo for each injury should be at the closest focal setting the camera can accommodate. Without special macro adapter lenses, most cameras cannot produce a focused picture when moved in closer than 2 feet.

If 35mm print film is used, it is recommended that the photographer use 12-exposure film. In this author's experience, 12 exposures are usually enough to document the average patient's injuries. If 24- or 36-exposure film is used, there is a tendency to want to "not waste film" by photographing two or more patients on one roll. This is contraindicated. One patient per roll of film is the forensic standard. If a patient has multiple trauma, use multiple rolls of 12-exposure film. For each injury, there should be at least one photograph with a scale present and one photograph without the scale. Scales include rulers and coins. Quality camera shops sell ruler scales that have standardized gray or color reference scales. When using standardized scales, the film developer should be notified *a priori* so that appropriate adjustments can be made during film processing to produce colors more true and accurate to that observed.

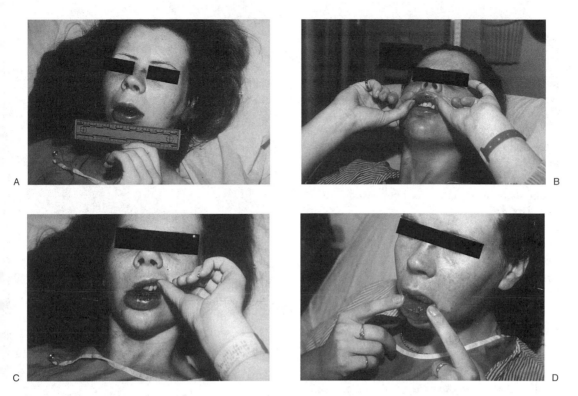

**FIG. 9-17.** Series of four photographs to illustrate how photographs can be used to demonstrate mechanisms of injuries. **A:** Victim has obvious facial trauma to her left eyelid, left lateral nose, and mouth. The left lateral nose contusion was caused by the nosepiece of her glasses being forcefully pushed into the nose from a punch injury to left eye. The patient's glasses absorbed much of the punch force and were broken (not pictured). Hence, the actual trauma to her left eye was limited to left upper eyelid. A second punch produced the mouth trauma. **B:** The force of the punch caused the upper teeth to leave patterned contusion, abrasion, and minor laceration trauma to oral mucosa. **C:** A few of the victim's upper teeth are shown to demonstrate the source of the trauma in the fourth photo. **D:** The victim has a patterned puncture wound to the lower oral mucosa that corresponds to the teeth shown in part C.

## SAFETY PLANNING AND DISCHARGE OPTIONS

Every battered female patient should be asked if she considers it safe to leave the treatment area or to return home. For many of the reasons discussed earlier in this chapter, battered women often choose to return to the abusive relationship. This author has found it clinically useful to do safety planning with every battered patient around four issues. Anticipatory teaching is done with each woman.

The woman is asked what she would do if her husband/boyfriend began hitting her a week, a month, or a year from now. Most women reply that they would call 911 and seek police assistance. Although this behavior is strongly encouraged, the woman is instructed to make her call for help a little more generic by stating that she needs police help because she is being beaten and/or threatened by a man. The woman is instructed that it is not necessary to state that the assailant is her husband or boyfriend. Although police officers are more highly trained in domestic abuse responses than in years past, domestic calls are still viewed as a waste of time by some officers. The victim may get a quicker police response if police think they are responding to a stranger assault.

A second safety planning technique is to ask the woman if her abuser always carries a weapon (knife or gun). There are several reasons for this question. First, the health-care provider needs to know if the abuser is probably armed with a weapon, especially if he is sitting in the waiting room or shows up in the treatment area. This knowledge can help protect the health-care provider, co-workers, and other patients. If the battered woman says her abuser is always or almost always armed with a weapon, she is instructed to share that information with the police anytime she makes an emergency call. This information may help to keep law enforcement personnel safer and may result in a multiunit, faster response time for the victim.

A third safety plan includes teaching a battered woman to prepack an emergency "flight bag" with important materials that she or her children might need were they to flee the home in danger. First, she needs to be asked if it is safe to have such a bag and where it can be safely hidden. Items to be included in the bag might include important documents (e.g., health, bank, court, birth, and citizenship records, and emergency family/friend contact telephone numbers); spare money (including change for pay phones); change of clothing, especially for the children; and a small toy for small children.

A fourth safety plan taught to every battered woman consists of inviting her to use the 24-hour accessible local emergency department as a short-term sanctuary for herself and her children. She is told that she can always return to the emergency department if she needs emergency safety. If necessary, she and her children can be assessed and treated. If no medical treatment is necessary, hospital and community social service and victim advocacy services can be obtained.

## ADULT MALTREATMENT SYNDROME

Every woman treated in a health-care setting for an abuse-related condition must be assigned one or more adult maltreatment syndrome diagnoses in the ICD 9 CM diagnostic code book. The diagnoses are as follows:

995.80 Adult maltreatment, unspecified
995.81 Adult physical abuse
995.82 Adult emotional/psychological abuse
995.83 Adult sexual abuse
995.85 Adult abuse and neglect/other

The use of adult maltreatment syndrome diagnoses will be an asset during Joint Commission on Accreditation of Healthcare Organizations site visits if battered-women client charts are needed for review (17).

## SUMMARY

Domestic violence identification and forensic documentation of histories and injuries by health-care professionals are critical in preventing further abuse. The provider must have an understanding of the barriers that prevent women from leaving abusive relationships, as well as an understanding of the necessity for asking routine abuse screening questions and for the assessing the level of harassment and potentially lethal danger. Written and photographic documentation of abuse, safety planning, and community referrals to abuse services by health care professionals are now considered to be the minimal standard of care. Failure to meet these standards not only places the abused patient and her children at further risk of abuse but also places the provider at risk of a tort for not meeting the standard.

## REFERENCES

1. Novella A. From the surgeon general, US Public Health Service. *JAMA* 1992;276(23):31–32.
2. Cruz JM, Firestone JM. Exploring violence and abuse in gay male relationships.*Violence and Victims* 1998; 13(2):159–173.
3. Renzetti CM. Violence in lesbian and gay relationships. In: O'Toole LL, Schiffman JR, eds. *Gender violence: interdisciplinary perspectives.* New York: New York University Press, 1997:285–293.
4. Coleman VE. Lesbian battering: the relationship between personality and the perpetration of violence. *Violence and Victims* 1994;9:139–152.
5. Loving N. *Responding to spouse abuse and wife beating: a guide for police.* Washington: Police Executive Research Forum, 1980.
6. Pizzey E, Shapiro J. *Prone to violence.* Feltham, Middlesex, England: Hamlyn Publishing, 1982.
7. Roy M. A current survey of 150 cases. In: Roy M, ed. *Battered women: a psychosociological study of domes-*

*tic violence*. New York: Van Nostrand Reinhold, 1977.

8. US Commission on Civil Rights. Battered women: issues of public policy. Washington, 1978.

9. Walker LE. *The battered woman*. New York: Harper-Colophon Books, 1979.

10. Buzawa ES, Buzawa CG. *Domestic violence: the criminal justice response. Studies in crime and law*, vol. 6. Thousand Oaks, CA: Sage Publications, 1990.

11. Edwards SSM. *Policing "domestic" violence: women, the law, and the state.* Thousand Oaks, CA: Sage Publications, 1989.

12. Drake VK. Battered women: a health care problem in disguise. *Image* 1982;14:40–47.

13. Lichenstein VR. The battered woman: guidelines for effective nursing intervention. *Issues Mental Health Nurs* 1981;3:237–250.

14. Lieberknecht K. Helping the battered wife. *Am J Nurs* 1978;78:654–656.

15. Parker B, Schumacher DM. The battered wife syndrome and violence in the nuclear family of origin: a controlled pilot study. *Am J Public Health* 1977;67:760–761.

16. Stark E, Flitcraft A, Frazier W. Medicine and patriarchal violence: the social construction of a private event. *Int J Health Serv* 1979;9(3):461–493.

17. Brockmeyer DM, Sheridan DJ. Domestic violence: a practical guide to the use of forensic evaluation in clinical examination and documentation of injuries. In: Campbell JC, ed. *Empowering survivors of abuse: health care for battered women and their children*. Thousand Oaks, CA: Sage Publications, 1998:214–226.

18. Campbell JC. Misogyny and homicide of women. *Adv Nurs Sci* 1981;3(2):67–85.

19. Campbell JC. Nursing assessment for risk of homicide with battered women. *Adv Nurs Sci* 1986;8(4):36–51.

20. Campbell JC. "If I can't have you, no one can": power and control in homicide of female partners. In: Radford J, Russell DEH, eds. *Femicide: the politics of woman killing*. New York: Twayne Publishing, 1992:99–113.

21. Grant CA. Women who kill: the impact of abuse. *Issues Mental Health Nurs* 1995;16:315–326.

22. Lynch VA. Forensic nursing in the emergency department: a new role for the 1990's. *Crit Care Nurs Q* 1991;14(3):69–86.

23. Lynch VA. Forensic nursing: diversity in education and practice. *J Psychosoc Nurs* 1993;31(11):7–14.

24. Sheridan DJ, Belknap L, Engel B, et al. *Guidelines for the treatment of battered women victims in emergency room settings*. Chicago Hospital Council.

25. Sheridan DJ. The role of the battered women specialist. *J Psychosoc Nurs* 1993;31(11):31–37.

26. Sheridan DJ. Family violence. In: Kitt S, Selfridge-Thomas J, Proehl JA, Kaiser J, eds. *Emergency nursing: a physiologic and clinical perspective*, 2nd ed. Philadelphia: WB Saunders, 1995:482–494.

27. Sheridan DJ. Forensic documentation of battered pregnant women. *J Nurse-Midwifery* 1996;41(6):467–472.

28. Campbell JC. Women's responses to sexual abuse in intimate relationships. *Women's Health Care Int* 1989; 8:335–347.

29. Eby KK, Campbell JC. Health effects of experiences of sexual violence for women with abusive partners. *Women's Health Care Int* 1995;14:563–576.

30. Campbell JC, Soeken K. Forced sex and intimate partner violence: effects on women's health. *Violence Against Women* 1999;5:1017–1035.

31. Pence E, Paymar M. *Power and control: tactics of men who batter*. Duluth, MN: Domestic Abuse Intervention Project, 1986.

32. Pence E, Paymar M. *Education groups for men who batter: the Duluth model*. New York: Springer Publishers.

33. Wilson M, Daly M. Spousal homicide risk and estrangement. *Violence and Victims* 1993;8(1):3–16.

34. Wilson M, Daly M, Daniele A. Familicide: the killing of spouse and children *Aggress Behav.* 1995;21:275–291.

35. Fishwick NJ. Health care encounters of women in abusive relationships: a process of protecting personal integrity. Unpublished dissertation, Case Western Reserve University, Cleveland, OH, 1993.

36. Landenburger KM. The process of entrapment and recovery from an abusive relationship. *Issues Mental Health Nurs* 1989;10:209–227.

37. Landenburger KM. Exploration of women's identity: clinical approaches with abused women. *Clin Issues Perinat Women's Health Nurs* 1993;4(3):378–384.

38. May BA. Abused women's cognition beliefs associated with readiness to terminate the relationship. Unpublished doctoral dissertation, Oregon Health Sciences University, Portland, 1990.

39. Sonkin DJ. *The counselor's guide to learning to live without violence*. Volcano, CA: Volcano Press, 1995.

40. Boulette TR, Andersen SM. "Mind control" and the battering of women. *Commun Mental Health J* 1985;21(2): 109–117.

41. Graham DLR, Rawlings EI. Bonding with abusive dating partners: dynamics of Stockholm syndrome. In: Levy B, ed. *Dating violence: young women in danger*. Seattle: Seal Press, 1991:119–135.

42. Graham DLR, Rawlings EI, Rimini N. Survivors of terror: battered women, hostages, and the Stockholm syndrome. In: Yllo K, Bograd M, eds. *Feminist perspectives on wife abuse*. Thousand Oaks, CA: Sage Publications, 1988:217–233.

43. Dutton DG, Painter SL. Traumatic bonding: the development of emotional attachments in battered women and other relationships of intermittent abuse. *Victimology: An Int J* 1981;1(4):139–155.

44. Dutton DG, Painter S. Emotional attachments in abusive relationships: a test of traumatic bonding theory. *Violence and Victims* 1993;8(2):105–120.

45. Fortune MM, Horman D. *Family violence: a workshop manual for clergy and other service providers. Domestic violence monograph series*, vol. 6. Rockville, MD: National Clearing House on Domestic Violence, 1981.

46. NiCarthy G. *Getting free: a handbook for women in abusive relationships*. Seattle: Seal Press, 1986.

47. Tolman RM. The development of a measure of psychological maltreatment of women by their male partners. *Violence Against Women* 1989;3:159–177.

48. Walker LE. *The battered women syndrome*. New York: Springer Publishers, 1984.

49. Biderman AD. Captivity lore and behavior in captivity. In: Grosser GH, Wechsler H, Greenblat M, eds. *The threat of impending disaster*. Cambridge, MA: MIT Press, 1964.

50. Raymond B, Bruschi IG. Psychological abuse among college women in dating relationships. *Percept Motor Skills* 1989;69:1283–1297.

51. Johnson MP. Patriarchal terrorism and common couple violence: two forms of violence against women. *J Marriage Family* 1995;57:283–294.

52. American Medical Association. *Diagnostic and treatment guidelines on domestic violence.* Chicago, 1992.

53. Helton A. *Protocol of care for the battered woman.* Houston: Houston Chapter of the March of Dimes, 1986.

54. Parker B, McFarlane J. Nursing assessment of the battered pregnant woman. *Matern Child Nurs J* 1991;16: 161–164.

55. McFarlane J, Parker B, Soeken K, Bullock L. Assessing for abuse during pregnancy. *JAMA* 1992; 267(3): 3176–3178.

56. Straus MA. Measuring intra-family conflict and violence: the Conflict Tactics (CT) scales. *J Marriage Family* 1979;41:75–88.

57. Hudson WW, McIntosh SR. The assessment of spouse abuse: two quantifiable dimensions. *J Marriage Family* 1981;43:(4):873–885.

58. Soeken KL, McFarlane J, Parker B, Lominack MC. The Abuse Assessment Screen: measuring frequency, severity, and perpetrator of abuse against women. In: Campbell JC, ed. *Empowering survivors of abuse: health care for battered women and their children.* Thousand Oaks, CA: Sage Publications, 1998: 195–203.

59. Sheridan DJ. Measuring harassment of abused women: a nursing concern. Unpublished doctoral dissertation, Oregon Health Sciences University, Portland.

60. Campbell JC. Homicide of and by battered women. In: Campbell JC, ed. *Assessing dangerousness: violence by sexual offenders, batterers, and child abusers.* Thousand Oaks, CA: Sage Publications, 1995:96–113.

61. Sonkin DJ, Martin D, Walker LE. *The male batterer: a treatment approach.* New York: Springer Publishers, 1985.

62. Hart B. Beyond the "duty to warn": a therapist's "duty to protect" battered women and children. In: Yllo K, Bograd M, eds. *Feminist perspectives on wife abuse.* Thousand Oaks, CA: Sage Publications, 1988: 234–248.

63. Limandri BJ, Sheridan DJ. Prediction of intentional interpersonal violence: an introduction. In: Campbell JC, ed. *Assessing dangerousness: violence by sexual offenders, batterers, and child abusers.* Thousand Oaks, CA: Sage Publications, 1995:1–19.

64. DiMaio DJ, DiMaio VJM. *Forensic pathology.* New York: Elsevier Science, 1989.

65. Gordon I, Shapiro HA, Berson SD. *Forensic medicine,* 3rd ed. Edinburgh: Churchill Livingstone, 1988.

66. Miller BF, Keane CB. *Encyclopedia and dictionary of medicine, nursing, and allied health,* 2nd ed. Philadelphia: WB Saunders, 1978.

67. Randall T. Clinician's forensic interpretations of fatal gunshot wounds often miss the mark. *JAMA* 1993; 269(16):2058–2061.

68. Vale GL, Noguchi TT. Anatomical distribution of human bite marks in a series of 67 cases. *J Forensic Sci* 1983;28(1):61–69.

69. Gold MH, Roenigk HH Jr, Smith ES, Pierce LJ. Evaluation and treatment of patients with human bite marks. *Am J Forensic Med Pathol* 1989;13(2):140–143.

70. American Board of Forensic Odontology. Guidelines for bite mark analysis. *J Am Dent Assoc* 1986; 112(3):383–386.

# 10

# Sexual Assault and the Criminal Justice System

DePriest W. Whye, Jr., and Sharon May

The individual who is alleged to have committed a sexual crime or any crime is innocent until proven guilty. This frequently recited but powerful phrase "innocent until proven guilty" is based on a set of constitutional principles that were designed to achieve a delicate balance between the maintenance of certain societal interests and the protection of individual civil rights. The government is responsible for the general welfare of the people, which includes their health and safety. On the other hand, the government must safeguard the individual's liberties, particularly when that individual is accused of a crime.

The Bill of Rights, comprising the first ten amendments to the United States Constitution, provides substantive and procedural due process for the individual charged with a crime. Substantive due process requires that the law be fair, equitable, and unambiguous. Procedural due process guarantees that the accused, among other things, can remain silent, must be advised of the charges against him, can demand the presence of witnesses, and can cross-examine his accusers. The accused must have a public trial, can select the mode of trial, and may not be retried for the same crime.

## SEX OFFENSES

Certain conduct involving sexual behavior is rooted in the common law legislated by each state. The phrase "sex crime" typically encompasses a spectrum of sexually related or sexu-

ally motivated crimes. Rape, sodomy, incest, and sexual assault or battery are commonly identified as sex crimes. Other sex crimes include obscenity, public nudity, and child pornography. Each state specifically defines the categories of sex crimes. Therefore, the legal requirements may vary somewhat from state to state. For example, a state law may classify one type of sex offense as rape in the first degree. The elements of that crime may be (a) vaginal intercourse, (b) against the will and without the consent of the victim, (c) by use of force or threat of force, and (d) while using a weapon, being aided by others, or inflicting strangulation, suffocation, or serious bodily harm. Each element of a crime must be proven for a jury to convict a defendant.

## OVERVIEW OF THE CRIMINAL JUSTICE SYSTEM

While basic constitutionally constructed and protected procedures within the criminal justice system remain constant from state to state, there are specific differences established by each state. Therefore, a discussion of the system is undertaken with the understanding that the particulars of criminal process and procedure are dependent on the geographic location of the crime.

The prosecution and punishment of a sexual assailant or predator require the effective interplay of multiple components of the criminal justice system. Law enforcement, the judicial branch of government, and the corrections system combine to process criminals effectively and fairly. The first component, law enforcement, serves as the charging and investigative arm of the criminal system. Investigative officers, police officers, or agents interview witnesses and suspects, seize and preserve tangible evidence, pursue leads in order to identify the alleged perpetrator(s) of a crime, and make arrests. Prosecutors review the evidence gathered by police, evaluate the sufficiency of the case against an accused, and present the evidence to the trier of fact. Police and prosecutors exercise significant discretion in performing their duties, but most comply with constitutional, statutory, and departmental regulations.

The courts represent the judicial branch and have the authority to hear facts and evaluate evidence within an accusatorial and adversarial legal model. In this model, the state must prove beyond a reasonable doubt that the defendant committed the crime. The defendant, if he so chooses, may refute that proof. Prosecutors, called district attorneys, state's attorneys, or United States attorneys, represent the state and federal governments. Defense attorneys represent the defendants. Criminal proceedings are presided over by a judge, who must ensure that the substantive and procedural rules are upheld by the prosecution and defense. During a jury trial, the judge decides what facts can be presented to the jury, maintains order, and instructs the jury as to its role in evaluating the evidence. Judges and the jury in some jurisdictions determine the sentence. A not guilty verdict means that a defendant must be released on those charges for which he was tried. A defendant convicted after a trial has the automatic right to an appeal. However, a defendant who pleads guilty may appeal on very limited grounds.

## ILLUSTRATION OF THE CRIMINAL JUSTICE PROCESS

A clearer impression of the structure and function of the criminal system is achieved by the following sequence of steps encountered from the time a crime is committed to the final legal disposition of the crime. Consider the following scenario and commentary: A sexual crime has been committed. A jogger was sexually assaulted while jogging in the park. The jogger was raped and battered. The police arrive on the scene and transport the victim to the nearest hospital or rape center for evaluation and treatment. After the evaluation by the medical staff, the police officers interview the victim and obtain a detailed description of the events. Critical in the interview is an accurate description of the assailant. The sexual assault nurse examiner collects forensic evidence from the victim. At the scene, police lab technicians from the crime scene and potential witnesses are interviewed. Detectives from the sex crimes unit are notified and dispatched to lead the investigation.

## INVESTIGATION

In order for the police to gather the vital evidence to support a successful conviction, the police must have the full cooperation of the victim. The officer will ask the cooperative victim to describe what transpired before, during, and after the assault. Questions concerning the use of force, threats, or weapons are asked. The victim must specify and articulate the exact acts of the assailant because different acts constitute different crimes. If the victim refuses to speak to the police, usually the police have difficulty continuing with the investigation and prosecution of the assailant cannot proceed. Sometimes a delay may occur in the victim's decision to cooperate with the police investigation. Obviously, this delay is problematic because memories fade and evidence is lost.

In addition to the medical evidence, the police collect physical evidence from the crime scene. It is very important that the crime scene be left undisturbed until the technicians can collect untainted evidence. Physical evidence includes fingerprints, hair, clothing fibers, body fluids, and any items that may contain trace evidence linking the assailant to the scene.

The police will interview the first person to have contact with the victim subsequent to the assault. In some jurisdictions, that first report of a sexual assault (i.e., the statement of the victim to a third party) is admissible at trial. Eyewitnesses who may have seen the crime or a suspicious person in the area provide valuable information to the police. The investigators prepare written reports detailing their findings. The crime lab analyzes the forensic evidence and documents their procedures and conclusions. All of this information is used to identify an accused and to develop the prosecution's case.

Several days after the assault on the jogger, police see a suspicious individual walking briskly from a small park after having heard a woman scream. He appears to be the only person in the vicinity from which the scream emanated. The police stop the suspect and ask for identification. The individual, whose clothing is unkempt and inappropriate considering the temperature, seems out of breath and fails to produce identification. He claims to live not far from the park. The police are suspicious and "pat the suspect down" for a weapon. Police need only to have an articulable suspicion to justify conducting a frisk. Given the aforementioned circumstances, police suspect criminal activity and fear for their own safety. They feel that the suspect may be armed. The suspect is protected by the Fourth Amendment of the Constitution against unreasonable searches and seizures. However, case law has determined that an individual may be stopped and patted down or frisked if the officer has reasonable suspicion that he can articulate regarding criminal activity by the person detained. An articulable suspicion, a lower threshold than probable cause, is predicated on extremely subjective observations, and permits the officer to stop, question, and possibly search the suspicious person if the officer believes that the individual may be carrying a weapon. During questioning or after a search of the individual, evidence may be discovered that raises the level of suspicion to the realm of probable cause. Probable cause indicates that the individual, based on answers to questions, a search, eyewitness identification, or other implicating information, is likely to have committed a crime. Under the facts of the scenario given here, the police do not have probable cause, so they ask the suspect if he is willing to go downtown for further questioning. The suspect, no stranger to the criminal justice sys-

tem, refuses to speak with the police any further. That ends the encounter for the moment because there is no basis for an arrest.

## ARREST

Continuing the assault scenario, a witness in the vicinity informs the police that the suspect walked hastily from the area where the screams originated and tossed an object into the bushes when he saw the police coming. The police search the bushes and recover a knife. The intended victim, who is still in the area, is brought by the police to where the suspect is being held. She shouts, "That's him. He attacked me with a knife." Now the officers have probable cause and inform the suspect that he is under arrest. Note that the courts do not view a one-on-one identification made shortly after the alleged crime as impermissibly suggestive.

Typically, police read the suspect his Miranda rights immediately, although the rights are not required until a custodial interrogation takes place. Blurts made by a suspect who has not been asked a question and not advised may later be ruled admissible. Responses to questions asked before the advice of rights and/or after a request for legal counsel are likely to be excluded at trial. Information or tangible evidence obtained through questioning of the suspect who was not advised appropriately will be excluded from use at trial. This is referred to as the exclusionary rule.

This arrest is warrantless because the suspect was apprehended at the scene of the crime based on evidence or observation, which supports a determination of probable cause. Since a felony was allegedly committed, the police were not required to request a warrant from a judge. (Had the crime been a misdemeanor, the police could only arrest without a warrant if the crime was committed in their presence. When the police do not witness the commission of the misdemeanor, the victim must go before a judicial officer, file charges, and take an oath that the allegations are true.)

When a suspect is not apprehended contemporaneously with the crime, the victim or witnesses may be asked to view a photo array or attend a line-up. In either of these identification procedures, the police and prosecutors must ensure that the "filler" individuals share very similar physical characteristics and clothing with the suspect. To do otherwise makes the procedure impermissibly suggestive and taints the identification, making it inadmissible at trial. When identification is to be made using a photo array, the police must follow strict departmental procedures including using either all-color or all-black-and-white mug shots. During a physical line-up, the participants may be asked by the police to repeat certain statements allegedly made during commission of the crime. This allows the victim to hear the voice of the alleged perpetrator and may be the sole basis for the identification in those instances when the victim or witness did not get a good look at the assailant. The line-up is conducted in a manner and place that prevents the suspect from seeing the witness.

## BOOKING

After being arrested by the police, the suspect is transported to the police station for booking. Booking is a police administrative process, which essentially records specific information about the suspect and describes the nature of the crimes committed. When booked, the suspect is fingerprinted and photographed. In those jurisdictions using modern technology, the suspect places each finger on a glass where his prints are read and recorded by the computer. His photograph is taken in color by a digital camera. Police check for outstanding warrants on the defendant. Typically, a suspect is permitted to make one phone call following the booking process.

In serious crimes against persons, such as sexual assault, a suspect may also be photographed to memorialize his overall appearance and particular physical characteristics as well as to record his clothing at the time of the arrest, which may be similar to that worn during the crime. In addition, police will get close-up shots of any injuries, which may be compatible with the victim's account of the crime.

After booking the suspect, police may get the court's permission to collect certain evidence

from the person of the suspect. For example, in a sexual assault, a sexual assault nurse examiner may extract head and pubic hairs, bodily fluids including those of the victim, as well as other evidence that may connect the suspect to the crime.

## COMPLAINT

The police officer files a complaint, which is the charging instrument. The complaint is a written statement of the facts demonstrating the existence of probable cause and forming the basis of the offense charged. When a warrant is requested, the complaint is presented to a judge in support of the warrant. In a warrantless arrest, the complaint serves as the charging document at the initial appearance or preliminary hearing.

## PROSECUTOR

The prosecuting attorney or prosecutor represents the government in all criminal cases within his jurisdiction. The prosecutor confers with police to review and assess the adequacy of evidence to support a decision to prosecute the case. The prosecutor makes the decision to proceed with the case, determines the prosecution strategy, negotiates plea bargains, and considers alternative dispositions of the case. The prosecutor evaluates the weight and admissibility of the evidence, the credibility of the witnesses, and the overall impression that the victim will make on the trier of fact. Further, the prosecutor must be convinced that the case against the defendant can be proven beyond a reasonable doubt. At any time before the case concludes, the prosecutor may withdraw or reduce charges. In some situations, the prosecutor and the defense may negotiate a plea. Finally, based on the weight of the available evidence, the prosecutor may decide not to prosecute.

## VICTIM

A victim's participation in the criminal process is not necessarily limited to testimony at trial. The victim may be asked to present evidence to a grand jury and testify at a preliminary hearing or a pretrial motion. With the permission of the court, a victim may testify at the sentencing of a defendant. Some jurisdictions allow victims to testify at parole hearings.

The victim affects the criminal prosecution in several ways. A victim who refuses to cooperate with the investigation may prevent the police from making an arrest. Even if an arrest has been made, the prosecutor may decline to proceed with prosecution despite a victim's desire to continue with the case. On the other hand, there may be special circumstances in which a trial can proceed even if the victim refuses to cooperate.

Some victims of sexual assault have resisted involvement in the criminal process because of either real or perceived insensitivity by the criminal justice system and law enforcement personnel. Efforts have been made to make the process more accommodating to the victim in order to encourage prosecution. For example, rape shield laws have been enacted to exclude mention of a rape victim's prior sexual history unless the prior sexual activity involves the defendant or could explain the victim's injuries or pregnancy.

## POLYGRAPH

The police or prosecutor may request that the sexual assault victim take a polygraph or some other truth verification device. The victim is free to refuse. Some sexual assault victim's advocates have unsuccessfully tried to gain passage of laws preventing the use of truth verification devices. The advocate's position grew out of some isolated instances when police refused to investigate cases in which the victim did not agree to take a polygraph within days of the assault. Investigators and prosecutors responded that the test is merely an investigative tool that may be appropriate to use when credibility questions arise late in the case. The prosecuting attorney may consider the results to decide whether to proceed with the case. In Maryland, polygraph results are inadmissible. However, if any state witness takes the test, that fact must be disclosed to defense counsel.

The defendant may ask to take a polygraph test to demonstrate his innocence. The results of the defendant's polygraph may impact the prosecutor's willingness to proceed against the defendant. In most jurisdictions, the results of the polygraph test as well as a defendant's willingness or refusal to take one is inadmissible in a criminal court. That is because the courts generally are not convinced of the reliability of truth verification devices. A few jurisdictions permit introduction of polygraph evidence if it is determined to be reliable.

## INITIAL APPEARANCE

Within a reasonable time after the arrest, the accused must be seen by a judicial officer for an initial appearance. At this proceeding, the judicial officer verifies the identity of the accused, informs him of the charges, and explains his right to counsel and to a preliminary hearing. If the defendant's charge is a felony, a preliminary hearing date is set. States vary on the time frame for that hearing, which could occur within 10 or 30 days of arrest.

The judicial officer then determines the defendant's eligibility for pretrial release based on such factors as the defendant's criminal record, the seriousness of the crime, the threat to public safety, the defendant's ties to the community, and his record for appearing for trial previously. The pretrial status of the accused is also affected by whether the judicial officer finds probable cause. If the judicial officer is a judge, the defendant may be ordered to do certain things, including reporting to pretrial release staff regularly or not having contact with the victim prior to trial. Bail can be revoked if this order is violated or if the defendant commits certain crimes while awaiting trial.

## PRELIMINARY HEARING

After the initial hearing before a judicial officer, the defendant is afforded a second hearing in more than half of the states. The preliminary hearing is a determination by an independent magistrate as to whether there is probable cause to allow the state to charge a felony defendant.

Probable cause examines the likelihood that a crime was committed and that the defendant is the perpetrator of that crime. If the preliminary hearing judge determines that sufficient evidence exists to hold the accused, then the State files a criminal information, which is a type of charging document.

At the hearing, the State presents witnesses whose testimony provides the probable cause for the arrest of the defendant. Hearsay, an out-of-court statement offered to prove the truth of the matter asserted, is permitted at a preliminary hearing. This means that a police officer may testify as to what the victim and other witnesses said, the crime lab's conclusions, the doctor's report, and so forth. The defendant or his attorney may ask questions but may not present evidence because the hearing is not a determination of guilt or innocence.

The State makes the decision to use either the preliminary hearing or a grand jury to evaluate probable cause. If a preliminary hearing is held, the defense can get a sampling of the State's case. The State does not have to present every piece of evidence that will be used at trial, but must only demonstrate that there is sufficient probable cause.

Some jurisdictions, such as California, prefer to use the preliminary hearing instead of the grand jury. After the preliminary hearing in the famous McMartin Day Care Center child abuse case lasted a full year, Californians voted to limit the length of such hearings.

## INFORMATION AND INDICTMENT

In order for the State to proceed against a felony defendant, the accused person must be formally charged using either a criminal information or an indictment. The prosecutor files an information when a judge has ruled that there is probable cause or when a defendant waives his right to a preliminary hearing. That waiver signals the defendant's acceptance that probable cause exists.

Bills of indictment are charging documents filed by a grand jury, which is a panel of citizens meeting in closed and secret probable cause proceedings. The prosecutor calls witnesses and presents evidence in support of probable cause.

A defendant is not entitled to be present but may choose to testify. If he does so, it is without the presence of his attorney. The attorney may be outside of the grand jury hearing room and may be consulted periodically by the defendant but cannot be inside with the grand jury. It is very unusual for a defendant to testify because of inherent dangers of which defense attorneys are aware. For example, Captain Jeffrey MacDonald, whose conviction for the 1970s murder of his wife and children was the subject of the book *Fatal Vision,* opted to testify before the grand jury. Later he was unable to overcome some serious contradictions between that testimony and his testimony at the trial.

The grand jury is empowered with broad investigative powers, including the power to compel witnesses to appear, to have witnesses testify under oath, and to compel witnesses to produce records and documents. Once the prosecutor has finished presenting evidence, the grand jury deliberates in secret and decides by a majority vote whether to indict. When an indictment is handed down, the grand jury issues an arrest warrant in those situations in which the accused has not already been apprehended.

Some authorities contend that the grand jury will "indict yesterday's newspaper" if the prosecutor says so. For this reason, they feel that the grand jury is superfluous.

## ARRAIGNMENT

At a proceeding called an arraignment, an accused is presented before a trial court judge to hear the formal information or indictment read. The defendant is informed of his right to an attorney if one has not already been obtained. The court appoints counsel if the accused is unable to afford counsel. There is no constitutional right to a separate arraignment proceeding. A defendant can be arraigned on the same day as his scheduled trial. Some jurisdictions arraign the accused separately to ensure that the defendant will have counsel on the appointed trial date. Arraignment can also be used to file on the record motions pertinent to the case.

At the arraignment, the defendant may enter a not guilty, guilty, "Alford," nolo contendere, or not guilty by reason of insanity plea at the arraignment. The first two types of pleas are self-explanatory and commonly understood. The third stems from a Supreme Court case, *North Carolina v Alford,* 400 US 25, 91 Sup Ct 160 (1970), which permits a defendant to acknowledge the sufficiency of the government's case to convict without admitting guilt. However, courts treat an Alford plea as a guilty plea.

A nolo contendere plea is not an admission of criminal conduct and not a conviction. The court has the discretion to allow or disallow the use of this plea. Once accepted, the Court treats this plea in the same manner as a guilty plea and can sentence accordingly. As is true with a straight guilty plea, a defendant waives any procedural defects in his case. One other unique feature of a nolo contendere plea is that it cannot be used against a defendant in a subsequent civil proceeding. The most famous nolo contendere plea in Maryland history is that of U.S. Vice President Spiro T. Agnew, who was accused of crimes committed while he was governor of Maryland. Eventually, Agnew was forced to resign as Vice President.

Another variety of guilty plea is "not guilty by reason of insanity" or "not criminally responsible." Use of this plea is an admission by the defendant that he has committed the crime, with the contention that because of a mental illness or defect he was unable to understand the criminality of his conduct and was unable to confine his behavior to the requirements of law. Unless the government agrees with the assessment that the defendant was not criminally responsible, the case proceeds to trial.

When a defendant enters a guilty plea, the judge must make certain that the accused is entering that plea freely, voluntarily, knowingly, and without coercion. The defendant must respond to a series of specific questions to demonstrate that he understands the rights he is waiving and the effect of the plea. Once the Court is satisfied, the government recites a statement of facts indicating the evidence that would have been presented against the defendant at a trial. If the facts are sufficient and sustain the charges, the Court will find the defendant guilty.

If the Court concludes that the defendant does not understand what he is doing or has been unduly influenced or subjected to duress, the judge may reject the plea. A not guilty plea is entered and the case is sent for trial.

## DISCOVERY

The attorneys on both sides learn more about the case through a process called discovery. Criminal discovery permits the exchange of information between the prosecution and the defense. The defense learns the nature of the evidence that the government has collected. Sometimes before and often after arrest, the suspect may have been required to undergo a variety of examinations including blood and saliva, DNA, and hair sample analysis. Results of those tests, physical evidence, hospital records, conclusions of experts, and any evidence tending to show the innocence or lessen the culpability of the defendant are turned over to the defense. The defendant informs the government of any alibi witnesses that will be called. In some states, such as California, discovery must be completely open, meaning that both sides must disclose everything that may be presented at trial. However, in other states discovery may be so restricted as to permit surprises at trial.

In some jurisdictions, defendants can be ordered by the court to submit to HIV testing before trial or after conviction. The results of that testing are given to the victim and the defendant only and cannot be used at trial or sentencing. Consequently, there is no discovery issue related to HIV test results.

## PRETRIAL MOTIONS

Between the arraignment and the trial, the prosecuting attorney and the defense attorney make several court appearances and argue various motions. Such motions include challenges to the validity or sufficiency of the charging document, requests for discovery, and motions to suppress evidence allegedly obtained illegally by the police.

Some criminal cases are resolved during pretrial motions. For instance, if the court grants a defense motion to suppress the use of seized drugs in a drug possession case, the case is ended. Possession, the key element of the charge, cannot be shown because the seizure and subsequent analysis of the drugs cannot be mentioned.

## PLEA NEGOTIATIONS

Plea negotiations can occur at any stage prior to the entry of a verdict. In less complex cases, the negotiations may occur at arraignment. The defendant is likely offered the best deal he will ever get in the case. At the completion of pretrial motions, the attorneys are well aware of the case's strengths and weaknesses. Frequently, discussions about a guilty plea take place. Plea negotiations have even taken place while the jury is deliberating. Neither side is willing to roll the dice and rely on the jury in this circumstance.

Usually both sides compromise during plea negotiations. The defendant agrees to plead guilty if the government will reduce the charges, call lesser counts, and/or recommend a lesser sentence. The prosecutor should discuss the plea with the victim but does not have to abide by his or her wishes. The Court must approve the plea agreement. Judges differ on whether it is appropriate for them to get involved in plea negotiations.

## TRIAL

The defendant possesses a constitutional right to trial by jury if he desires. For those defendants who plead not guilty, the right to a trial by an impartial jury is guaranteed by the Sixth Amendment. When imprisonment for more than 6 months may result, this requirement has been interpreted as an absolute right in some jurisdictions.

The defendant makes the election to be tried by the Court or by a jury. The prosecutor and defense select the jury panel through a process called *voir dire,* a French term meaning "to bring forth the truth." The Court must be satisfied that the jurors can be fair and impartial in their evaluation of the evidence. The Court and/or attorneys question the jurors about their prior knowledge of the case pretrial publicity, personal incidents or attitudes, and anything else that may cause them not to be fair and impartial. For various reasons, potential jurors are dismissed by the Court or challenged by counsel.

After the jury is seated, the jury takes an oath to well and truly try the defendant. That oath represents the attachment of jeopardy in a jury trial. In a court trial, jeopardy attaches when the first witness is sworn.

Opening statements by the counsel outline their theories of the case and establish what the evidence will show. Defense counsel has the option of speaking directly after the prosecutor or can reserve remarks until the start of the defense's case.

The government presents its case in chief first. Typically, though not always, the victim is the first witness and is followed by others who have information to present to the trier of fact. Defense counsel cross-examines each of the government's witnesses following direct examination. Cross-examination is often painstakingly thorough to highlight weaknesses in the witness's testimony.

At the conclusion of the state's case, the defense moves for a judgment of acquittal based on the insufficiency of the state's case. If the motion is granted, the trial ends and the case is dismissed. If the motion is denied, the case proceeds. The defense may present a case if it chooses. The defense may offer evidence to challenge the prosecution's case and to generate reasonable doubt. A defendant's right to remain silent includes his right not to testify and his prerogative not to present any evidence. Knowing that the burden of proof is on the state to prove the defendant's guilt, a daring defense attorney may decide not to present a defense if the prosecution's case is glaringly weak. The defendant is not required to testify in his own behalf and can never be called by the state.

In sexual assault cases, the most common defense is consent. Defendants have been known to deny culpability and knowing or meeting the victim pretrial. However, when DNA results conclude that the defendant had sex with the victim, suddenly the defense becomes consent.

At the conclusion of the defense's case, the prosecution may put on rebuttal evidence, but only if a defense was presented. The rules of evidence require that rebuttal can only refute evidence developed during the defense. The state may not present as rebuttal completely new evidence unrelated to the defense's case.

At the conclusion of the prosecution and defense cases, the defense renews its motion for judgment of acquittal in hopes of gaining a dismissal of some or all charges. Depending on the jurisdiction, either instruction by the judge to the jury or final argument comes next. Procedural rules differ among the states as to the order of closing arguments. In some states, the government argues first and last, whereas other jurisdictions allow only one argument per side.

Jury deliberations by the entire panel excluding alternates are held in private. Unless the defendant agrees to a less than unanimous verdict, all panel members must agree and reach a verdict as to each count of the indictment or information. If the jury is unable to return a verdict, then the court will declare a hung jury. That panel is dismissed and the government has the option of trying the case again.

If the jury finds the defendant not guilty, the decision is final and the verdict may not be appealed. The not guilty verdict does not necessarily indicate that the defendant was innocent. It merely signifies that the state did not prove its case beyond a reasonable doubt. The defendant is released and may not be retried on the same charge in state court because of the protection against double jeopardy.

The defendant may be tried anew in federal court if his acts violated federal law regardless of how the state case ended. This is not deemed violation of the double jeopardy provision. For example, state and federal courts have concurrent jurisdiction in bank robbery cases. The state court may try a defendant of robbery under state law. Since banks fall under federal protection, the same defendant can face federal robbery charges as well. As a practical matter, however, this is not done often.

If the verdict is guilty, usually the defense submits a motion for new trial, alleging some procedural error or that the verdict was against the weight of evidence. Such motions are not often successful. When they are successful, a new trial date is set. The motion is sometimes set on the same day as sentencing. If the motion is denied, the judge then imposes sentence.

## SENTENCING

Judges possess the ultimate responsibility of imposing sentences. In the case of felonies, the judge orders a pre-sentence report prepared by the probation department. The report summarizes the criminal's personal and social background, criminal history, adjustment to probation and institutionalization, employment, health, and mental stability. The report often includes a victim impact statement. The purpose of the pre-sentence report is to assist the judge in pronouncing an appropriate sentence by presenting aggravating and mitigating circumstances while incorporating the public policy goals of retribution and rehabilitation. The judge has some restrictions imposed by the criminal code, such as minimums and maximums. Nevertheless, the court retains a significant degree of flexibility in considering sentences. Generally the judge may impose a suspended sentence, a fine, probation only, a split sentence combining jail and probation, or incarceration. A defendant facing a death sentence chooses whether he wants the judge or the jury to decide if the sentence should be death or life.

## POST-CONVICTION PROCEDURES

Defendants can typically ask the sentencing court or an independent panel of judges to reconsider the sentence. In order not to penalize a defendant for exercising his rights, the sentence can be reduced but never increased.

The admissibility of evidence, the instructions given to the jury, prosecutorial misconduct, and other procedural rulings are appropriate issues for appellate review. A defendant convicted in state court may be able to get his case reviewed by all state courts of appeal. He may only get into federal court if he has exhausted the state appellate process and if constitutional issues are involved.

Another mechanism for reversing a conviction is habeas corpus. The term means, "you have the body." The habeas corpus writ orders the person who has custody of the prisoner, usually the warden, to bring the detainee before the Court. The prisoner may utilize this writ to gain freedom from unlawful detention or imprisonment. Federal habeas corpus is used to challenge state court convictions. If the defendant asserts that his federal constitutional rights were violated in state court, the conviction may be attacked through the federal habeas corpus process. A state defendant must exhaust state remedies within 5 years of sentencing to be eligible for federal habeas corpus relief.

Some states have a process called post-conviction relief for certain defendants. Post-conviction relief is a collateral attack on the verdict and provides relief on limited grounds, such as incompetence of trial and appellate counsel. Should post-conviction relief be granted, the defendant may get permission to file a belated appeal, a belated reconsideration of sentence, or even receive a new trial.

## INCARCERATION

The prisons exist to insulate society from the threat posed by criminals. Because efforts to rehabilitate criminals have been a dismal failure, the focus of incarceration has shifted to longer sentences and the building of more prisons. States are passing more laws to keep violent criminals incarcerated for longer periods. Many states have "three-time loser statutes" or mandatory sentences for career criminals. Washington State has a law that allows law enforcement authorities to imprison an individual for his status. For instance, a prisoner released from confinement on a child abuse sentence can be returned to prison for being a child molester. The person does not have to commit a new offense for this to occur.

## PAROLE

Depending on the state's sentencing system, prisoners are given either a mandatory release after serving their time or a discretionary release based on the decision of the parole board. In most states, the parolee is required to remain under supervision until his sentence has expired. States vary in their laws concerning when a prisoner is eligible for parole and to what crimes parole may apply. For example, Maryland law provides for prisoners to receive 5 days per month off their sentence for good behavior and permits a court to sentence certain criminals to a term without the possibility of parole. Maryland prisoners convicted of violent crimes must serve half of their sentence before they are eligible for parole. By sharp contrast, Texas prisoners given life sentences may be released after only 5 years behind bars.

## SUGGESTED READINGS

Allison JA, Wrightsman LS. *Rape: the misunderstood crime.* Thousand Oaks, CA: Sage Publications, 1993.

Bailey FL, Rothblatt HB. Investigation and preparation of criminal cases. Rochester, NY: The Lawyers Co-operative Publishing Co., 1970.

Cole GC. *The American system of criminal justice,* 5th ed. Pacific Grove: Brooks/Cole Publishing Company, 1989.

Hall DE. *Criminal law and procedure,* 2nd ed. Albany: Delmar Publishers, 1996.

Hall R. *Rape in America: a reference handbook.* Santa Barbara, CA: CLIO, 1995.

Hrones S, Czar C. *Criminal practice handbook,* 2nd ed. New York: Mathew Bender, 1999.

Hohenhaus S. Patterned injury and court testimony in a sexual assault. *J Emerg Nurs* 1998;24:614.

Hohenhaus S. SANE legislation and lessons learned. *J Emerg Nurs* 1998;24:463–464.

Lasater M. Sexual assault: the legal framework. In: Warner CG, ed. *Rape and sexual assault management and intervention.* Germantown, PA: Aspen Publishers, 1980: 231–263.

Lowey AH, LaFrance AB. *Criminal procedure arrest and investigation.* Cincinnati: Anderson Publishing, 1996.

McGregor MJ, Le G, Marion SA, et al. Examination for sexual assault: is the documentation of physician injury associated with the laying of charges? A retrospective cohort study. *Can Med Assoc J* 1999;160(11): 1565–1569.

MD DPSCS PCT MCCPI Sexual Assault (Maryland Community Crime Prevention Institute) (http://ns1.dpsc.state.md.us/pct/ccpi/sex.htm) (10/11/99).

National Institute of Law Enforcement and Criminal Justice: Law Enforcement Assistance Administration. Forcible rape police, vol. 3. Washington: US Government Printing Office, 1978.

National Institute of Law Enforcement and Criminal Justice: Law Enforcement Assistance Administration. Forcible rape police, vol. 4. Washington: US Government Printing Office, 1978.

National Institute of Law Enforcement and Criminal Justice: Law Enforcement Assistance Administration.

Forcible rape: an analysis of legal issues. Washington: US Government Printing Office, 1978.

Paquin GW. Legal aspects of acquaintance rape. In: Wiene VR, Richards AL, eds. *Intimate betrayal. An understanding and responding to the trauma of acquaintance rape.* Thousand Oaks, CA: Sage Publications, 1995:88– 107.

Pentilla A, Karhumen PJ. Medicolegal findings among rape victims. *Med Law* 1990:9:725–737.

Reed M. The judicial system and laws. In: *Sexual assault forensic examiner training manual.* University of Maryland Department of Surgery, Division of Emergency Medicine, 1998; Sec. 7:1–59.

Review of state sexual assault laws, 1998 Legislative Codes. (http://www.ilj.org/sa/review_of_state_sexual_asault_1.htm) (10/10/99)

Selkin J. *The child sexual abuse case in the courtroom*, 2nd ed. Denver: James Selkin, 1991.

Sexual assault in America (AMA), Nov 6, 1995. (http://www.ama-assn.org/public/releases/assault/action.htm.) (10/11/99).

Soules MR, Stewar SK, Brown KM, et al. The spectrum of alleged rape. *J Reprod Med* 1978;20(1):33–39.

Stuckey GB, Roberson CR, Wallace H. *Procedures in the justice system*, 5th ed. Upper Saddle River, NJ: Prentice-Hall, 1997.

Temkin J, ed. *Rape and the criminal justice system.* Brookfield: Dartmouth Publishing Company, 1995.

West Virginia Sexual Assault Legal Guide.(htp:www.lectlaw.com/files/sex11.htm.) (10/10/99).

# 11

# Testifying

DePriest W. Whye, Jr., and Sharon May

## ROLE OF THE SEXUAL ASSAULT HEALTH-CARE EXAMINER

The sexual assault health-care examiner, be it a physician, nurse, physician's assistant, or sexual assault nurse examiner (SANE), is frequently the first health-care practitioner to have contact with the sexual assault victim in the aftermath of the attack. In addition to attending to the emotional needs of someone who is understandably distressed and distraught over a vicious, dehumanizing, and demoralizing event, the health-care practitioner is responsible for assessing the extent of injury and providing the necessary treatment and support for the acute injuries and anticipated health hazards. Although the first priority is directed to identify physical and psychological injury and render medically indicated therapy, the practitioner's responsibilities necessarily extend to the collection of evidence and the accurate recording of the victim's history, physical findings, and the results of laboratory and radiographic studies. The ability to prosecute the assailant hinges on the accuracy and precision of assembling the historical data, physical findings, and crucial forensic evidence. Deficient or defective intervention by the practitioner at the preliminary stage of this investigative process can lead to the inability to charge an alleged attacker criminally or the failure to convict a defendant. Similarly, the effective collection of pertinent forensic evidence can potentially exculpate an innocent suspect.

Consequently, the indispensable role of the practitioner in a sexual assault encompasses two distinct duties. First is the irrevocable legal duty to render reasonable medical care. Second, a professional duty exists to gather evidence that will assist the authorities in determining whether a crime has been committed and in establishing the identity of the perpetrator. Ultimately, the practitioner must be prepared to report the sexual assault examination findings in a professional and unbiased manner to an official fact-finding tribunal. Understanding that the practitioner bears an enormous responsibility to the victim and to society at large, the practitioner must be intensely vigilant and attentive to detail in handling sexual assault cases to ensure that competent and reliable decisions can be achieved regarding the criminal disposition of cases.

Effective involvement of the health-care practitioner in sexual assault cases requires a fundamental understanding of the process and procedure of criminal prosecution. The prosecution of a defendant is the process whereby a legal representative of the state—the prosecutor—investigates and then attempts to prove in a criminal court that the defendant committed an act in violation of criminal law. For example, a typical penal code defines first-degree rape as follows. A person is guilty of rape in the first degree if (a) the person engages in vaginal intercourse with the victim, (b) by force or threat of force against the will and without the consent of the victim, and (c) employs a deadly or dangerous weapon, or (d) inflicts suffocation or strangulation, or (e) is aided and abetted by others, or (f) commits the act during the course of a burglary. To convict the defendant, the prosecution must amass evidence that proves beyond a reasonable doubt that the defendant committed the crime.

Traditionally, the crux of rape conviction centers on constructing a case in which the evidence exhibits overwhelmingly that the victim did not consent. Without supportive evidence of physical force from which to infer lack of consent or forensic evidence to assist in the identification of the attacker, the prosecution's task becomes much more challenging. In the absence of such probative evidence, the prosecution must rely on the testimony and credibility of the victim, the attendant circumstances of the crime, and the perception of the defendant's lack of credibility in order to build a case. Thus, evidence collection and analysis are pivotal to the prosecution of a sexual assault case.

The defense attorney is duty bound to counter or neutralize the prosecution's case effectively by attacking weaknesses particularly through cross-examination of the state's witnesses or by offering contradictory evidence during the presentation of the defense. One of the defense's objectives is to demonstrate that the prosecution has failed to present evidence of each element of the crime. The defense relies on several strategies to achieve this end. The defense attorney may argue that his or her client could not have committed the crime based on an alibi, which places the defendant at another location at the time the crime was perpetrated. Alternatively, the defendant may assert that the victim consented. An example of a defense strategy published in a recent report involved the introduction of photographs that showed the defendant's penis with a ring at the base of the glans. The defense claimed that the traumatic genital injuries recorded and reported by the SANE were the result of consensual intercourse with the penis ring in place. Accurate records, photographs, and grueling hours of SANE testimony enabled the jury to convict the defendant of the crime based on the fact that the orientation of the ring was inconsistent with the location of the vaginal laceration.

## THE SEXUAL ASSAULT EXAMINER AS EXPERT WITNESS

The evidence presented at trial may be complex, technical, and beyond the comprehension of the average juror. Therefore, professionals who possess the requisite level of expertise and good communication skills are indispensable in the legal process. The presence of the expert witness helps the jury understand and connect the evidence in order to make a measured inference that the defendant committed the crime. An expert witness, in contrast to a lay witness, is permitted to express an opinion on relevant issues pertaining to the facts and falling within his or her professional expertise.

The lay witness, on the other hand, may testify only to what he or she saw, heard, felt, or smelled. The lay witness must have direct knowledge of the event rather than secondary knowledge. A second distinguishing feature of the lay witness is that he or she is not qualified to express an opinion or speculate about the meaning of testimony. The exception here is that the lay witness can testify to ordinary observations, such as stating that "the car was going fast." The expert witness is needed to say how fast the car was going or whether the speed is reasonable and prudent for that particular location.

Having an array of expert witnesses is possible in a sexual assault case depending on the nature and complexity of the case. The sexual assault examiner or health-care practitioner is routinely requested to testify as to the medical findings. Many jurisdictions have certified SANEs as experts for judicial purposes. In a recent nationally publicized sexual assault investigation in New York City, evidence was submitted to the grand jury to determine whether the accused perpetrators would be indicted for the crime. The evidence encompassed the testimony of the doctors who examined the victim, the testimony of FBI experts who analyzed the forensic evidence gathered from the rape kit, and other physical evidence gathered during the investigation. The grand jury received testimony from two forensic pathologists who reviewed the FBI reports and the medical reports concerning the victim's condition. Forensic psychiatrists formulated opinions and testified to the likelihood that a sexual assault was committed based on a review of the medical records. Using the evidence supplied during that proceeding, the grand jury declined to indict the alleged attackers.

Routinely, the examining health-care practitioner asks the sexual assault victim questions about the attack to determine how to treat the patient. Although the examining practitioner's testimony as to what the victim related during the examination is technically hearsay and therefore inadmissible, the examiner may be permitted to testify concerning historical information under an exception to the hearsay rule. A treating practitioner may testify as to what the victim/patient said so long as it is relevant to the treatment of the medical and psychological condition. If the victim reported to the physician or nurse that she was bitten several times on her back and that her arm was twisted, the physician or nurse may testify to this statement. Generally, the physician is not permitted to testify to statements of identity or culpability. If the victim told the physician, "John, my friend's brother, forced me to the ground and assaulted me," the portion of the statement that identifies the assailant would possibly be inadmissible. As a practical matter, identification can be elicited through the victim's direct testimony at trial. The examining practitioner may testify as to the mental state of the victim upon arrival at the health-care facility. The victim's demeanor may be important in categorizing the response as consistent with a traumatic event. Obviously, this assessment is prone to subjectivity and therefore may not be a reliable determinant.

Based on the testimony of the examining practitioner, the jury may decide based on the statements of the victim concerning physical force or injury and the corroborating evidence on the physical exam and laboratory results that the sexual encounter was not consensual. Clearly, any complaints of pain and any corroborative evidence of injury, such as abrasion, bruises, bite marks, lacerations, bleeding, sprains, strains, broken bones, closed head injuries, penetrating trauma, or injury to the genitalia, perineum, or rectum, bolster the probability of a violent act that was nonconsensual.

In the absence of persuasive physical evidence, the practitioner's impression of the victim's demeanor, state of mind, affect, or emotional status remains integral evidence of a potential assault. The victim may be tearful, excited, angry, withdrawn, anxious, or distraught. All of these emotions are stereotypical reactions that a layperson may expect when the victim has been exposed to a traumatic event. By contrast, the victim who is smiling, calm, engaging, conversational, or indifferent does not fit the conventional impression of how a victim should respond after a sexual assault. An attempt to categorize or label the response as consistent or inconsistent with a sexual assault is fraught with danger. Because the victim did not respond in the subjectively conventional mode does not negate the probability that a crime occurred. The examiner should be familiar with the spectrum of recognized posttraumatic responses accompanying a sexual assault and should not permit the biases or incorrect assumptions regarding the patient's emotional presentation to influence the interpretation of the evidence. The examiner is qualified to opine whether the injuries and presentation observed were consistent with exposure to physical force or sexual assault. The examiner should be prepared to answer this question confidently.

## CONSTRUCTING THE MEDICAL REPORT

The medical record should contain a variety of information. A sexual assault victim may be transported to the emergency department or some other health care facility by ambulance; in the automobile of a friend, family member, or stranger; or the victim may ambulate to the nearest facility. The method of transport should be recorded in the medical record. After a preliminary assessment in the trauma assessment mode, a comprehensive history is obtained. This history should include:

- A description of the incident
- Location where the assault took place
- Identity of the assailant, if known
- Home and workplace of the assailant, if known
- Method by which the assailant left the scene
- Whether a weapon was used to coerce the victim
- Whether drugs or alcohol were utilized before or during the attack
- Whether the patient has changed clothes, showered, voided, or douched since the incident

- Complaints of pain or injury
- Date of the victim's last consensual intercourse
- Date of the victim's last menstrual period
- Any birth control measures used

The physical examination includes a survey of the entire body for evidence of physical injury. Gynecologic and genital examinations in a female are mandatory unless the victim refuses. An anal exam must be included to document evidence of penetration injuries. The increasing use of a colposcope with a camera attachment to assist in gathering forensic evidence is having enormous implications in providing relevant evidence in a prosecution. A Wood's lamp may be used to identify semen stains on the victim. A swab of the external genitalia, the cervix, and the anal canal may reveal motile sperm.

A clinician or SANE will be asked to report in painstaking detail any findings that corroborate or dispute that the sexual assault took place. In this role, the examiner is providing firsthand impressions as an expert witness. The examiner records the victim's complaints and photographs physical findings. The victim's history, physical exam, studies, and lab results are introduced via oral testimony and through the medical records.

Recognizing the intensity with which the medical report will be scrutinized, the examiner must address the evaluation and management of a sexual assault victim with an unrelenting compulsion. A complete examination and management are indicated. Meticulous medical record documentation constitutes the foundation of the medical evidence presented at trial. All records and materials are transmitted to the prosecuting attorneys and turned over to the defense. Medical records, including ones recorded by other physicians in addition to those performing the initial rape examination, may be introduced into evidence. Any notes that were written by the examining physician will be included as part of the medical record. Thus, the medical record must be neat, understandable, accurate, and consistent. The record will be utilized to refresh the practitioner's memory and will be combed extensively by the defense to uncover shortcomings in the evaluation.

## CHAIN OF CUSTODY

The forensic evidence that is collected by the examiner may provide the most powerful evidence in identifying the suspect or perpetrator of the crime. Each item must be meticulously collected and maintained. Samples, which can deteriorate, need to be preserved properly. Handling of the evidence must be accurately documented in order to establish and safeguard the integrity and competence of the evidence. The examiner must demonstrate that the gathering, preservation, sealing, and storage of collected evidence were done in such a manner as to prevent tampering. Documentation should include the name of the law enforcement official who received the rape kit and any other collected evidence along with the date and time.

## SUBPOENA

A subpoena strikes fear in the hearts and minds of men, women, and physicians who recognize that as a result of this written instrument they have temporarily lost free will. For those who are unfamiliar with the power of a subpoena, it represents nothing more than a traffic citation. A frequent response to the subpoena is to ignore it. Both of these approaches should be erased from a witness' mindset.

A subpoena is a written legal document issued by a court at the request of a party to a civil or criminal legal proceeding. It directs a named witness to appear at a designated place for a designated reason. A subpoena is issued under court authority and directs the witness to obey and respond to the order. If the witness fails to comply with the subpoena, he or she may be arrested. Furthermore, subpoenaed witnesses who have moved out of state are not relieved of their responsibility to appear. There are procedural mechanisms in every state that allow the court where the witness resides to demand that the witness show cause why he or she should not appear in the requesting state. A properly executed and properly served subpoena cannot be ignored.

Service of a subpoena issued by a court of competent jurisdiction must be made upon the person named or to an agent authorized by appointment or by law to receive service for the named person. The subpoena may be served by a sheriff or by a person who is not a party and who is at least 18 years old. Some states may have specific rules that allow service by mail.

The top of the subpoena identifies the case. A criminal case is captioned as State v. John Doe. A civil case is captioned Smith v. Brown. The names may mean very little to the named witness. SANE personnel most likely will only have had contact with the victim, whose name is not usually on the subpoena in a criminal case. The subpoena should give the date and time that the witness is commanded to appear. The place, including a room number, should be printed on the subpoena. In addition, the document should indicate whether the state, plaintiff, or defense is calling the witness to testify. The expert witness should contact that party to verify specifically which case is going to trial and what is expected.

A subpoena for records requires the production of certain documents, such as medical records. The person to whom this type of subpoena is directed may not necessarily be required to appear, but may need only to produce the documents on a designated date at a particular place. A subpoena duces tecum requires the summoned witness to appear on the given date and bring certain specified documents or objects. Again, any witness who receives a subpoena of any variety should contact the summoning party for further information and instruction.

## ORIENTATION OF THE COURTROOM

One bit of information that the subpoenaed witness can get by contacting the summoning party is an orientation of the courtroom. The design of the courtroom varies from venue to venue. However, a prototypical form tends to prevail. The judge's bench is situated in front of the courtroom and is elevated, giving the judge a view of the entire space. The witness box is generally to the left or right of the judge's bench, but it may be on a lower level. The prosecution and defense tables are situated across from, but

facing, the judge's bench and witness box. The jury box is located perpendicular to the judge's bench or in the front and to one side of the courtroom. The party with the burden of proof sits at the table nearest the jury box. In a criminal case, the prosecution sits closest to the jury. In a civil case, the plaintiff sits closest.

Additional courtroom personnel sit just forward of the judge's bench. These individuals include the courtroom docket clerk, who notates procedural steps on the court file and keeps track of tangible evidence. The stenographer often sits close to the witness box in order to record the testimony verbatim. Typically, a sheriff or other law enforcement official sits between the judge and the attorney's tables poised to dissuade outbursts from the displeased and to take custody of prisoners.

In front of the witness box, there sometimes is a podium, which the attorneys may be required by the court to use when examining witnesses and addressing the jury. When the attorneys are confined to the podium, they usually have their trial notes before them as a guide.

The courtroom atmosphere is typically stern and sterile. An expectation exists that all the participants comply with courtroom decorum and demonstrate the utmost respect for the process. The practitioner expert witness, although respected for her expertise, receives no preferential treatment in the process of seeking the truth. The judge, prosecution, or defense may vigorously challenge the expert.

## QUALIFYING AS AN EXPERT

The advent of the SANE as a specialist has advanced the capacity to collect and preserve evidence to assist with the prosecution of assailants and, in some instances, the exoneration of the falsely accused or the erroneously implicated. The SANE has been trained to collect forensic evidence following the correct chain of custody procedure while facilitating the psychological, physical, and medical needs of the victim. The quality of evidence collection is tremendously high because the SANE is focused and performs sexual assault examinations regularly. Because of the skill and expertise of the nurse, SANEs have been qualified as expert witnesses in the majority of jurisdictions in which they serve.

Again using the process called *voir dire,* the attorneys ask a series of questions to demonstrate and test the witness's expertise. If the witness is being called by the state, the prosecutor will ask the witness about employment, duties, education, training, professional experience, and the number of works published, if any. In addition, the SANE will be asked how many sexual assault exams she has done either independently or with the aid of another practitioner. Finally, the prosecutor will elicit whether the witness has ever qualified as an expert in sexual assault forensic examination previously, how many times, and in what courts.

Defense counsel may, if he or she so chooses, apply voir dire to the witness. Very specific questions about sexual assault, studies in the field, definitions of certain terms, and the use of certain techniques or medications may be asked in the hope that the witness will get stumped on something. Once the questioning by both sides is concluded, the prosecutor then offers the witness as an expert in the field of sexual assault forensic examination. Opposing counsel may object. Depending on the answers given by the witness, the court may or may not declare that the witness is an expert.

The decision to request qualification should not be made when the witness is on the stand. A denial of the state's motion to qualify may undermine the case and will most certainly diminish the witness and the prosecution in the eyes of the jury. Well before the trial date, the witness and the party calling that witness need to discuss whether the witness will actually be treated as an expert (i.e., be allowed to render a scientific or medical opinion). At the outset, the attorney should be given a copy of the witness's resume. This alerts the attorney to the appropriate areas that ought to be covered during voir dire. The attorney should be made aware of how many times the witness has in fact qualified as an expert and where. If the pending case is the first time, the attorney will assess whether it is even appropriate to attempt qualification. The decision to offer a witness as an expert is based on experience in the discipline, the information

being solicited, and whether any other person can testify to the same information. Every expert has a first time to be so qualified in court.

## TESTIFYING ON DIRECT

As a consequence of the specialization of the sexual assault crisis process, increasingly the testifying experts are seasoned veterans when it comes to courtroom testimony. Nonetheless, rape crisis programs and sexual assault examiners are not ubiquitous. Therefore, the uninitiated physician or nurse practitioner must be prepared to testify. The experience of testifying can be a terrifying encounter. Obviously, with time, practice, and experience, the encounter can be less intimidating. Like any other experience in which the individual has to perform before an audience, preparation is the best antidote for anxiety surrounding an anticipated courtroom appearance.

Because the stakes are high, the practitioner should expect to undergo an interrogation about the medical findings by both the prosecution and defense. Both will want to meet with the clinician before trial to review the evidence and the testimony. This is an important exercise for the witness and the attorney. The practitioner should take the initiative by contacting the attorney who has summoned her. Usually this is the prosecutor. The practitioner, especially one who has limited or no experience as a witness, never wants to appear in court unprepared.

For the witness to achieve success, first and foremost, he or she must have a command of the facts. The examiner should have a thorough knowledge of the circumstances of the assault, the history including physical complaints, and the physical findings, particularly from the genitalia examination. Laboratory results and radiographic studies should be memorized. The expert witness must be thoroughly familiar with her testimony, which means significant time has to be spent before trial reviewing the medical record and anticipating questions. The expert should study and prepare for the presentation as if preparing for an exam or a formal lecture. The expert witness will greatly impress the jury with a smooth presentation. The witness should sound as though the label "expert" is an accurate one.

Once mastery has been achieved regarding the facts of the case, the witness must be able to communicate the salient information to the jury in a credible and unbiased manner. The expert witness is reminded that her role is not to take sides but to convey her findings to the jury objectively and allow the jury to make a decision based on the credibility of the evidence delivered. The expert witness may be asked whether the evidence suggests that a physical assault took place. The witness should answer this question within the limits of his or her medical judgment.

It is critically important that the witness tell the truth and not feel obligated to help one side or the other. This means that certain social biases and prejudgments must be divorced from the oral testimony. The oral communications should reflect a clinical approach devoid of emotion or embellishment. Direct questions should be answered systematically and methodically. The expert must speak loudly and clearly so that all the jurors can hear without straining. The expert should explain answers in simple, easy-to-understand language. The sexual assault practitioner should avoid using slang or profanity. A trial is not the time to entertain the jury with a few well-placed jokes or punch lines. The witness should use a natural voice with an even and smooth delivery and not attempt to dramatize or reach a theatrical, Perry Mason-like climax. It is important to make eye contact with the examining attorney and with the judge as appropriate. The expert witness should appear confident and competent, professional, and courteous to all counsel. The witness must not argue or pontificate with the attorneys.

The expert witness will be asked a series of questions, which will develop a pattern of facts that the prosecution is asserting. The witness must listen to the questions intently and answer as concisely and precisely as possible. The witness should remember his or her answers because on cross-examination those answers will be revisited and likely challenged. A frequent ploy is for the defense attorney to misstate an answer in an effort to confuse the witness and the jury. Consequently, the witness should listen closely to the question. The witness should be prepared to reassert a prior response in a self-assured yet nonbelligerent manner. A witness who has misspoken should not be afraid to say so and correct the error.

The witness's courtroom decorum is equally important because the jury frequently determines credibility of the witness by simple observations such as dress, mannerisms, voice quality, and delivery. As a consequence, the witness must engage in conduct, which will enhance credibility rather than diminish it. A suit is appropriate dress for a male witness and a suit or conservative proper length dress is suitable for a female witness. Conservative colors, such as blue, gray, black, or brown, are appropriate.

The following pointers may be helpful. The witness should sit upright and face the person asking the questions. Because the testimony is recorded, the witness should avoid covering his or her mouth. All answers must be verbal. Nods cannot be recorded by a stenographer and may not be discernible on a video. In addition, the witness should not eat or chew gum while on the stand. Nervousness is natural, but the witness should make every effort to appear calm. A few deep breaths should help to limit a halting speech pattern. Usually, as the testimony progresses, the witness will begin to relax. The witness should control his or her temper no matter how irritating counsel becomes. The screaming surgeon in the operating room routine is ineffective and inappropriate.

Occasionally, counsel may ask the expert witness to leave the witness box and either approach the jury or move closer to audiovisual equipment. The witness will do this when demonstrating how something occurred or while using an item of demonstrative evidence to explain a particular point. For instance, the witness may use an enlarged diagram of the female genitalia to show exactly where the victim's injuries were located. Such demonstrations must necessarily be planned in advance by the expert in consultation with the attorney who calls the expert.

## CROSS-EXAMINATION

Cross-examination frequently is the true measure of a lawyer's trial skill. After one side has presented a witness to recite evidence to bolster its case, the opposing counsel is given an opportunity to clarify or dismantle the testimony. The goal of the defense in a criminal case is to plant doubt in the minds of the jury concerning the witness, the testimony, or the evidence presented. Defense counsel wants to damage the expert witness's credibility. Even though defense counsel may have lost on a motion to prevent qualification of the witness as an expert or may have readily agreed to the qualification, counsel may still ask questions designed to attack or undermine the witness's status as an expert. The defense attorney may attack how the exam was performed or how the evidence was collected. The defense attorney may also challenge the conclusions drawn from the evidence by eliciting admissions that contradict the principal conclusions made by the expert. The defense tries to discredit the expert or lead the expert to provide an opinion helpful to the defendant.

On cross-examination, the witness must be particularly attentive to the questions asked. The attorney may be pleasant, courteous, nonthreatening, and conciliatory at the outset in order to lull the witness into a false sense of security. The next series of questions will go to the heart of the matter. Unlike direct examination, cross-examination is composed almost exclusively of leading questions, which characteristically contain the answer within the question and can usually be answered with a simple yes or no. For example, "Isn't it true that the injuries sustained by the victim could have been caused by vigorous intercourse?" The intent of such a question is for defense to provide a plausible explanation other than force for the victim's injuries.

To reduce the likelihood of falling prey to trick questions, the witness must listen very carefully to each component of a question. If an individual part of the question is incongruous or inaccurate, the witness should point that out immediately. This forces the attorney to revise or retract the question. Furthermore, the witness should take care to answer only what is asked. Waxing eloquent with long, scholarly explanations provides the opposition with fodder to dismantle the expert's findings and opinions.

Opposing counsel may attempt to short-circuit answers that go beyond yes or no. The court may admonish the cross-examiner to allow the witness to complete the answer. If not, the longer explanation may be elicited by the state on redirect.

Hypothetical questions present various combinations of facts and circumstances similar to or distinctive from the facts of the pending case. The expert is asked to draw a conclusion. "Suppose a woman has been using drugs and drinking alcohol before the incident. Isn't it possible that she would not recall accurately and precisely everything that happened?" Before answering, the witness must make certain that the hypothetical is factually consistent and contains enough facts for a reasonable conclusion to be drawn.

The witness should take as much time as necessary before answering and have the question repeated if necessary. A thoughtful answer requires some measuring and deliberation. A response that is too quick may be erroneous or unclear. At the same time, a protracted pause before an answer is given raises suspicion that the expert lacks knowledge or that the answer is fabricated. It is acceptable for the witness to respond truthfully. It is appropriate for the witness to admit that he or she does not know the answer, cannot recall a particular fact, needs to have the question repeated, or does not understand what is being asked. However, overuse of any answer can irritate the jury and diminish the witness's credibility. The witness, unless an objection is sustained, must answer every question.

Finally, boilerplate jury instructions include the advice from the court that the jury may use a witness's manner of testifying to evaluate her credibility. This means that the manner of speaking, words used, demeanor, presence or lack of ease, and even the facial expression of the witness are appropriate factors to determine whether to believe all, some, or none of the testimony. The expert witness should keep this instruction in mind while on the stand.

## SUGGESTED READINGS

Allison JA, Wrightsman LS. *Rape. The misunderstood crime.* Thousand Oaks, CA: Sage Publications, 1993.
Bailey FL, Rothblatt HB. *Investigation and preparation of*

*criminal cases.* Rochester: The Lawyers Co-operative Publishing Company, 1970.

Ceci SJ, Hembrooke H, eds. *Expert witness in child abuse cases.* Washington, DC: American Psychological Association, 1998.

Ernoehazy W, Murphy-Lavoie H. Sexual assault. (http://www.emedicine.com/emerg/topic527.htm.) (10/11/99).

Hall R. *Rape in America. A reference handbook.* Santa Barbara, CA: ABC CLIO, Inc., 1995.

Hohenhaus S. Patterned injury and court testimony in a sexual assault. *J Emerg Nurs* 1998;24:614.

Hohenhaus S. SANE legislation and lessons learned. *J Emerg Nurs* 1998;24:463–464.

Hrones S, Czar C. *Criminal practice handbook*, 2nd ed. New York: Mathew Bender, 1999.

McGregor MJ, Le G, Marion SA, et al. Examination for sexual assault: is the documentation of physician injury associated with the laying of charges? A retrospective cohort study. *Can Med Assoc J* 1999;160:1565–1569.

Paquin GW. Legal aspects of acquaintance rape. In: Wiene VR, Richards AL, eds. *Intimate betrayal. An understanding and responding to the trauma of acquaintance rape.* Thousand Oaks, CA: Sage Publications, 1995.

Pentilla A, Karhumen PJ. Medicolegal findings among rape victims. *Med Law* 1990:9:725–737.

Poynter D. *The expert witness handbook. Tips and techniques for the litigation consultant.* Santa Barbara, CA: Para Publishing, 1997.

Reed M. The judicial system and laws. In: Jackson C, ed. *Sexual assault forensic examiner training manual.* University of Maryland, Department of Surgery, Division of Emergency Medicine, 1998; Sec. 7, 1–59.

Report of the grand jury concerning the Tawana Brawley investigation: a courtroom TV document. (http:208.229.230.57/legaldocs/newsmakers/tawana/part4.html) (10/11/99).

Selkin J. *The child sexual abuse case in the courtroom*, 2nd ed. Denver: James Selkin, 1991.

Taslitz AE. *Rape and the culture of the courtroom.* New York: New York University Press, 1999.

Temkin J, ed. *Rape and the criminal justice system.* Brookfield: Dartmouth Publishing Company, 1995.

Warner CG, ed. *Rape and sexual assault: management and intervention.* Germantown, PA: Aspen Publishers, 1980.

West Virginia sexual assault legal guide (htp:www.lectlaw.com/files/sex11.htm.) (10/10/99).

# 12

# Law Enforcement

Richard C. Fahlteich, Sr.

The roles of a law enforcement officer and other law enforcement personnel vary from jurisdiction to jurisdiction. Therefore, police officers, investigators/detectives, criminologists, and technicians *must* follow the policies and procedures of their respective agencies.

In this chapter, we will discuss the following:

- The primary officer (duties and responsibilities)
- The victim
- The crime scene
- The investigation
- The suspect
- The prosecution

In most cases, a uniformed police officer is the first person in the criminal justice process encountered by a victim of sexual assault. The officer is also the first person whom the victim tells what happened. It is therefore of great importance that the officer listen to not only what the victim says but also the way in which he or she describes the incident.

Victims of crime, especially those who have been physically and/or sexually assaulted, are frequently apprehensive when making their first statement about what occurred. Officers must be patient and understanding; at the same time, they must make the victim confident that they are going to help her through the process. The officer must also explain, briefly, what is going to occur (i.e., the physical examination, interviews by the officer or an investigator, questions by both administrative and medical staff at the hospital). The victim must be told that she might have to tell "her story" several times to several people, but that it is a very important part of the entire

fact-finding process in a criminal matter. Police personnel must remain professional and attentive throughout the entire investigational process. The officer must be compassionate and not insensitive. An authoritative yet calm manner must be maintained with the victim.

Some victims are more comfortable and communicate more freely with a female police officer. In this situation, if the first responding officer is male, a female officer can be brought into the process as long as agency guidelines are respected and the integrity of the investigation is maintained. In some police departments, the entire investigation must be conducted by the first responding uniformed officer. In other departments, the case may be taken over, almost immediately, by a detective/investigator. In yet other departments, both uniformed officers and detectives will have particular roles in the overall investigation. Regardless of the procedure a department follows, the purpose is the same:

1. To establish that a crime was committed
2. To identify the suspect(s)
3. To successfully prosecute the person(s) charged with the crime

## MEDICAL NEEDS OF THE VICTIM

The first police officer arriving at the scene of a reported sexual assault must ascertain the victim's condition. If the victim is injured, the priority is to have her taken immediately to the nearest hospital. This need may create a dilemma if the nearest hospital does not have the capabilities to perform the detailed sexual assault/rape examinations that are needed to support the criminal aspects of the case. However, the primary concern must be the well-being of the victim, even if some evidence may be lost in the process of treating the victim. Certainly, under *no* circumstances should officers or investigators overlook the victim's treatment needs for the purpose of "the case."

If the victim is transported to a hospital in an ambulance, an officer may want to accompany her to the medical facility. This may become important months later if a criminal case goes to trial because there could be a "chain of custody" issue in the defense argument. This matter will be covered in greater detail later in this chapter.

After assessing the medical needs of the victim, with the appropriate action taken, the officer's next area of concern should be the suspect. The officer should obtain as much information as possible from the victim, as quickly as possible, and relay that to other law enforcement personnel who can begin looking for the suspect. However, the primary officer/investigator *should not* conduct a detailed interview of the victim. The detailed interview should be conducted on the following day or a couple of days after the incident. This gives the victim some time to calm down and to think about the incident in greater detail than was possible shortly after it occurred. The reactions of rape victims vary; the emotional and psychological reactions are as different as the victims.

Many sexually assaulted victims know or are acquainted with the suspect. In these cases, the officer/investigator has more time to gather and disseminate a description of the suspect than in cases in which only an unknown suspect is being sought.

## LOCATING AND PRESERVING THE CRIME SCENE

The responding officers must ascertain from the victim where the assault took place. Once this is determined, the primary officer must ensure that the crime scene is preserved. Unlike eyewitness evidence, physical evidence located in a crime scene can never be intrinsically wrong. The evidence located and then properly collected at a crime scene can make the difference between a guilty or not guilty verdict.

In a rape or other sexual assault investigation, it must be remembered that the victim is also "evidence of the crime." Evidence must be collected from the victim with the same care, caution, and proper methodology as that collected at the crime location. Medical personnel must be accurate in recovering the physical evidence from the victim and in marking and documenting the containers, envelopes, and other packaging used for the evidence. When the police officer or investigator is given the evidence by the medical personnel, he or she must ensure that all evidence is marked correctly and initialed by the person who collected the items. Rape evidence kits are now used in most emergency departments where sexual assault victims are examined.

The location of the crime must be protected and preserved so that the evidence is not lost, moved, altered, contaminated, or destroyed. The officer responsible for protecting the scene must make certain that *only* those persons necessary to the investigation enter the scene. A log must be maintained with the name and assignment of each person who enters the scene.

Officers must have a working knowledge of the processing of a crime scene: from the initial photographing or videotaping by the mobile crime lab technician, to sketching of the scene, to collection of all items known to be or thought to be evidence in the crime. The procedures for evidence collection are beyond the scope of this chapter.

## REPORTING

### Field Notes

The primary officer, as well as other officers on the scene, must maintain legible, accurate field notes. These notes should answer the six basic questions that must be answered in every type of case. The questions are as follows:

- WHO (victim, suspect, witnesses)
- WHAT (nature of crime)
- WHERE (location of the scene)
- WHEN (date, time; occurred, reported)

- HOW (way in which the crime was committed)
- WHY (reasons for the offense)

Within each of these primary questions are numerous related questions. The officer should attempt to answer as many of these as possible in the field notes. These notes are the primary source for the officer to write the necessary detailed offense report of the incident. They are also useful at other stages of the investigation and prosecution of the suspect.

### Formal Reports

Officers must prepare detailed, thorough, accurate reports documenting the offense that was committed. These reports become the basis for everything that happens in the case, from the initial reporting through the investigation. Incomplete or incorrect reports can be the reason for a suspect not being identified or for the case being lost in court. The reporting officer must never rush through the reporting aspects of his or her duty. As a general rule, short sentences and short paragraphs make the report much easier to understand and less likely to be misinterpreted by the reader. Officers should also keep in mind, particularly in rape/sexual assault cases, that the fewer formal medical terms they use, the better. The medical terminology will be used by doctors and nurses in their reports. The reporting officer should state the doctor's determination, such as "the victim had injuries to her vaginal and rectal area, indicative of rape." The formal medical report will give all other necessary details.

### Additional Reports

The primary officer or the investigating detective is responsible for coordinating and collecting reports from the other units involved in the case. These include the mobile crime lab reports, the trace analysis lab reports, DNA reports, and hospital reports. All documents should be collected and placed in the case folders, which is used as the primary repository for the incident. The case folder should also contain printed copies of any photographs taken in the case. In some jurisdictions, copies of all laboratory reports, photographs, drawings, and sketches are sent directly to the prosecutor's or state attorney's office at the same time they are sent to the case investigator. It is the responsibility of the investigator to make certain that all parties have the same documents.

### INVESTIGATION

Most detectives and investigators have been police officers for several years and therefore have developed the necessary level of experience and ability to conduct detailed investigations. There are essential qualities that an investigator must have. The investigator must be patient: good investigations often take time to develop and bring to a successful outcome. A good investigator must also be thorough: in many investigations even the smallest detail can make the difference as to whether the case is solved or remains open. Some would argue that luck plays a large part in the success of a detective or investigator. At times there is an element of luck, but more often cases are solved by inductive reasoning and the open-minded approach an investigator brings to the case. Detectives and investigators must be confident and well disciplined. They must also refrain from being opinionated. Tunnel vision can end an investigation before it starts.

A rape/sexual assault investigator must be compassionate, understanding, and sensitive when interviewing the victim. The investigator must elicit as much detail as possible about the incident without causing additional emotional distress for the victim. From the preliminary stages through the trial of the defendant, the detective/investigator must build and maintain a solid professional relationship with the victim that, above all, reassures the victim. The victim must be reassured that she is important, respected, and supported by the investigator and the entire criminal justice process.

The rape/sexual assault investigation begins with the first officer on the scene and continues until the suspect (s) are apprehended and tried. The detective/investigator assigned to the case will initially make certain that the crime scene is processed correctly by mobile crime lab personnel. In most agencies, the detective/ investigator meets the victim at the hospital where the rape examination is being done. This is the time when the victim's trauma and emotions are still very intense. The initial interview would be made after the detective/investigator has received the basic information from the first officer(s) on the scene. As previously mentioned, the detective/investigator should not conduct a lengthy detailed interview at this time. If the investigator is a man, he may wish to have a woman present to help the victim feel more at ease; however, this should be the victim's decision. The investigator must not interfere with or interrupt the medical examination. In fact, it may be better for the investigator to wait and get preliminary medical findings from the hospital staff before interviewing the victim. This is not to be confused with previously mentioned suggestions that the primary officer obtain basic information from the victim about the incident and the suspect. In rape/sexual assault cases it is extremely important that the interviewing detective/investigator avoid accusatory statements and questions such as, "Why were you dressed like that?" or "Why did you go to the suspect's apartment?" Such questions will cause greater distress for the victim and will quite possibly "shut down" any further dialogue with the victim.

As is the case with all types of criminal investigations, the detective must look at *all* of the evidence. This includes the victim's statements, any witness information, suspect statements, and the physical evidence that is known in the case. The totality of these data with the proper interpretation by the case investigator will lead to a successful conclusion.

## THE SUSPECT

The perpetrators who commit crimes of violence, including rape/sexual assault, are discussed in Chapter 2. In this chapter, we will limit our discussion to what the detective/investigator should and must do from the investigational perspective.

If a suspect is arrested almost immediately after the crime has been committed, the investigator must make certain that *all* clothing the suspect is wearing is seized and submitted as evidence. Certainly, all preservation-of-evidence procedures must be followed and the items submitted to the laboratory for examination. As a general rule, it is not necessary to obtain a court order or a search and seizure warrant to collect the suspect's clothing when an immediate arrest has been made. But, as previously stated, the rules and regulations of the department must be followed in these matters to avoid problems when the case goes to trial.

The suspect must be advised of his constitutional (Miranda) rights before any interrogation is conducted. The exception held valid by the courts is that if the suspect voluntarily talks about the case, without having been asked by the police, the remarks are admissible in trial. To be on the safe side of the law, it is usually wiser to advise the suspect of his rights and to have him read, initial, and sign an explanation of rights form, documenting that the suspect waived his rights, before beginning any formal interrogation. An interview of an individual who is not yet a suspect does not require that Miranda rights be given.

When interrogating a suspect, the investigators should have already established a firm working knowledge of the crime scene and the condition of the victim. Open-ended questions should be asked and the suspect should be allowed to answer without interruption. Even when the detective/investigator knows that the suspect is being less than honest, it is more productive to let him tell "his story" and then use that information later in the interrogation. All statements made by the suspect must be documented because they can be crucial evidence for use later in the trial.

The interrogation should be conducted in an area that is private, quiet, and free from interruption. The room should be empty except for a table and chairs. If an audiotape or a videotape of the interrogation is being made, the suspect must state that he is aware of the taping and has been advised of his constitutional rights, which he has waived.

Some agencies require that two investigators conduct the suspect interrogation. It is recommended that one investigator ask the questions while the other takes notes of what the suspect says, highlighting any inconsistencies that can be used later in the interrogation.

If the suspect writes his statement or confession, it should be expressed in his own words. It is unlikely that a suspect would actually state, "When I arrived at the scene my intent was to sexually assault the victim." The suspect should not be coached. Even the perception that the suspect was led in his statement can have a devastating negative result in court.

During the interrogation of the suspect, everything that the detectives/investigators do should be documented. If the suspect is taken to the bathroom, given food or a drink, or allowed to stand and walk around the room, it must be documented. In addition, if the suspect is photographed or if a laboratory test such as gunshot residue (GSR) test is conducted, the times when it began and when it was completed must be documented. All of this information must be kept in the case folder.

Upon completion of the interrogation, if the suspect is to be immediately charged with the crime, all charging documents should be prepared and the suspect then transported to the detention facility. When the suspect is sent to the detention facility, photographs of him should be taken and placed in the case folder. This documentation simply shows that the suspect was not injured when he left the interrogation.

## THE PROSECUTION

Case preparation for trial is a critical part of the investigation. It is the time when the detective/investigator reviews all of the facts of the case with the prosecuting attorney. The pretrial process varies from jurisdiction to jurisdiction. Essentially, it is now the time that the case moves to the next tier of the criminal justice process. Everything that was done in the case will be reviewed. From the report of the first officer on the scene of the assault to the last report that has been written, the prosecuting attorney *must* see everything.

This is usually the time that the victim and the prosecutor meet for the first time. Because of the unique nature of sexual crimes, many jurisdictions have a specific unit in the prosecutor's office that handles these cases. Generally, this group of attorneys has been selected not only for their legal ability but also for their ability to make the victim comfortable during the trial.

It is extremely important that the primary detective/investigator work with the prosecutor at this stage of the case. Months may have passed since the incident occurred. The victim may suffer again from the emotional trauma that was experienced when the crime occurred.

## SUMMARY

The police are the first part of the criminal justice system to interact with the victim of rape/sexual assault. The impressions of the first officer and investigator will have a lasting effect on the victim. Professional law enforcement personnel have a duty to do everything possible to help the victim. From obtaining immediate medical attention through the prosecutorial process, officers must make certain that they are compassionate and sensitive to the victim. The officers' attitude must help the victim understand that they are concerned but that they also have a mandate to gather information and facts, which may at times make her more uncomfortable. The victim has to know that the officers' ultimate goal is the arrest and conviction of the person(s) responsible for the crime. For the police to do less would only make the rape/sexual assault victim feel further victimized.

## SUGGESTED READINGS

Geberth VJ. *Practical homicide investigation,* 3rd ed. Boca Raton: CRC Press, 1996.

Ogle RR Jr. *Crime scene investigation & physical evidence manual,* 2nd ed. Vallejo, CA: 1998.

Spitz WU, Fisher RS. *Medicolegal investigation of death,* 2nd ed. Springfield, IL: Charles C. Thomas Publishers, 1992.

# 13

# Forensic Photography in the Emergency Department

Patrick E. Besant-Matthews and William S. Smock

To the list of individuals who take pictures, professionals who do so for a living and amateurs who do so for fun, must be added occupational, semiprofessional, or functional photographers.

Emergency physicians fall into this last category. The physician in an emergency department (ED) may use photography as often as weekly or daily but may never have had the benefit or luxury of any formal photographic instruction. The purpose of this chapter is to inform and educate the emergency physician on the principles and practices of forensic photography in the ED.

## WHY USE PHOTOGRAPHY IN THE EMERGENCY DEPARTMENT?

We use photography in the ED because a well-composed picture is worth *at least* a thousand words. In the ED, photography is generally used for one of two reasons: forensic or educational. The term *forensic photography* implies that the photograph, when properly obtained, may be used in legal proceedings (1). Traditionally, the use of forensic medical photography has been limited to crime scene locations and autopsy suites.

Now, and with ever-greater frequency, forensic medical photography is finding its way into EDs in the United States. Cameras are being used to document wounds on individuals who survive their injuries. This change is being brought about primarily by the development of new fields of expertise, such as sexual assault nurse examiner (SANE) programs, child abuse and domestic violence units, and clinical forensic medicine programs.

The reasons for employing a camera to aid in addressing the forensic needs of living patients in the ED are numerous and include the following:

1. To record and document injuries and evidence that cannot be preserved indefinitely or left untouched, given the treatment which is medically indicated.
2. To act as a future reference or aid to memory.
3. To document lesser features and details of a situation, which would not otherwise be practical or important for the purpose of medical treatment.
4. To permit the court and jurors to see things as they were and, in effect, check the testimony being presented to see if it makes sense in context.
5. To document injuries or conditions, and record what they looked like before and after medical treatment.
6. To demonstrate malice or criminal intent.
7. To show the condition of evidence or injuries at the time of discovery or examination.
8. To demonstrate the absence of injury or alleged findings.
9. To illustrate and supplement the written medical record.
10. To teach medical students and residents.

From the standpoint of photography's educational merits, the rationales are self-evident. The ability of the emergency physician to photographically document a patient's injury, wound, lesion, or rash or to obtain a radiograph will ensure that the patient's information can be shared with other health care professionals for educational purposes.

## CONSENT FOR FORENSIC PHOTOGRAPHY

After death, the patient capitulates the right of refusal and the investigating agency makes decisions and follows an accepted course of practice; however, living persons and patients must give consent for photography, unless they are unconscious, under arrest, and/or there is a court order for pictures to be taken, or unless they are photographed from a public place, such as a street or sidewalk. The physician is obligated by law to obtain consent, either implied or informed, from the living patient before photographs are taken for educational or forensic purposes. Informed consent involves explaining to the patient the purpose of taking the forensic or educational photograph. An awake and alert patient may refuse to be photographed, just as a patient may refuse to undergo a medical procedure or test. The physician must explain the reason for the photograph and the associated risks and benefits, if any. When approached in a respectful and polite manner, most patients permit the photographic documentation of their injuries or wounds, especially when it can be of benefit to their criminal case. Likewise, most patients agree to have their lesions, injuries, or rashes photographed for educational purposes when it is explained that future students will benefit from their generosity. The consent form (Fig. 13-1) must become part of the patient's permanent medical record.

Implied consent is a legal construct used to secure consent from an individual who is unconscious or so seriously injured as to be incapable of comprehending the consent request or responding to it. Consent in this context is construed as a course of action that a reasonably prudent person would adopt. A reasonably prudent person would allow the photographic documentation of injuries when the photographs will aid in the subsequent evaluation and treatment.

The photographic documentation of injuries may be vital to the conviction of those individuals who perpetrated a crime or inflicted a wound. Conversely, such documentation may help to ensure that suspects are not wrongfully charged (2). For example, an unconscious victim of an assault presents with a soot-covered gunshot wound (Fig. 13-2, see Colorplate following page 144). The physician may obtain photographs based on the assumption that a reasonably prudent person would permit photographic documentation of injuries or evidence that would be destroyed or altered in the course of medical treatment (Fig. 13-3). When implied consent has been used, the physician must obtain at some later time consent from either the patient or the next of kin.

Hospitals may include consent for photography language on operative consent or admission forms (Fig. 13-4), such as: "I consent to photographing of the operation/procedure, including portions of the body for medical, scientific, or educational purposes, provided my identity will not be revealed by the pictures or descriptive text accompanying them" (3). If photography language is not included in the routine surgical consent form, then a separate form with wording similar to the above is required. Wording may vary slightly from state to state (such as in Louisiana, where slightly different laws exist because of the French influence many years ago), so make sure any proposed form is reviewed by your hospital.

The following is an example of a draft for a separate consent to medical photography form:

> In connection with the medical services which (name of patient, next of kin, child, or ward) is to receive at (name of hospital), I hereby consent that photographs, videotapes, motion pictures, or illustrations may be made of him/her by members of the staff or other personnel working with or for the hospital, or any

**FIG. 13-1.** Sample consent-for-photography form from the University of Louisville Hospital. The consent form becomes a permanent part of the patient's medical record. The photographer should also maintain a copy for his records.

## University of Louisville Hospital

### PHOTOGRAPH/INTERVIEW CONSENT

Medical Record No.

Name

Unit/Bed

| Date | Unit | Name of Patient |
|------|------|-----------------|
|      |      |                 |

I, _____ ; authorize the party named

below to photograph, video tape and/or interview _____

while a patient at University of Louisville Hospital. I release University of Louisville Hospital from any and all liability

which may arise from the use of these photographs, tapes or interviews. I waive all rights I may have for any claims

for payment in connection with any exhibition, televising or publication of said photographs.

| X | TYPE OF CONSENT | YES | NO |
|---|-----------------|-----|-----|
|   | 1. Interview    |     |     |
|   | 2. Photograph   |     |     |
|   | 3. Video Taping |     |     |

Please indicate location where photographs/tapes will be stored (cannot be stored in Medical Records)

| X | PURPOSE OF CONSENT | YES | NO |
|---|--------------------|-----|-----|
|   | 1. Public Relations Purposes (newspapers, radio, television) |     |     |
|   | 2. Legal Purposes  |     |     |
|   | 3. Educational Purposes |     |     |
|   | 4. Personal Reasons |     |     |

| Name of Person Conducting Photo/Taping/Interview Session | Title of Person | | | |
|---|---|---|---|---|
| Name of Organization Being Represented | | | | |
| Address of Organization | City | State | Zip Code | Telephone No. ( ) |
| Signature of Patient/Legal Guardian | Date | Relationship to Patient | | |
| Witness | Title | | Date | |

ULH/600-113(10/96)

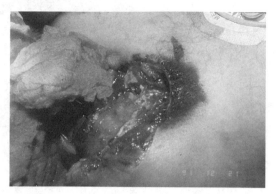

**FIG. 13-2.** The soot present on this close-range shotgun wound is short-lived. When the wound is scrubbed, debrided, and closed, the soot, which indicates a close range of fire, will have been destroyed.

hospital staff member, for the following uses and subject to the following conditions: (a) that photographs, or excerpts therefrom, may form part of the medical record, or be used for illustrative purposes in lectures and medical publications being shown, published and republished in any manner which the hospital and medical staff shall deem proper; (b) that best efforts will be made to prevent or limit

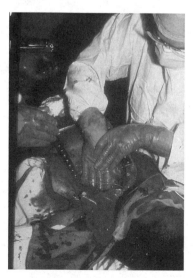

**FIG. 13-3.** The opening of the chest wall can alter a wound's size and characteristics. If possible, wounds and fragile evidence should be documented prior to surgical intervention.

personal identification and recognition. I expect no compensation or other remuneration. This consent as to any use of said photographs, videotapes, motion pictures, or illustrations, shall act to expressly release from liability the photographer, videographer, or illustrator, the attending physicians, the hospital and affiliated corporations, the authors, editors and publishers, if any, their officers and members.

The form should include the name of the physician and be signed and dated by the patient.

## ADMISSIBILITY AND SUBSTANTIVE EVIDENCE

A photograph must be an accurate and objective depiction of its subject to be accepted as evidence in a court of law (4). The photographer and the photograph must be able to withstand legal challenges as to the photographic authenticity, integrity, and credibility, or the judge has an obligation to disregard it as demonstrable evidence.

A photograph is not usually substantive evidence. This means that a photograph cannot be submitted in court as evidence and stand alone without an advocate for it. Someone is going to have to verify it, and attest to it, and say that they either took it or saw it be taken. The court will expect to hear from the photograph's advocate that it is indeed a fair and accurate representation of the situation at the time it was taken.

A photograph will probably be admitted as evidence by a judge if:

1. It shows the original appearance or findings, and "fairly and accurately depicts" what the health professional saw.
2. It assists in the identification or characterization of the wound or injuries.
3. It is not unduly gruesome or inflammatory.
4. It is of sufficient value to warrant its inclusion.
5. It will aid the court or jury in obtaining an intelligent or dispassionate evaluation or conclusion.
6. It is well composed, and most of the picture area is filled with the wound or injury in question.

**Consent:**

The above has been explained to me by Dr. _____. I have had a chance to ask questions and I have the information I need to make a decision about this procedure. I consent to this procedure. I agree to let the hospital use or dispose of tissue removed from me. I consent to photographing of the operation/procedure including portions of the body for medical, scientific, or educational purposes provided that my identity will not be revealed by the pictures or descriptive text accompanying them. **I have answered the doctor's questions about my health truthfully.**

I would like a copy of this consent form.  ☐ YES  ☐ NO

_____

Patient's Signature                               Date                               Time

**Witness and/or Interpreter:**

_____

Witness to Patient's Signature                        Interpreter              Date       Time

0919001 (11/99)                                    **(OVER)**

**FIG. 13-4.** Operative consent form, which includes language about educational intraoperative photography.

7. The feature or wound is clearly visible.
8. The picture is nicely exposed and about the right color.
9. The picture is in focus.
10. The photograph has a small ruler in the plane of the wound, to show the wound size (in inches and/or centimeters) (Fig. 13-5).
11. The photograph corresponds closely to the verbal description given by the emergency physician.
12. The photograph does not contain extraneous matter such as surgical instruments or bloody dressings (Fig. 13-6).

The nurse or physician must also be ready for legal challenges regarding the admissibility of the photographs. The questions and challenges may include:

1. Exactly where and when the photograph was taken.
2. Exactly what the photo depicts (use lay terms for the benefit of the court, attorneys, and jurors).
3. The exact anatomical location (supplement with lay terms).
4. The type of camera and film used.
5. If filters were used on the lens.

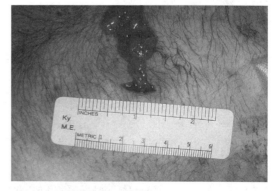

**FIG. 13-5.** The abdominal stab wound from a single-edged blade is nicely composed with the ruler parallel to the wound. The scale is in the plane of the wound and would accurately depict the size of the stab wound.

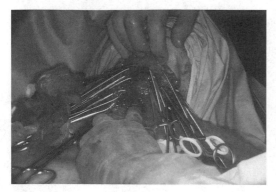

FIG. 13-6. The presence of extraneous surgical instruments or bloody dressings will detract from the significance of the photograph.

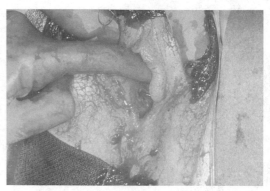

FIG. 13-7. A large vaginal laceration that occurred as a result of sexual assault. The presence of blood and the graphic nature of the injury resulted in the judge ruling the photograph inflammatory and not admissible.

6. Whether the photograph was obtained by informed or implied consent.
7. Where the film was developed and if it represents the hospital's standard protocol.

The issue of a photograph's potentially inflammatory content will be questioned. If a photograph is so gruesome and "inflammatory" (4) that it may cause "undue prejudice" (5) toward the accused on the part of the jury, the judge may exclude it from evidence.

Suppose that an elderly woman seen in the ED suffered a severe vaginal laceration from a sexual assault and her accused assailant is on trial. The emergency physician who examined the patient is testifying about a victim's injuries. The physician describes lacerations (a blunt force, torn, crushing injury) of the vaginal wall, consistent with forced vaginal penetration. The district attorney or commonwealth attorney, who called the treating physician as a witness, produces a photograph (Fig. 13-7, see Colorplate following page 144) and asks, "Doctor do you recognize this photograph?" The physician replies, "Yes, it was taken in the emergency department. The photo depicts the victim's vaginal laceration." After asking several more questions of a legal nature, the lawyer shows the photograph to the defense attorney, offers the photograph in evidence, and hands it to the judge. The defense attorney rises and says that he objects to the introduction of the photograph. His principle concern

is that its introduction will be prejudicial to his client. The judge, whose role it is to see that the trial is conducted according to the accepted rules of law, proceeds to examine the photograph and its suitability for use as evidence. The judge sustains the objection and the photo is not admitted on the grounds that the severity of the laceration and the presence of blood would be inflammatory and prejudicial.

In general, a judge probably will *not* admit the photograph if:

1. The composition is absurd because the photograph was taken at such a distance from the wound that the wound occupies only a fraction of the image. The remainder of the image area is taken up with parts of the resuscitation or autopsy table, on which are a number of potentially offensive and objectionable items, such as bloody sponges, dressings, pools of partly dried blood, scissors, or clumps of hair (Fig. 13-8).
2. The wound is out of focus and hard to see.
3. The picture is overexposed and "washed out." There is a reflection of the on-camera flash in the middle of the wound. The color is not right. There is also a distracting greenish reflection of the overhead fluorescent lights in the metal surface of the resuscitation table.

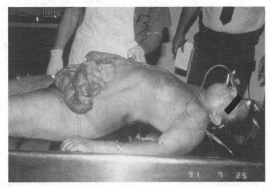

**FIG. 13-8.** Photographs taken from a distance are important for an overview or general shot but may not be admissible in court on the grounds that they are not specific, detract from the significance of the injury, or include unnecessary information.

4. Poor "scale" technique is used:

   a. Only a section of a plastic ruler is used, cut so that numbers begin at 2 on the inch side and 5 on the centimeter side.

   b. An equipment maker's name is on the scale.

   c. The scale is covering part of the wound.

   d. The scale is not in the plane of the wound but at an angle to it, meaning that since part of the wound is nearer the camera than the scale, any measurement derived from it will be in error by several percentage points.

5. The physician has just described the wound as being vertical, and clearly it was with respect to the standard anatomical position, but the wound appears horizontal in the photograph.

6. The photograph was not taken at 90 degrees to the wound and perspective distortion is present (Fig. 13-9).

A recent Kentucky ruling determined that "there was no reason to exclude photographic evidence by claiming the photographs were unduly gruesome when the crime itself was brutal and gruesome. The Commonwealth cannot be prevented from proving the commission of a crime that is by its nature heinous and repulsive. Gruesome photographs alone cannot be the basis for the exclusion of such evidence" (4).

## BASIC FORENSIC PHOTOGRAPHY

The physical care of the patient is always paramount. As important as they are, photographic documentation and evidence collection are secondary concerns. In practice, it is possible to perform forensic photograph evidence collection without compromising patient care (2).

Individuals who intend to take forensic photographs should have some basic working knowledge of photographic theory. Even if providers are utilizing a "point-and-shoot" camera, they will need some background information to understand what goes into making an acceptable forensic photograph. For the purposes of discussion, the author assumes that the reader will be using a 35-mm single-lens reflex (SLR) camera. The "35-mm" camera is so named because the film it utilizes is 35 mm wide.

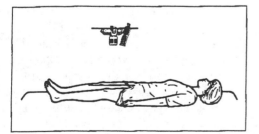 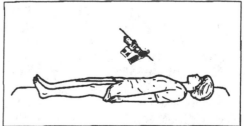

**FIG. 13-9.** The emergency department photographer should maintain the lens at 90 degrees to the subject. Angles less than 90 degrees introduce perspective distortion, which renders the scale inaccurate. (Reprinted from Smock WS. Forensic photography. In:. Stack L, Storrow A, Patton D, eds *Physician's handbook of clinical photography.* Philadelphia: Hanley & Belfus, 2000, with permission.)

## LENS CHARACTERISTICS

The lens is a clear window of glass, or high-tech plastic, made and positioned so as to gather and focus light onto the light-sensitive film inside the camera when the shutter is opened. The lens controls the magnification of the object photographed and other characteristics (sharpness, contrast, color, etc.) of the image. In conjunction with the shutter, it also controls the amount of light that reaches the film or light-sensitive device.

The focal length of a lens is the distance from a point called the optical center to the point behind the lens at which rays of light from a distant subject are brought to a focus. If a lens brings rays of light from a far distant object to a focus in a distance of 50 mm (just under 2 in.), then this is the focal length of the lens. In effect, it is the magnifying power of the lens.

If one takes the 50-mm lens off the camera and replaces it with another that has a focal length of 100 mm (just under 4 in.), then the subject will appear twice as large in the viewfinder and on the film. It is as though we put a telescope on the camera and made everything look nearer. We see less of the subject in the viewfinder but what we do see appears twice the size. Ignoring various technicalities of optics, people frequently refer to such a lens as a telephoto.

Now suppose we replace the 50-mm lens with another that has a focal length of 24 mm (just under 1 in.) and look though the viewfinder again. We will see a much wider field, with more things in the field of view, but each object appears about half the size. We are now using what is called a wide-angle lens.

So you can either stand at a distance of 4 feet and photograph the whole upper part of a patient on a stretcher with your 50-mm lens, or you can put on your 105-mm lens and, from the same working distance, concentrate on the head of an injured person, which is now about twice as big in the viewfinder as it was before.

Now you understand that the value of a "longer" lens (longer or greater focal length) is that it gives you more distance to work with. In surgery or in the emergency department, a 200-mm lens (instead of a regular 50-mm) will enable you to:

1. Stand four times as far away from the patient and get the same size image,
2. Stand at the same distance but get an image four times larger, or
3. Stand twice as far away and get twice as large an image, simultaneously.

In general, there is a direct relationship between focal length and working distance. If you double the focal length, the camera-to-subject distance doubles, for the same image size. If your work entails extensive close-up photography, you should buy a lens that is specially designed for that purpose. These are commonly called macrolenses and they're specially designed to give:

1. Excellent sharpness in the close-up range, including sharpness from edge to edge of the image, not only at the center.
2. Flat undistorted fields, meaning no curved lines when copying graph paper, diagrams, and printed matter.
3. Excellent contrast.
4. The ability to focus down to half life size, or even life size, without any additional attachments.

In fact, the best macrolenses are so good that they will resolve more detail than many ordinary films can record (Fig. 13-10). They are also very good for general subject matter. As you might expect, they tend to be more expensive because they're sold in smaller numbers, but if you plan to do a significant amount of close-up work, they are well worth the cost.

Macrolenses are commonly available in three different focal length ranges:

1. 50–60 mm (1), excellent for copying flat materials.
2. 100–105 mm (2), a very popular range (there are a few at 90 mm) with twice the working distance. These are great for general patient, injury, and autopsy photography. If in doubt, this is the type you should buy first, unless a very large part of your work involves copying flat objects or the like.
3. 180–200 mm ($1\frac{3}{4}$–2). These lenses are a bit more specialized. They're understandably popular with nature and wildlife

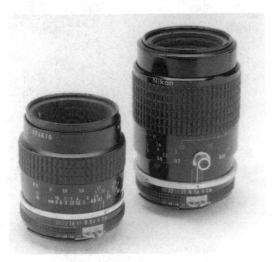

**FIG. 13-10.** Micro-Nikkor 55-mm, f2.8 and Micro-Nikkor 105-mm lenses permit the emergency department photographer to take close-up photographs with good depth of field.

photographers who want to leave subjects, such as insects, undisturbed or need to keep their distance from dangerous animals. They are also excellent for operating room photography and for patient photography (e.g., when one doesn't want to get too close to a nervous child or to a recent victim of sexual assault).

Just in case you haven't yet fully grasped the concept of working distance, a macrolens with a longer focal length—say 100 mm—will in general enable you to obtain the same image from twice as far away as a 50-mm lens, or of course twice the image size from the same distance. In biomedical and forensic work their increased working distance is invaluable:

1. In the operating room over the surgeon's shoulder.
2. In the ED when a belligerent alcoholic in restraints is trying to hit you.
3. At a crime scene, enabling you to "reach" the hair and blood on the windshield of the vehicle while resting your arms on the back of the front seat.
4. In outdoor circumstances, facilitating the recording of evidence on the ground with a minimum of kneeling and bending over.

What is a zoom lens? It is a lens that offers continuously variable magnification (focal length). Zoom lenses have a collar or ring that can be turned, or slid lengthways, thereby moving the lens elements to give the image the magnification you desire.

## APERTURE

Now that the meaning of focal length is understood, lens aperture becomes quite easy because the f/- numbers are derived from the effective aperture and the focal length of a lens. In theory, if a lens has an opening of 2 in. and it brings parallel rays to a focus in a distance of 4 in., then its aperture is $\frac{2}{4}$ or, as photographers say, f/2. Likewise, if a lens has a 1-in. opening and brings light to a focus in a distance of 4 in., it has an aperture of $\frac{1}{4}$ or f/4. This is the reason why the size of the hole admitting light, and the amount of light that gets through a given lens, goes down as the f/- number goes up, and vice versa.

What the ED photographer should know is simply that every time you move from one full f/- number to another, the amount of light entering the camera is halved or doubled, depending on the direction in which you are going.

## SHUTTER SPEEDS

The fact that lens apertures move in steps of two is equally important because when you look at your camera you will see that the shutter speeds also go up and down in steps of two. Examine your shutter speed control. It reads something like 2, 4, 8, 15, 30, 60, 125, etc., which is an abbreviation for $\frac{1}{2}, \frac{1}{4}, \frac{1}{8}, \frac{1}{15}, \frac{1}{30}, \frac{1}{60}, \frac{1}{125}$, etc., of a second.

## EXPOSURE

Now we are in a position to control the amount of light reaching the film, by adjusting either the size of the aperture, or the time the shutter is open. In particular, we have the option of being able to trade lens aperture against shutter speed. For instance, if we double the amount of light coming through the lens, and cut the shutter time in half, we will end up with the same amount of light reaching the film.

This is one of the most basic and useful concepts in photography. Suppose there is enough light to get a proper exposure with a shutter speed of $\frac{1}{125}$ second and a lens opening of f/8. By simply doubling the aperture (f/8 to f/16) and halving the shutter speed ($\frac{1}{125}$–$\frac{1}{60}$), we can still obtain the correct exposure.

For all practical purposes, any of the above combinations will admit the same amount of light, so we can now choose whatever pair we desire. This gives us flexibility and control.

If we wish to "catch" or "stop" a moving object such as a high jumper, it would be desirable to use a short shutter opening of $\frac{1}{1,000}$ second or less with a big lens opening, whereas if we wanted to create a blurred, artistic image of water coming over a waterfall, we might choose $\frac{1}{2}$ second or longer with a small lens opening.

Now you see why understanding that lens aperture and the shutter speeds progress in steps of two is so valuable. Simply stated, we use whatever combination of aperture and shutter time we need to obtain the photograph we want.

## SHUTTER PRIORITY

Shutter priority means that you select the shutter speed for the job at hand, and the camera will calculate the right lens aperture at the moment you make the exposure.

- Use this mode when you have to control action. For instance, freeze moving cars on a freeway with a short shutter time, or blur the water of a waterfall by use of a longer opening.
- Be alert to the possibility that if the shutter is only open for a short period and the lens opens up, the depth of field may be too shallow.

## APERTURE PRIORITY

Aperture priority means that you select the lens opening to give you the depth of field you require, and the camera will determine the proper shutter time when you make the exposure.

- Use this when it's important to use a small aperture for greater depth of field or a large aperture to throw a background out of focus, and thereby emphasize a nearer subject.
- Be alert to the possibility that a long shutter opening may lead to blurring of anything that may move during the exposure.

## PROGRAM

Then there may be a third setting called something like "program." This means that the camera has been preprogrammed by the manufacturer to make a reasonably good choice between both shutter speeds and apertures, depending on the distance of the subject and the amount of light available when the camera is used. For instance, the manufacturer is likely to have programmed the camera to avoid very long shutter openings during which the hands of the user might shake and thereby cause smearing of the image. All will be well with the "program" setting if, and only if, the subjects you are taking match the built-in instructions reasonably well. This is why good cameras allow you to switch from one option to another.

## DEPTH OF FIELD

Depth of field is determined by the size of the aperture set on the lens (the f/- number). The depth of field means the nearest and farthest distances between which things will appear acceptably sharp or in focus.

If our close-up lens is wide open at f/4.0 and we focus on a subject 5 feet away from us, the lens will yield sharp focus from about 4 feet 11 in. to 5 feet 1 in. If we now change the aperture to f/22 and again focus on a subject at 5 feet, the lens will yield a sharp image from about 5 feet $7\frac{1}{2}$ in. to 5 feet 5 in. That is to say, as the aperture becomes smaller the lens provides a greater depth of sharpness, called *depth of field,* in front of and behind the point at which the lens was theoretically in perfect focus.

This has great practical value. We can use a wide aperture to capture an image separate from its surroundings, or use a small aperture to get the surroundings sharp on the near and far side of our focal image.

Although it may seem at first glance that we should always keep the lens closed down to get the greatest depth, this is not necessarily true. At small apertures, there may be loss of sharpness due to a physical effect called *diffraction*. Also, at small apertures, one has to compensate for lack of light with faster (more sensitive) film or longer exposures (risking the blur due to camera motion). At very wide apertures, optical shortcomings (lens aberrations) may reduce sharpness.

In summary, the following should be remembered regarding lenses:

1. The focal length of a lens is in essence its magnifying power. The smaller/shorter the focal length is, the wider the angle the lens will "see" and, conversely, the larger/longer the focal length the nearer and bigger objects will appear.
2. Moving from one full f/- stop to another will double or halve the amount of light that reaches the film, depending on the direction in which you're going.
3. As the f/- number increases, the amount of light that can reach the film decreases and vice versa.
4. Smaller apertures (larger f/- numbers) yield greater depths of acceptable sharpness than larger apertures (smaller f/- numbers).

## LIGHTING

Lighting is the key to photography. Anyone can take a reasonable photograph if the lighting is good, but not when it is bad. You must devote some thought to light and how it behaves. A general principle is to mimic or add to existing light or to create your own lighting according to preference and the kind of subject.

Photographic lighting is the practical and artistic application of scientific principles:

- There must be enough light to expose the film properly.

- The color of the light should be right for the film selected.
- Contrast (range of brightness between darkest shadows and brightest highlights) should be within the capability of the film.

Roughly speaking, the eye can handle a brightness range of about 1000:1, film about 100:1, new video systems about 30:1, and old video systems about 20:1. Translated this means that film can, at best, handle a brightness range of about $6\frac{1}{2}$ f-stops. Normally a ratio of 3:1, 4:1, or 5:1 is best.

In the ED and in a forensic setting we too must be concerned about lighting. Flash is convenient, but we must control it, get the exposure right, eliminate unwanted shadows, and draw attention to the subject.

When living persons are your subject matter and the flash is too close to the lens, you may see the phenomenon called "red eye." Simply stated, light travels into the eye of a person, picks up the color of blood at the retina, and is reflected back to the camera lens. It is prevented by making the pupil of the eye close down, and/or by moving the light source away from the line along which the lens of the camera sees.

Many of the newer cameras have a red-eye reduction mode. This provides up to 15 flashing bursts to reduce the diameter of the pupil.

What about the little flash units that are built into many of the midrange single lens reflex cameras? They don't have enormous power (guide numbers of about 40–55 for feet are common) but are pretty good. They're mainly intended for taking photographs of people at a distance of about 10–12 feet. They are useful for patient photography, photography of small crime scenes, and recording of the interiors of vehicles. They will certainly get you off to a good start. They are often capable of filling shadows outdoors in bright light, but you will eventually need a larger, more powerful, add-on flash for larger, remote, or difficult subjects.

To obtain the best results with flash photography, you must move the flash away from the camera lens and position it above the lens axis, on a bracket attached to the base of the camera or on a separate stand nearby. The pocket-size "point-and-shoot" cameras, with a flash built in next to the lens, will be perfectly satisfactory for amateur and pleasure purposes, and to get you started in biomedical or crime scene photography, but as you advance they cannot give you optimal lighting for scientific work. As you progress you will want to add a separate flash unit and buy a cord to go between it and the camera to give you the option of moving the light farther away and/or choosing its position with respect to the lens so as to pick up texture.

Another basic concept of lighting is the size of the light source in relation to the subject. If we place a small bright light in a suitable place and try to photograph a patient, we will get shadows with very well-defined or sharp edges. Photographers call this "hard" lighting. From this we should learn that on-camera flash is only a convenience; it does not necessarily provide the best lighting.

Therefore, as your skill increases, you will need a special cord to go between your camera and the flash unit to enable you to put the light source where you want it while retaining all of the helpful features, such as automatic exposure. In my opinion, an off-camera cord is one of the few "must have" accessories, such as the Nikon SC17 (Fig. 13-11A, B) or the Canon Off-Camera Shoe Cord 2.

Several manufacturers produce useful and imaginative light sources called ring lights or ring flashes (Fig. 13-12). They are small flash tubes formed into a circle to fit around the camera lens so as to produce light on all sides of the subject and thus shadow-free illumination. They are ideal for close-up (within 18 in.) detail shots, such as gunshot wounds in the mouth, bite marks, teeth, and vaginal injuries, or for the rapid recording of small items, such as bullets, and trace evidence (Fig. 13-13A, B, see Colorplate following page 144). But they are not a cure-all for biological subjects. The problem is not with the lights but rather with the subject being photographed. So much medical and biological subject material is wet or shiny. Ring flashes result in glare under these conditions, often in the middle of the most important thing in the photograph. Ring flashes should be regarded as a tool and therefore helpful in some—but not all—situations.

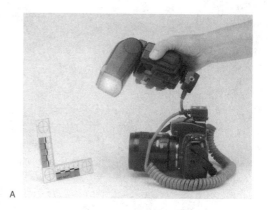

A

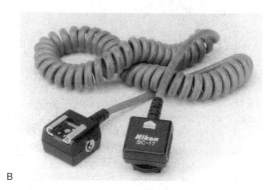

B

**FIG. 13-11.** The flash extension cord permits the emergency department photographer to divert the flash out toward the subject.

Note that some of the best so-called ring lights have two separate flash tubes, one on either side of the lens that can be operated together or independently for better results. You can achieve much the same by covering parts of a ring light with some opaque adhesive tape or a card, provided you allow for the loss of light.

## BACKGROUND

What background is desirable for photography of an injured person? Will the background detract from the subject of the photo (e.g., a crowded resuscitation room with ten medical providers surrounding the patient)? What color of paper or paint or curtains will you place behind the injured warm-skinned persons you are photographing? If possible, look at your background to determine if unwanted or extraneous material will detract from what you need to document.

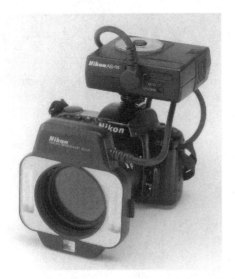

**FIG. 13-12.** The lens-mounted ring flash (Nikkor SB-21) permits good close-up lighting from 1 to 18 in. The flash tubes on either side of the lens may be fired independently to give the subject more definition. If the flash tubes are fixed simultaneously, they will produce a flatter appearance.

## EQUIPMENT FOR FORENSIC PHOTOGRAPHY IN THE EMERGENCY DEPARTMENT

Any photograph is better than no photograph, so the ED photographer may be tempted to purchase a "point-and-shoot" camera; however, the 35-mm SLR is considered the standard for forensic ED photography. The SLR has multiple advantages over the point-and-shoot models:

- Through the lens viewing (TTL) permits the photographer to see exactly what the film sees.
- Interchangeable lens, 55 mm to 105 mm, macro.
- Ability to control shutter speed and aperture settings.
- Ability to have off-camera flash.

### CAMERA BODY

The camera body is the "brains" of the photographer. There are a number of camera manufacturers that produce adequate photographic equipment for work in the ED (Table 13-1). In particular, Nikon and Canon have an excellent selection of equipment dedicated to medical photography. Expect to spend at least $300.00 for the body.

### LENS

The evidence photographer must have a lens capable of rendering clean images with fine details at close range, as well as sharp images of larger subjects at varying distances. The macrolens (also called microlens) provides these features because it can produce a wide range of reproduction ratios (1:1 to infinity.)

Very little about the human body is flat. When imaging wounds on a rounded surface, the photographer will need a lens with very

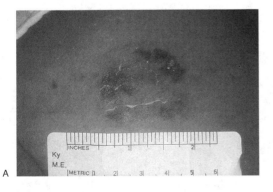
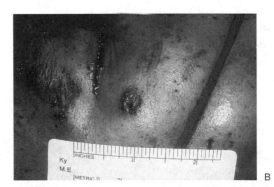

A                                                                      B

**FIG. 13-13. A:** Healing bite mark to breast. **B:** Gunshot entrance wound with the associated abrasion collar. The injuries are well lighted by the ring flash.

**TABLE 13-1.** *Suggested equipment list for the emergency department*

Nikon camera body: FE2, FA, F100, N60, N70, N90s, N100, 6006, F3, F4s, F5
Canon camera body: EOS Rebel 2000, EOS-A2, EOS-3, EOS-1
Nikkor-Micro 55 mm/f2.8, AF-Micro 60 mm/f.28D
Nikkor-Micro 105 mm/f2.8, AF-Micro 105 mm/f.28D
Lester-Dine ring/point flash or Nikon ring flash SB-21
Nikon SB-23, SB-26, SB-27, SB-28 top-mounted flash
Canon 540EZ, 550EX top-mounted flash
Nikon Databack (varies with camera model)
Nikon flash extension cord SC-17
Nonglare, rigid scale (without advertisement)
Background towel or drape
Adhesive scale for wound/subject size determination and on which the patient's name and record number can be clearly written

small aperture capabilities (f/22 to f/45) to increase depth of field. When using smaller aperture settings (larger f-number), depth of field is increased, giving an expanded breadth of focus. This is essential for images on curved surfaces such as bite marks on the hand or wrist (Fig. 13-13A, see Colorplate following page 144). The most popular lenses for medical and forensic photography are manufactured by Nikon and include the Micro-Nikkor 55 mm, f/2.8, the Micro-Nikkor 60 mm, f/2.8; the Micro-Nikkor 105 mm, f/2.8 (Fig. 13-10); and the Medical-Nikkor 120 mm, f/4. Other camera manufacturers also produce macrolenses with similar features. The 105-mm and 120-mm lenses have an increased focal length when compared with the 55-mm lens and enable the photographer to double the film to subject distance and obtain the same image. This increased focal length may be advantageous when attempting to take photographs over the back of the treating medical staff during a resuscitation or in the operating room.

## CAMERA BAG

In a busy ED, a camera bag is essential to protect your equipment. The bag should be large enough to leave some space for other items, such as lens shades, flash, batteries, an off-camera cord, a note pad, and spare film.

In general, the older looking and less attractive your bag is, the less likely your equipment is to be stolen. Some photographers have been known to carry expensive equipment in diaper bags! A lockable drawer or cabinet in the ED is ideal.

## ELECTRONIC FLASH

An electronic flash is required equipment for any medical or forensic photographer. The photographer will be able to capture essential details if the flash has enough power to illuminate subjects when using f-stops in the 22–32 range. Preferably, the flash should be a dedicated electronic flash with TTL metering. TTL metering permits the camera to communicate with the flash to modify flash intensity given a selected shutter speed or aperture.

The well-designed camera and flash combination positions the flash several inches above the lens. This causes shadows to fall below and behind the average subject, and eliminates hard shadows on the right or the left.

Ideally, the flash should be attached to the camera by a bracket that enables the light to come from 8–10 in. above the lens and slightly off to the side. This unfortunately makes the camera somewhat bulky and is not well designed for hospital situations. The built-in and top-mounted flash units are suited to effectively illuminate subjects 24 in. to 15 feet from the photographer. These flash options are inadequate as much of forensic photography is performed at a distance of less than 24 in.

The forensic photographer must have the ability to photograph at distances ranging from several inches to infinity. The light generated by a built-in or a top-mounted flash will not adequately illuminate a subject at distances less than 24 in. due to the angle of the flash (Fig. 13-14). A lens-mounted ring flash unit (Fig. 13-12) or a flash with a cord extension (Fig. 13-11A, B) directs the flash on the subject and corrects for this close-up deficiency of top-mounted flashes.

A ring flash and the combination ring/point flash units mount directly on the end of the lens. These flash units properly illuminate a

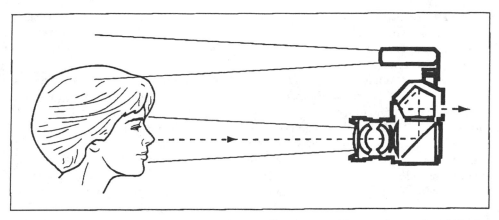

**FIG. 13-14.** Top-mounted electronic flashes may not illuminate subjects adequately within 6 in. of the lens. The light passes over the subject, leaving an underexposed photograph. (Reprinted from Smock WS. Forensic photography. In: Stack L, Storrow A, Patton D, eds. *Physician's handbook of clinical photography.* Philadelphia: Hanley & Belfus, 2000, with permission.)

subject within inches of the lens. Most lens-mounted flash units work well in the range of 1–18 in. from the subject. A ring flash creates its own set of challenges. It generates a round reflection on shiny surfaces and produces a flat image without shadows on areas with depth.

A point light source attached to the camera by a synchronization cord allows the flash to be hand-held at an angle to the subject (Fig. 13-11B). This casts shadows, giving the image depth. The point source has a smaller reflection than a ring flash and imposes less distraction from the image.

### Databack

A databack (Fig. 13-15) is an electronic device that replaces the standard camera back and enables the photographer to imprint the date, time, or frame number onto the slide or negative. This imprint assists the photographer and the court to determine the date, time, and order in which the photographs were taken. Newer databacks perform advanced functions, such as exposure bracketing, timed photography, and automatic shutter release when a subject enters a predetermined focal position. The databack should be standard equipment for the forensic photographer.

### FILM

The ED photographer must decide whether to utilize print, slide, or digital film. Each of these offers advantages and disadvantages.

In the amateur markets, print film is by far the most popular, reportedly accounting for 90% of film sold. Forensic pathologists, physicians, and functional photographers tend to use more slide (transparency) film. Which should the ED photographer choose? To oversimplify,

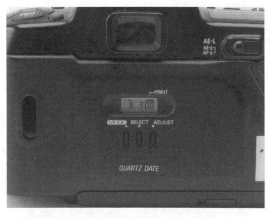

**FIG. 13-15.** A databack imprints the date, time, or sequence number on the film. This option assists the emergency department photographer in dating the photograph.

if you usually want prints, use negative film. You can always have slides made from selected negatives if the need arises. If you usually want slides, use slide film. It is possible to make good-quality prints from slides in a single step, if the slides are good. For the best possible results, it is still advisable to have an internegative made. Table 13-2 provides some pointers to help decide between the two types of film. In general, most police departments and investigative agencies use negative (print) film.

Film is rated by speed or ASA (American Standards Association) or ISO (International Standards Organization), which describes its sensitivity to light. For forensic purposes, the film must deliver sharp resolution and proper color. A "slow" film, with a lower ISO number, responds slowly and needs a lot of light to produce a satisfactory image. A "fast" film, with a higher ISO number, is more sensitive to light and therefore needs less light to do its job.

If you occasionally need large prints (poster size), you are probably better off using properly exposed slow-speed (ISO 25–100) negative film and having the prints made from negatives rather than from slides, but it can be done either way.

ASA (ISO) ratings between 50 and 200 support the function of ED photography to document wounds and injuries. These speeds will give the photographer the sharpest images and saturated color.

You may see the letters "DX" on a film box and notice that the metal film cassette has some small light silvery squares on it. This is so-called DX (Digital indeX) coding, which in many cameras sets the camera mechanism to the film speed automatically as soon as the film is inserted. This is helpful because it makes it harder to change film speed and then forget to reset the camera meter; however, good-quality equipment incorporates a means of adjusting the exposure up and down to allow for deviations, manufacturing tolerances, personal preferences, etc. If you insert a film cassette that has no DX code into a camera that looks for it, the camera will

**TABLE 13-2.**  *Slide versus negative film*

| Slide (color reversal, transparency) films | Negative (print) films |
|---|---|
| Projecting slides onto a screen gives the best color and range of brightness. | Prints have less brightness range and less inherent sharpness. |
| An original slide can be used to check the quality and color of any copy made from it. | You cannot compare a negative to the original by eye. |
| Slides are easy to see with a magnifier, and easy to evaluate for exposure, color, and sharpness. | Negatives are harder for most people to evaluate because of the distracting yellow-orange backing. |
| Slides are easy to sort, store, file, and shuffle to make up, or alter, a presentation. | Negatives aren't as easy to number and file. |
| Slides have a paper or plastic mount on which information and case number(s) can be written or added by means of an adhesive label. | Negatives have to be marked on their edges, or be filed in an envelope or sleeve, from which they may become separated. |
| There is a wide choice of slide films, each with its own capabilities and way of depicting color. | There is a choice of negative films, some of which are good at certain things (e.g., skin color in portraiture), but it is not as extensive as slides. |
| Slides cost less per image for film processing and mounting. | Prints generally cost more per image for film processing plus printing, much more when large prints are made. |
| Slides are less tolerant of errors in exposure and therefore help to evaluate the performance of automatic exposure systems. | Negative films are more tolerant of errors in exposure and therefore help to ensure image acquisition. There is even a color negative film that has an extra wide exposure latitude by design. |
| Prints can be made from slides, but the process has some technical limitations. For instance, if a slide has contrast or is in some other way less than ideal, it may be necessary to make a special internegative from which to derive prints. | It is easy to print negatives on an automatic machine, and many amateurs make prints at home with good results. It is generally less expensive to make custom prints from color negatives than from slides. |

usually default to a film speed of ISO 100, but some point-and-shoot cameras will default to ISO 25. The DX code also tells the camera something about the exposure latitude of the film and has a bar code adjacent to it, which can be scanned by the photofinisher to identify the type of film and number of exposures.

Kodak and Fuji produce both commercial and professional grade slide film. The commercial grade films are more than adequate to meet the needs of the forensic photographer in the hospital. Professional grade films also produce excellent results but require constant refrigeration and are less forgiving when exposure mistakes are made. Each type of film has a slightly different color balance and may be affected by ambient light in the hospital. The photographer should select the type and speed of film that most accurately represents the wounds and injuries seen at the time the images were obtained.

For slides/transparencies, in daylight or with electronic flash, start with:

Fujichrome Astia 100 (accurate skin and fabric tones)
Fujichrome Provia 100F (very fine grain)
Fujichrome Sensia II 100 (excellent color)
Kodak Ektachrome 100S

Then compare:

Fujichrome Velvia 50
Kodak Ektachrome Elite II, ISO 100
Kodak Ektachrome 64 Professional
Kodak Ektachrome 100 Plus (EPP)
Kodak Ektachrome 200 Professional (EPD)

For slides under tungsten lighting indoors (Type B film, 3200°K)

Kodak Ektachrome 64T, Fujichrome 64T type II

For color negatives and prints, start with:

Kodak Gold 100, Portra 160, or Fuji Reala 100 then compare:
Agfacolor Ultra 50. (Use for brilliant colors and real "snap".)
Agfacolor Portrait 160. (Designed for portrait work, has good skin tones.)
Kodak Royal Gold 100, 200 and 400. (Good skin tones.)

Fujicolor Reala 100. (Great color rendition, very good in high contrast lighting.)
Fujicolor Super G 100, 200 and 400.
Fujicolor NPS 160 (portrait film), NPL 160, NPH 400, and NGHII 800.
Fuji Superia in 100, 200, 400, 400 X-TRA (800). 100 is excellent for normal lighting.

Kodak is replacing most professional negative films with speeds between 100 and 400 with Portra 160NC and 400 NC (natural color), 160 black and white VC, and 400VC (vivid color) for slightly enhanced color.

Kodak Vericolor III (VPS), a professional favorite for portraits, may not last very long.

Ideally, in order to stop slide film from degrading, it should be stored in a refrigerator. This is particularly important for professional film. This type of film is generally not designed for ED use.

On the other hand, films marked "professional" are generally manufactured to closer tolerances and aged until they have reached an optimum color balance. They are then refrigerated, and delivered to critical professional users. They must be kept cold until just before use, allowed to warm up, exposed and developed almost immediately. In this way the critical user is more likely to obtain optimal color balance. Storage at 50–55°F or less is suggested.

Likewise, color printing papers will also maintain their color balance better if stored in the cold. All films store better away from heat and humidity.

Regardless of type, you must let film warm up before you unwrap it or open the plastic container. As a guide, allow 1 hour for 35-mm cassettes to warm up after refrigeration, and $1\frac{1}{2}$ hours after freezing. Keep a 35-mm cassette in its plastic container until it has warmed up, to prevent unwanted condensation. To prevent cardboard boxes from getting soggy, store them in plastic bags with desiccant inside. You can take film in and out of a refrigerator or freezer repeatedly without harming it, provided the container remains sealed to exclude moisture.

In general, it is usually safe to use film that has been well stored about 6 months past, refrigerated film 12 months past, and film frozen at or near 0°F about 24 months past the printed expiration dates. Note that this is only a guide for ordinary outdoor and indoor applications, not for recording subtle changes of color on the human body or in the laboratory. The point is that there is no reason to discard a roll of film because it is a few days outdated.

Two of the greatest threats to undeveloped film are heat and humidity. Therefore, do not leave unprocessed film or your camera in the glove box or trunk of your car on a hot sunny day, where the temperature can easily reach 140°F and lead to visible color shifts. Inside a car in the sun the surface temperatures are even higher, often approaching 200°F.

## PROCESSING

Photographs or slides from the ED or clinical forensic facility should be developed utilizing a standard protocol for your department. You will have films from important cases, many of which are sensitive and may depict unpleasant scenes, or scenes and subjects beyond the daily experience of the average person. With sensitive subject matter such as sexual assault photographs, an in-hospital, medical school, or professional laboratory is preferred. You want to avoid explaining to your local police or drug store why you have photographs of a sexual assault victim or gunshot wounds. The point is that you are not dealing with family snapshots but serious subject matter, so your films should be treated accordingly.

You should anticipate the possibility of questions about chain of custody during processing and whether standard processing methods were used. If you selected negative film and the last half of a dozen frames were left unexposed at the end, will you discard them, and risk being asked questions about lost or concealed photographs? It is for such reasons that some EDs prefer to record a case card or serial number at the beginning and end of each sequence. It doesn't matter greatly what sort of procedure you decide to follow, so long as you do the same thing all the time and can easily show and testify that it is your routine. Simply stated, be prepared for the opposing attorney who will be looking for every opportunity to throw doubt on your procedures, opinions, or credibility.

## SCALES OF SIZE AND FRAMES OF REFERENCE

If a photograph is to be used for forensic purposes to demonstrate the exact size of a wound, it is necessary to include a scale (Figs. 13-16 and 13-17). If you take a very-close-up photograph of a bullet wound on a chest, it will be difficult to know if the wound was $\frac{3}{8}$ or $\frac{3}{4}$ in. in

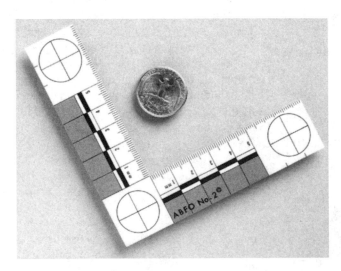

**FIG. 13-16.** An ABFO No. 2 is an excellent scale and provides measurements in two dimensions. The quartered circles permit the photographer to check for perspective distortion.

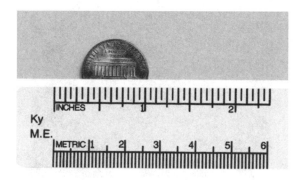

**FIG. 13-17.** Adhesive scales permit the photographer to write identifying information, such as medical record number, date, or name. On a curved surface the scale may be bent out of the plane of focus.

greatest dimension, unless there is a familiar object or scale (Fig. 13-18). Pictures of wounds and injuries need a scale of size to show or determine months or years later how big the various features were.

When you get through documenting an injury, the photographs should show where it was located on the body surface, how big it was, and what it looked like. This is usually achieved by:

1. A view to show its location and orientation, sometimes called an overall, staging, or orientation photo (Fig. 13-19A).
2. A second but nearer view to show location and identify the wound (Fig. 13-19B).
3. A third close-up photo including a scale of size to show the details (Fig. 13-19C).

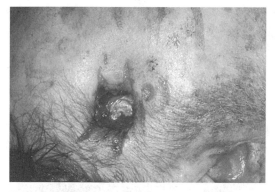

**FIG. 13-18.** Failure to place a scale in this photograph of a contact gunshot wound to the right temple will prevent the photographer or the court from determining the exact size of the wound or injury.

If a traditional ruler or scale is not available, then a familiar object with a standard size, such as a coin (Fig. 13-20), may be placed in the photograph.

Remember that if you don't put a scale in a photograph, an attorney might complain, and if you do include one, it might be possible for him to claim that it was covering something important. So be sure that your photographs are taken both with and without a scale. For instance, the overall positioning shot might have a scale at the bottom, but not next to the wound in question, and then the close-up would include a scale next to the wound. In that way nobody can claim that another feature of injury was covered by the scale because there is always another view showing the subject without a scale.

The following are general guidelines for using scales of size:

1. The scale should be sized in proportion to the subject. Perhaps an inch or two in length (3–5 cm) for cartridges and small wounds, 6 in. or so for people, a couple of feet for tires, and about 6 feet for car doors, and so forth.
2. The numbers representing inches or centimeters must be large enough to read in the end product. Many scales use very small numbers, which are not easy to read in a print.
3. The scale must be in the plane of interest, not behind it (further away from the camera) or in front of the plane (nearer to the camera). In either event, errors will arise when measurements are derived based on comparison with the scale.
4. The units must be familiar. Familiar means inches for most jurors in the United States

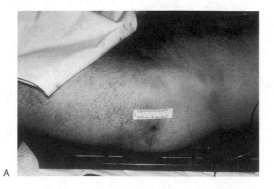

A

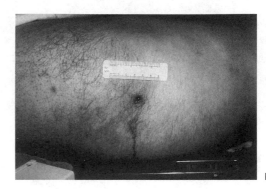

B

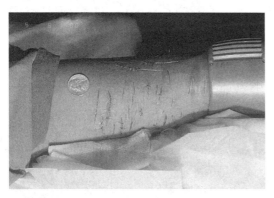

C

**FIG. 13-19. A:** The orientation or overall shot demonstrates the anatomical location of the wound, such as a gunshot wound to the left hip. **B:** A closer view, which identifies the wound. **C:** A close-up that depicts the gunshot wound at entrance with an abrasion collar.

and centimeters in most other parts of the world. It must be absolutely clear whether inches or centimeters was used. If in doubt use both, provided they don't take up too much space with a small subject.

5. None of the numbers or letters should be upside down with respect to the subject matter or other numbers. In other words, do not use the kind of ruler that has one set of numbers down one edge, and then along the other edge in reverse, upside down. When you hold the scale in your hand, everything should be in a single orientation, the right way up for reading.

6. The placement of the scale should be in a natural orientation, so that it is in a normal reading position as you look at the subject just before you take the picture.

7. The scale should not cover part of the subject. If for any reason it does, it is usually desirable to take another photograph without the scale.

8. Ideally, there should be no advertising material of any kind on the ruler or scale (Fig. 13-21). There should be room on the scale for essential identifying data, such as the case number and/or date and/or initials of the photographer. Write these numbers carefully, for a professional appearance, because they may be magnified in the final print.

**FIG. 13-20.** Placement of a coin can serve as a reference if a scale is not available.

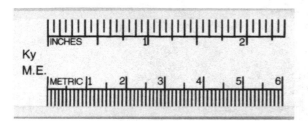

**FIG. 13-21.** The adhesive scale lacks any advertisement and has the identifying ring data written on label.

9. The scale of size should not compete with the subject matter for attention and should be aesthetically pleasing (Fig. 13-22, see Colorplate following page 144). For instance, the use of bright red is probably inadvisable.

10. The scale should be generally helpful to you and to your co-workers. For instance:

- It should not be unduly shiny or reflective
- It should not be curved or bent unless you wish it to be
- It should be easy to clean and dispose of
- It should be easy to position
- It should be darker if the subject is dark, and lighter if the subject is light, to avoid exposure problems.

Scale sources include:

1. The Lightning Powder Company, 1230 Hoyt Street, S.E., Salem, OR 97302-2121. (503) 585-9900, (800) 852-0300.

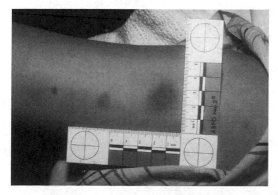

**FIG. 13-22.** A photograph with a scale and without perspective distortion permits accurate measurement of a wound. These fingertip contusions on the upper left arm are from a domestic assault.

2. Shamrock Scientific Specialty Systems, Inc., P.O. Box 143, Bellwood, IL 60104. (312) 992-1187. (1989)

## ADHESIVE LABELS

Lynn Peavey Company, P.O. Box 14100, Lenexa, KS 66285-4100. (800) 255-6499, Fax 24-hrs (913) 888-1066.

## BACKGROUND CONTROL

The ED photographer must take steps to limit the amount of extraneous material or information contained in the photograph. The presence of bloody clothes, dressings, or medical instruments will distract the viewer and may be deemed inflammatory by a judge rendering an opinion as to a photo's admissibility to evidence. The placement of surgical drapes or towels behind the subject or over the dressings is the easiest way to mask the distractions if it is not possible to physically remove the objects (Fig. 13-23).

## FILTERS

Regarding filters, there are two schools of thought: (a) Anything placed over the lens is another potential source of reflection, dirt, or image degradation, and should therefore be avoided. (b) Lenses are expensive and it's a good idea to protect the front lens element with something that can be replaced at low cost. Use of a filter is a very good idea in a dirty or gritty environment, like the ED. If you do decide to protect your lens with a filter, and intend to leave it on, make sure its optical quality is as good as the camera lens or you will inevitably lose

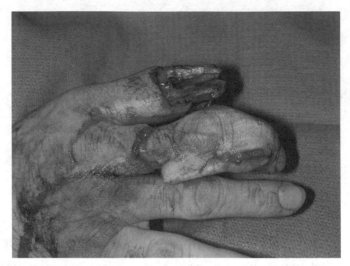

**FIG. 13-23**. The placement of surgical drops clarifies the subject of the photograph and covers extraneous details.

sharpness. There is no sense in using an uncoated $5 filter on the front of a $500 lens.

When using color film, the apparently clear haze and UV filters remove ultraviolet, which we cannot see. The very slightly pink-looking skylight filter removes UV as well as a little blue. In general terms, a so-called skylight filter removes the least UV, then a Haze no. 1, then a UV filter, and finally a Haze no. 2. Manufacturers vary somewhat in their use of names, so purchasers should check if the difference will matter. If the fabric brightener in the white bed sheets causes them to look blue, the cure is to put a UV filter over your flash so the flash will not affect the fabric brightener.

Filters are used to increase apparent sharpness, intensify colors (e.g., enhance foliage), and reduce glare.

Filters for color films fall into several categories. Individuals who are just getting into photography often find them confusing.

- *Conversion* filters are placed over the lens to let you switch from one kind of light to another. An example would be use of tungsten (indoor) film in daylight.
- *Balancing* filters make small changes for lighting color, such as between noon and the redder light of sunrise or sunset.

- *Neutral-density* filters cut down on the amount of light but, in theory, do not alter the color at all. They look gray.
- *Color-compensating,* or CC, filters correct the exposure in one color layer (yellow, magenta, or cyan) only
- *Polarizing* filters are used to reduce reflections from nonmetallic objects to increase color saturation and to reduce haze when taking distant objects. Other common applications include copying, reducing glare from road surfaces when recording skid marks, and taking photographs through glass windows. Good-quality polarizing filters do not appreciably alter color, but inexpensive ones may do so to a limited extent.

Note that the light metering systems of some cameras are adversely affected by the use of polarizing filters. Many see the reduced light intensity and adjust correctly, but others, which use beam splitters to send light to the photocells, are unable to react properly when a linear polarizer is used. This may result in very large exposure errors. Check the instruction manual for the make and model of your camera to see which type is best. When in doubt, put a polarizing filter on your camera and focus on a sheet of plain white paper or suitable directionally lit subject.

Then rotate the filter. A slight change in the exposure reading is normal as reflections are controlled, but if there is a sudden large change in the exposure indication you will probably need a circular polarizer (a linear polarizer combined with a $\frac{1}{4}$-wave plate).

## DIGITAL PHOTOGRAPHY

With the emergence of digital cameras and the precipitous decline in their prices near-film quality images are possible (Fig. 13-24). Only a year ago, obtaining a three million pixel photograph would have required a $5,000 camera. Today the Nikon CoolPix 990 provides this degree of detail for less than $1,000.

The digital camera does offer some advantages over traditional slide-and-print films, particularly for educational purposes. Digital images are easily stored, e-mailed, and exported into multimedia presentations. The photographer knows within seconds if the image is in focus, well illuminated, well composed, and displays what the photographer intended. The digital image can also be easily converted to a slide or print.

The digital image is easily manipulated or altered, and this has been an early concern for many lower courts. These alterations in digital images may be impossible to detect. Such factors as backgrounds, perspective, and poor lighting are just as much of a problem, and a question about who can authenticate an image may arise at any time. Basic principles still apply, and a fair and reasonably accurate depiction is still required in legal applications. Some alterations or enhancements are acceptable that do not involve change of content and are similar to accepted darkroom techniques. They include:

1. Making improvements in contrast by slightly darkening or lightening areas with a view to improving the printing or reproduction characteristics, or making selected details a little easier to see.
2. Dodging or burning in areas to lighten up a face or bring something out, such as a license plate.
3. Correcting technical defects, such as dust spots or a skipped scan line in a TV picture.
4. Making slight changes in color to reduce adverse effects of artificial lighting, or errors in processing.

Unacceptable alterations, unless everyone has agreed to and is fully aware of them, include:

1. Removing objects from a photograph.
2. Making radical changes in color, for instance the color of a car, or of human skin.
3. Adding new or repeated images by cloning of pixels.

The bottom line will be the integrity and honesty of the photographer when he or she states in court that the image is not radically manipulated.

Within the next 5 years, improvements in digital photography technology may result in the digital camera's completely replacing the 35-mm camera.

There are several broad categories of digital cameras:

- Today's amateur point-and-shoot, pocket size, under $500, allowing prints up to 3 × 5 in.
- Yesterday's top-of-the-line, reduced to $500–800, allowing prints up to 5 × 7 in., with 2 million pixel.
- Today's top-of-the-line, $1,000, with more than 3 million pixels (Fig. 13-25), allowing 8 × 10 in. prints.

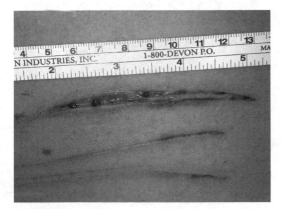

**FIG. 13-24.** Superficial self-inflicted incised wounds taken with a digital camera with 3.14 million pixels.

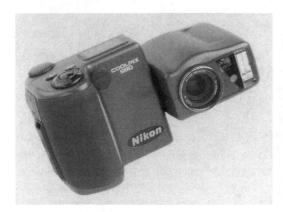

**FIG. 13-25.** The Nikon CoolPix 990 produces a near-film-quality photograph with a 3.14 million pixel image.

- Professional grade, single-lens reflexes, over $5,000 like the Nikon D1 (Fig. 13-26) and Canon D-2000.
- Scanning backs for professional grade medium- and large-format cameras. Expensive!

Until mid-1999, the chips in point-and-shoot digital cameras didn't have enough pixels (picture elements) to capture sufficient detail to make a large print. They were more than capable of putting a low-resolution image on the Web or showing a potential house buyer what a home looked like, but many digital cameras didn't have the resolution to compete with film. Until

recently, one could generalize by saying that low-priced digital cameras had about one third the resolution of film. The situation is improving and we may be approaching half the resolution of film (6 million pixels), but to get a system that is close to film one still has to spend several thousand dollars.

The sensitivity (ISO/ASA) range of the common chips is less than that of film. One of the best digital cameras that has 6 million pixels only works in the range between 80 and 200 ISO, whereas film cameras and films range from single digits to 1,600 ISO off the shelf. Furthermore, the majority of chips are slow. Any apparent increase in sensitivity is attained by amplification, which by definition introduces "noise."

The major disadvantages of present-day digital imaging for legal and scientific applications are image quality and resolution, image storage, and image authentication (proving reality and lack of modification.)

Until legal admissibility of digital image has been adequately dealt with in the higher courts, it is advisable not to rely entirely on digital image capture for legal and scientific work.

Is an image that was compressed for storage and then decompressed truly original, however slight the changes may be? Is the compression system truly error-free down to the last pixel? Which pixel(s) might have been improperly reproduced after the storage and retrieval process?

How will you deal with image archiving, storage, and chain of custody? One of the best Kodak digital cameras has a chip with about 6 million pixels that gives rise to a proprietary image file of about 18 megabytes. So if you have a 4-gigabyte hard drive on your computer you will be able to store about 220 images—the equivalent of about 6 rolls of film. Of course, you can compress the images, but when decompressed will they be truly accurate?

If an original image is copied and a copy is given to someone, are you prepared for questions about minor differences that might be present between the original and the copy?

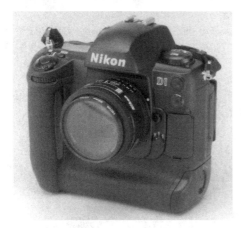

**FIG. 13-26.** The Nikon D1 is a high-end digital SLR camera that produces film-quality images.

Slide and print films still have about the highest resolving power available today. In addition, one can take a slide or print almost anywhere and get it printed, duplicated, enlarged, made into an overhead transparency, or scan it into a computer at far higher resolution than any affordable digital camera can deliver. A 35-mm slide, properly made with 100- or 200-speed film, reportedly contains enough information to scan and convert a 30- to 40-megabyte image file. Find the cost of a digital system that will record that much detail, and see how portable and practical it is. Some archivists believe that paper, and in our case conventional film, may still be the best medium for preserving a record of the present, but relatively early, digital times.

Obviously, capture of still images by digital means is a great innovation, and it's "coming on strong" while still evolving. It is the author's opinion that digital photography isn't quite ready to stand alone for general, legal, and scientific use. It has certainly reached the point where it can be used as an adjunct to film, and one may find it satisfactory in its own right for certain uses in the ED. If rapid image capture, high image quality, long-term storage and established legal acceptability are necessary, continue to use film.

## NUMBERING AND IDENTIFYING PHOTOGRAPHS

Always write identifying information, such as the case number, hospital number, patient number, and/or the name and initials, on the slide mounts, or negative envelopes, immediately after your films are developed. This will facilitate retrieval at a later date on a case-by-case basis.

## COURTROOM PRESENTATION

Never purport to be or permit yourself to be qualified as an expert in photography when in a court of law. Even people who do or teach photography for a living are reluctant to allow this. Instead, be qualified as someone who is experienced and uses photography a great deal. Acknowledge that you have taken some instruction and have knowledge over and above that of the general public. Be qualified as a practitioner, if that is appropriate, as opposed to an expert, and stay well within your field of expertise, just as you would in medicine.

## SUMMARY

Your success as a functional ED photographer depends in large part on your ability to look critically at your own photographs, learn from your mistakes, improve with experience, do better the next time, and thereby slowly improve your technique. Do not confuse good technique and common sense with the acquisition of technical information.

"A good photograph, I think, is one which conveys to the observer something which he has not seen, known, or thought of before."— *Andreas Feininger*

## ADDITIONAL RESOURCES

1. Vetter JP. Biomedical photography. Stoneham, MA: Butterworth-Heinemann, ISBN 0-240-80084-2, TR708.B55,1992, 610'.28-dc20 91-31077.

2. Warren B. *Photography.*:West Publishers, ISBN 0-314-92914-2 (soft cover) TR146.W27, 1992, 771-dc20  91-37913.

3. Williams RA, Williams GF. *J Biol Photogr Assoc*(now the Biocommunication Association).

Pt 1: Introduction and reflected ultraviolet techniques: Vol. 61, No. 4, Oct 1993:115–132.

Pt 2: Fluorescence photography: Vol 62, No.1, Jan 1994:3–19.

Pt 3: Reflected infrared photography: Vol. 62, No. 2, April 1994:51–68.

4. The Kodak Information Center (800) 242-2424. (8 a.m. to 8 p.m. EST). Web site: http://www.kodak.com (on-line information) and http://www.kodak.com/go/professional. Information by mail: Eastman Kodak Company, 343 State Street, Rochester, NY 14650-0519.

5. The Fujifilm Sensitized Products Technical Hotline is (800) 788-3854, ext. 73.

The Fuji ProNet(tm) Hotline is (800) 332-FUJI, and Fuji ProNet(tm)

Fuji Web site access: www.fujifilm.com

Fuji consumer information: (800) 800-FUJI.

6. Polaroid Corporation Technical Support line (800) 225-1618, Customer Care (800) 343-5000.

7. Pasqualone GA. Documentation in the ED: forensic RNs as photographers. *J Psychosocial Nurs* 1996;34(10):47–51.

8. The Nikon School of Photography, 300 Walt Whitman Road, Melville, NY 11747-3064. Telephone number (516) 547-8666 between 8:00 a.m. and 4:30 p.m. Monday through Friday EST, Fax number (516) 547-0309. http://www.nikonusa.com.

9. Former chief of law enforcement photography markets for Eastman Kodak: R. T. "Dick" McEvoy, President, Imaging, Inc., P.O. Box 597, Victor, NY 14564-9998. Telephone number (716) 924-9410; Fax number (716) 924-8854.

10. Evidence photographers International Council (EPIC). Robert F. Jennings, Executive Director, 600 Main Street, Honesdale, PA 18431-0351, Telephone number (717) 253-5450, (800) 356-3742; Fax number (717) 253-5011.

11. Polaroid Corporation has two Web sites with a forensic orientation. They are: www.polaroid.com/at-work/law-enforcement and www.polaroid.com/at-work/familyviolence. The U.S. law enforcement marketing manager is Barbara Poremba, (800) 811-5764, ext. 734.

12. Kerr N. *Lighting techniques for photographers,* 3rd ed. Amherst Media, Inc.

## REFERENCES

1. Gove PB, ed. *Webster's third new international dictionary of the English language,* Unabridged. Springfield: Merriam-Webster, 1986.
2. Smock WS. Clinical forensic medicine. In: Rosen, ed. *Emergency medicine: concepts and clinical practice.* St. Louis: Mosby, 1998:243–262.
3. University of Louisville Hospital, Operative Consent Form, Louisville, Kentucky, 1999.
4. Osborne TL. Demonstrative evidence. In: Osborne TL, ed. *Trial handbook for Kentucky lawyers,* 2nd ed. Rochester, NY: Lawyers Cooperative Publishing, 1992.
5. *Kentucky rules of evidence, Kentucky rules of court.* St. Paul: West Group, 1999.

# Subject Index

Note: Page numbers followed by *f* indicate figures; those followed by *t* indicate tables.

## A

AAS (Abuse Assessment Screen), 211, 212*f*, 213*f*

Abandonment, of elderly, 177, 177*t*, 184*t*, 199*t*

Abdominal trauma, from child abuse, 153–154

Abduction, child, 12–13

Abrasion(s)
  from domestic abuse, 216–218, 219*f*, 220*f*. *See* Colorplate following page 144
  fingernail, 75, 77*f*
  ligature, 75, 77*f*
  muzzle, 67, 67*f*, 68*f*. *See* Colorplate following page 144
  pattern, 75, 77*f*

Abrasion collar (abrasion margin, abrasion rim, abrasion ring), 70–71, 70*f*, 71*f*, 276*f*
  false, 72, 72*f*

Abuse Assessment Screen (AAS), 211, 212*f*, 213*f*

Acquaintance perpetrators, of child abuse, 49

Acquaintance rape, 33

Acquired immunodeficiency syndrome (AIDS). *See* Human immunodeficiency virus (HIV)

Acyclovir, for genital herpes, 142

Adhesive labels, 277

Admissibility, of photography as evidence, 260–263, 261*f*–263*f*. *See* Colorplate following page 144

Adolescent(s)
  especially vulnerable, 124–125
  health care access by, 122
  pregnancy of, 145–146
  and puberty, 121, 124–126, 120*f*, 122*f*
  service delivery systems for, 122–123, 123*f*
  as sex offenders, 146
  sexual abuse and sexual assault of, 119–147
    consent and confidentiality issues in, 121, 122, 127–128
    defined, 119
    with developmental disabilities or mental retardation, 124
    of drug and alcohol users, 124
    epidemiologic considerations in, 119–121
    evidentiary laboratory tests for, 143
    of gay youth, 124

  with history of childhood sexual abuse, 124, 145
  history taking for, 128–129, 122*f*, 123*f*
  of males, 124
  mental and social consequences of, 144–146, 128*f*
  nondisclosure and delayed disclosure of, 120
  parental notification of, 127
  and parents with mental health or substance abuse issues, 124
  physical examination for, 129–134, 131*f*
  in poverty, 124
  pregnancy tests for, 143
  relationships with parents and, 121–122
  reporting of, 119–120, 143
  risk taking behavior and, 121
  sexually transmitted diseases from, 134–143, 135*t*
  in special subpopulations, 124–125
  turmoil in, 122
  unique vulnerabilities of, 121–123, 122*f*

Adult(s), interviewing of, 60–61

Adult maltreatment syndrome, 226

Adult protective services (APS), 181, 193, 194, 197–199

Advocacy for Women and Kids in Emergencies (AWAKE), 42

Advocate, during female sexual assault examination, 97

Ageism, 187

Aggravated sexual abuse, 32

AIDS. *See* Human immunodeficiency virus (HIV)

Alcohol users, adolescent
  sexual assault of, 124

"Alford" plea, 234–235

Alopecia, traumatic, 223

Alzheimer's disease, interviewing of victims with, 61

Anal ampulla, 113

Anal examination
  of female sexual assault victim, 96–97, 96*f*, 102–103. *See* Colorplate following page 144
  of male sexual assault victim, 110
    adolescent, 132, 133–134

Anal fold, 113

Anal rugae, 113